Families and Social Policy: National and International Perspectives

Families and Social Policy: National and International Perspectives
has been co-published simultaneously as *Marriage & Family Review*,
Volume 39, Numbers 1/2 and 3/4 2006.

Monographic Separates from *Marriage & Family Review*™

For additional information on these and other Haworth Press titles, including descriptions, tables of contents, reviews, and prices, use the QuickSearch catalog at http://www.HaworthPress.com.

Families and Social Policy: National and International Perspectives, edited by Linda Haas and Steven K. Wisensale (Vol. 39, No. 1/2/3/4, 2006). *Examination of current research on the impact of government policy–and lack of government policy–on family life in developed and developing societies.*

The Craft of Teaching About Families: Strategies and Tools, edited by Debra L. Berke and Steven K. Wisensale (Vol. 38, No. 2/3/4, 2005). *"A superb resource for all who teach about families, this collection offers concrete examples focusing on how to teach family policy, research, and clinical techniques effectively. The breadth of coverage is impressive. . . . This book offers an exciting array of ideas and suggestions–all grounded and tested in real classrooms with real students. . . . Should be read cover-to-cover by all of us concerned with teaching the next generation of family scholars, advocates, and practitioners." (Eileen Trzcinski, PhD, Professor and Director of Social Work, Wayne State University)*

Challenges of Aging on U.S. Families: Policy and Practice Implications, edited by Richard K. Caputo, PhD (Vol. 37, No. 1/2, 2005). *Examines the policy and practical implications of the aging United States population, the changes within the family structure, caregiving by various family members, and the overall economic impact.*

Parent-Youth Relations: Cultural and Cross-Cultural Perspectives, edited by Gary W. Peterson, Suzanne K. Steinmetz, and Stephan M. Wilson (Vol. 35, No. 3/4, 2003; Vol. 36, No. 1/2/3/4, 2004). *A comprehensive examination of how culture interconnects with parent-child relationships.*

Emotions and the Family, edited by Richard A. Fabes, PhD (Vol. 34, No. 1/2/3/4, 2002). *"An exciting collection. The contributors insightfully unfold the nature of emotions as relational processes in marriage and parenting, and illuminate how emotional communication, competence, and regulation color family life. Chapters on siblings, stepfamilies, economic stress, and family therapy add richness to the collective portrayal of how emotions infuse marital and parent-child relationships. Scholars of marital and family life will find this a valuable resource." (Ross A. Thompson, PhD, Carl A. Happold Distinguished Professor of Psychology, University of Nebraska)*

Gene-Environment Processes in Social Behaviors and Relationships, edited by Kirby Deater-Deckard, PhD, and Stephen A. Petrill, PhD (Vol. 33, No. 1/2/3, 2002). *"During recent years there have been somewhat fruitless battles on whether family influences or peer influences are more important in children's psychological development. This book is both innovative and helpful in seeking to bring the two sets of influences together through a range of studies using twin, adoptee, and stepfamily designs to assess how genetic and environmental influences may work together in bringing about individual differences in children's emotions, behavior and especially social relationships. The different research approaches provide some new ways of thinking about, and investigating, how interpersonal relationships develop and have their effects." (Michael Rutter, MD, FRS, Professor of Developmental Psychopathology, Institute of Psychiatry, King's College, London)*

Pioneering Paths in the Study of Families: The Lives and Careers of Family Scholars, edited by Suzanne K. Steinmetz, PhD, MSW, and Gary W. Peterson, PhD (Vol. 30, No. 3, 2000; Vol. 30, No. 4, 2001; Vol. 31, No. 1/2/3/4, 2001; Vol. 32, No. 1/2, 2001). *The fascinating autobiographies of 40 leading scholars in sociology, family studies, psychology, and child development.*

FATHERHOOD: Research, Interventions and Policies, edited by H. Elizabeth Peters, PhD, Gary W. Peterson, PhD, Suzanne K. Steinmetz, PhD, MSW, and Randal D. Day, PhD (Vol. 29, No. 2/3/4, 2000). *Brings together the latest facts to help researchers explore the father-child relationship and determine what factors lead fathers to be more or less involved in the lives of their children, including human social behavior, not living with a child, being denied visiting privileges, and social norms regarding gender differences versus work responsibilities.*

Concepts and Definitions of Family for the 21st Century, edited by Barbara H. Settles, PhD, Suzanne K. Steinmetz, PhD, MSW, Gary W. Peterson, PhD, and Marvin B. Sussman, PhD (Vol. 28, No. 3/4, 1999). *Views family from a U.S. perspective and from many different cultures and societies. The controversial question "What is family?" is thoroughly examined as it has become an increasingly important social policy concern in recent years as the traditional family has changed.*

The Role of the Hospitality Industry in the Lives of Individuals and Families, edited by Pamela R. Cummings, PhD, Francis A. Kwansa, PhD, and Marvin B. Sussman, PhD (Vol. 28, No. 1/2, 1998). *"A must for human resource directors and hospitality educators." (Dr. Lynn Huffman, Director, Restaurant, Hotel, and Institutional Management, Texas Tech University, Lubbock, Texas)*

Stepfamilies: History, Research, and Policy, edited by Irene Levin, PhD, and Marvin B. Sussman, PhD (Vol. 26, No. 1/2/3/4, 1997). *"A wide range of individually valuable and stimulating chapters that form a wonderfully rich menu from which readers of many different kinds will find exciting and satisfying selections." (Jon Bernardes, PhD, Principal Lecturer in Sociology, University of Wolverhampton, Castle View Dudley, United Kingdom)*

Families and Adoption, edited by Harriet E. Gross, PhD, and Marvin B. Sussman, PhD (Vol. 25, No. 1/2/3/4, 1997). *"Written in a lucid and easy-to-read style, this volume will make an invaluable contribution to the adoption literature." (Paul Sachdev, PhD, Professor, School of Social Work, Memorial University of Newfoundland, St. John's, Newfoundland, Canada)*

The Methods and Methodologies of Qualitative Family Research, edited by Jane F. Gilgun, PhD, LICSW, and Marvin B. Sussman, PhD (Vol 24, No. 1/2/3/4, 1997). *"An authoritative look at the usefulness of qualitative research methods to the family scholar." (Family Relations)*

Intercultural Variation in Family Research and Theory: Implications for Cross-National Studies, Volumes I and II, edited by Marvin B. Sussman, PhD, and Roma S. Hanks, PhD (Vol. 22, No. 1/2/3/4, and Vol. 23, No. 1/2/3/4, 1997). *Documents the development of family research in theory in societies around the world and inspires continued cross-national collaboration on current research topics.*

Families and Law, edited by Lisa J. McIntyre, PhD, and Marvin B. Sussman, PhD (Vol. 21, No. 3/4, 1995). *With this new volume, family practitioners and scholars can begin to increase the family's position in relation to the law and legal system.*

Exemplary Social Intervention Programs for Members and Their Families, edited by David Guttmann, DSW, and Marvin B. Sussman, PhD (Vol. 21, No. 1/2, 1995). *An eye-opening look at organizations and individuals who have created model family programs that bring desired results.*

Single Parent Families: Diversity, Myths and Realities, edited by Shirley M. H. Hanson, RN, PhD, Marsha L. Heims, RN, EdD, Doris J. Julian, RN, EdD, and Marvin B. Sussman, PhD (Vol. 20, No. 1/2/3/4, 1994). *"Remarkable! . . . A significant work and is important reading for multidisciplinary family professionals including sociologists, educators, health care professionals, and policymakers." (Maureen Leahey, RN, PhD, Director, Outpatient Mental Health Program, Director, Family Therapy Training Program, Calgary District Hospital Group)*

Families on the Move: Immigration, Migration, and Mobility, edited by Barbara H. Settles, PhD, Daniel E. Hanks III, MS, and Marvin B. Sussman, PhD (Vol 19, No 1/2/3/4, 1993). *Examines the current research on family mobility, migration, and immigration and discovers new directions for understanding the relationship between mobility and family life.*

American Families and the Future: Analyses of Possible Destinies, edited by Barbara H. Settles, PhD, Roma S. Hanks, PhD, and Marvin B. Sussman, PhD (Vol. 18, No. 3/4, 1993). *This book discusses a variety of issues that face and will continue to face families in coming years and describes various strategies families can use in their decision-making processes.*

Publishing in Journals on the Family: Essays on Publishing, edited by Roma S. Hanks, PhD, Linda Matocha, PhD, RN, and Marvin B. Sussman, PhD (Vol. 18, No. 1/2, 1993). *This helpful book contains varied perspectives from scholars at different career stages and from editors of major publication outlets, providing readers with important information necessary to help them systematically plan a productive scholarly career.*

Publishing in Journals on the Family: A Survey and Guide for Scholars, Practitioners, and Students, edited by Roma S. Hanks, PhD, Linda Matocha, PhD, RN, and Marvin B. Sussman, PhD (Vol. 17, No. 3/4, 1992). *"Comprehensive. . . . Includes listings for some 200 social science journals whose editors have expressed an interest in publishing empirical research and theoretical articles about the family." (Reference & Research Book News)*

Families and Social Policy: National and International Perspectives

Linda Haas
Steven K. Wisensale
Editors

Families and Social Policy: National and International Perspectives
has been co-published simultaneously as *Marriage & Family Review*,
Volume 39, Numbers 1/2 and 3/4 2006.

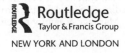

Routledge
Taylor & Francis Group

NEW YORK AND LONDON

First published by

The Haworth Press, Inc., 10 Alice Street, Binghamton, NY 13904-1580 USA

Transferred to Digital Printing 2010 by Routledge
270 Madison Ave, New York NY 10016
2 Park Square, Milton Park, Abingdon, Oxon, OX14 4RN

Families and Social Policy: National and International Perspectives
has been co-published simultaneously as *Marriage & Family Review*,
Volume 39, Numbers 1/2 and 3/4 2006.

The development, preparation, and publication of this work has been undertaken with great care. However, the publisher, employees, editors, and agents of The Haworth Press and all imprints of The Haworth Press, Inc., including The Haworth Medical Press® and Pharmaceutical Products Press®, are not responsible for any errors contained herein or for consequences that may ensue from use of materials or information contained in this work. With regard to case studies, identities and circumstances of individuals discussed herein have been changed to protect confidentiality. Any resemblance to actual persons, living or dead, is entirely coincidental.

The Haworth Press is committed to the dissemination of ideas and information according to the highest standards of intellectual freedom and the free exchange of ideas. Statements made and opinions expressed in this publication do not necessarily reflect the views of the Publisher, Directors, management, or staff of The Haworth Press, Inc., or an endorsement by them.

Cover design by Karen M. Lowe

Library of Congress Cataloging-in-Publication Data

Families and social policy : national and international perspectives / Linda Haas, Steven K. Wisensale, editors.
      p. cm.
      "Families and social policy: national and international perspectives has been co-published simultaneously as Marriage & Family Review, Volume 39, Numbers 1/2 and 3/4 2006."
      Includes bibliographical references and index.
      ISBN-13: 978-0-7890-3239-3 (hard cover : alk. paper)
      ISBN-10: 0-7890-3239-2 (hard cover : alk. paper)
      ISBN-13: 978-0-7890-3240-9 (soft cover : alk. paper)
      ISBN-10: 0-7890-3240-6 (soft cover : alk. paper)
      1. Family–United States. 2. Family policy–United States. 3. United States–Social policy.
4. Family policy–Cross-cultural studies. 5. Social policy–Cross-cultural studies. I. Haas, Linda.
II. Wisensale, Steven K., 1945- III. Marriage & family review.
HQ536.F33352 2006
306.8509–dc22

                                                                          2006011437

Indexing, Abstracting & Website/Internet Coverage

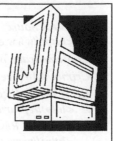

This section provides you with a list of major indexing & abstracting services and other tools for bibliographic access. That is to say, each service began covering this periodical during the year noted in the right column. Most Websites which are listed below have indicated that they will either post, disseminate, compile, archive, cite or alert their own Website users with research-based content from this work. (This list is as current as the copyright date of this publication.)

Abstracting, Website/Indexing Coverage . . . . Year When Coverage Began

- *Abstracts in Social Gerontology: Current Literature on Aging* **1993**
- *Academic Abstracts/CD-ROM (EBSCO)* **1993**
- *Academic ASAP (Thomson Gale)* **1989**
- *Academic Search Elite (EBSCO)* **1993**
- *Academic Search Premier (EBSCO) <http://www.epnet.com/academic/acasearchprem.asp>* **1993**
- *AgeLine Database (AARP) <http://research.aarp.org/ageline>* **1991**
- *AGRICOLA Database (National Agricultural Library) (AGRICultural OnLine Access) A Bibliographic database of citations to the agricultural literature created by the National Agricultural Library and its cooperators <http://www.natl.usda.gov/ag98>* **1992**
- *AGRIS/CARIS <http://FAO-Agris-Caris@fao.org>* **1992**
- *Applied Social Sciences Index & Abstracts (ASSIA) (Cambridge Scientific Abstracts) (Online: ASSIA via Data-Star) (CDRom: ASSIA Plus) <http://www.csa.com>* **1993**
- *AURSI African Urban & Regional Science Index. A scholarly & research index which synthesises & compiles all publications on urbanization & regional science in Africa within the world. Published annually* **2004**

(continued)

(continued)

(continued)

- *Sage Family Studies Abstracts (SFSA)* 1992
- *ScienceDirect Navigator (Elsevier)*
  <http://www.info.sciencedirect.com> 2002
- *Scopus (See instead Elsevier Scopus)*
  <http://www.info.scopus.com> 2002
- *Social Science Source: Coverage of 400 journals in the social*
  sciences area; updated monthly; EBSCO Publishing 1996
- *Social Scisearch <http://www.isinet.com>* 1992
- *Social Services Abstracts (Cambridge Scientific*
  Abstracts) <http://www.csa.com> 1990
- *Social Work Abstracts*
  <http://www.silverplatter.com/catalog/swab.htm> 1992
- *SocioAbs <http://www.csa.com>* 1990
- *Sociological Abstracts (Cambridge Scientific Abstracts)*
  <http://www.csa.com> 1990
- *Special Educational Needs Abstracts* 1992
- *Studies on Women and Gender Abstracts <http://www.tandf.co.uk/swa>* .. 1992
- *SwetsWise <http://www.swets.com>* 2001
- *Violence and Abuse Abstracts: A Review of Current Literature*
  on Interpersonal Violence (VAA) 1995

*Exact start date to come.

Special Bibliographic Notes related to special journal issues
(separates) and indexing/abstracting:

- indexing/abstracting services in this list will also cover material in any "separate" that is co-published simultaneously with Haworth's special thematic journal issue or DocuSerial. Indexing/abstracting usually covers material at the article/chapter level.
- monographic co-editions are intended for either non-subscribers or libraries which intend to purchase a second copy for their circulating collections.
- monographic co-editions are reported to all jobbers/wholesalers/approval plans. The source journal is listed as the "series" to assist the prevention of duplicate purchasing in the same manner utilized for books-in-series.
- to facilitate user/access services all indexing/abstracting services are encouraged to utilize the co-indexing entry note indicated at the bottom of the first page of each article/chapter/contribution.
- this is intended to assist a library user of any reference tool (whether print, electronic, online, or CD-ROM) to locate the monographic version if the library has purchased this version but not a subscription to the source journal.
- individual articles/chapters in any Haworth publication are also available through the Haworth Document Delivery Service (HDDS).

Families and Social Policy: National and International Perspectives

CONTENTS

ABOUT THE EDITORS

Linda Haas is Professor of Sociology and Adjunct Professor of Women's Studies at Indiana University in Indianapolis, USA. She regularly teaches courses on gender, family policy and families and work. Her research interests focus on the linkages between gender, family and work in post-industrialized societies. Publications include *Equal Parenthood and Social Policy* (SUNY Press, 1992) and *Organizational Change and Gender Equity* (with P. Hwang and G. Russell, Sage, 2000).

Steven K. Wisensale is Professor of Public Policy in the School of Family Studies at the University of Connecticut. His research and teaching interests are in social welfare policy with a particular focus on family policy and the politics of aging. He has published extensively in major professional journals and is the author of a recent book, *Family Leave Policy: The Political Economy of Work and Family in America* (M.E. Sharpe, 2001).

Introduction

Steven K. Wisensale

Linda Haas

The year 2005 marked the 70th anniversary of the signing of the Social Security Act and the 40th anniversary of the enactment of both Medicare and Medicaid. Not forgotten entirely, but barely remembered, was another milestone in the history of American social policy that can be associated with the anniversary year 2005. Twenty-five years before, in 1980, the nation held its first and only White House Conference on Families (WHCF).

Held just months before President Jimmy Carter's loss to Ronald Reagan in the 1980 election, the WHCF is still viewed by many as one of the major watersheds in the developmental history of family policy (Cherlin, 1996; Dempsey, 1981; Steiner, 1981). More than a thousand delegates met in three separate cities (Baltimore, Minneapolis, and Los Angeles) during the summer and early fall of 1980 to address a variety of family-oriented issues and, ultimately, to present to the President a checklist of policy recommendations and legislative proposals designed to strengthen and support the nation's families. While some consensus was reached on proposed solutions to problems confronting the aged and handicapped, there was little agreement on other family-oriented issues, such as the prevention of teen pregnancy, gay rights, the Equal Rights Amendment, and abortion. All told, thirty-four of sixty-two proposals were eventually adopted, but only seven were supported by more than 90 percent of the conference delegates (Dempsey, 1981).

[Haworth co-indexing entry note]: "Introduction." Wisensale, Steven K., and Linda Haas. Co-published simultaneously in *Marriage & Family Review* (The Haworth Press, Inc.) Vol. 39, No. 1/2, 2006, pp. 1-9; and: *Families and Social Policy: National and International Perspectives* (ed: Linda Haas, and Steven K. Wisensale) The Haworth Press, Inc., 2006, pp. 1-9. Single or multiple copies of this article are available for a fee from The Haworth Document Delivery Service [1-800-HAWORTH, 9:00 a.m. - 5:00 p.m. (EST). E-mail address: docdelivery@haworthpress.com].

In the end, the contentious conference gatherings produced little in terms of significant policy initiatives that were eventually enacted into law. However, in addition to providing a glimpse into the future of the "family values debate," the conference did produce at least two other important outcomes. First, for the first time in history, the family had been placed on the national agenda and a new policy question was posed: Where should the line be drawn between what the family is expected to do and what government has been created to do? And second, perhaps equally significant, the WHCF raised the consciousness of America, forcing many people to think beyond policy proposals geared primarily to individuals, and to consider instead the general health and well-being of families. Almost immediately after the closing session of the conference, an onslaught of books and articles on family policy began and has continued for a quarter of a century since. So too has there been a growth industry in research centers, think tanks, and advocacy organizations devoted to family issues. And not to be forgotten, interest in families has gone global, with the United Nations convening the first International Year of the Family conference in 1994 and then again in 2004.

As the editors of this collection of sixteen excellent articles on family issues, we recognize the importance of benchmarks in providing some degree of historical perspective as we attempt to understand the complexity of the social, economic, and political forces that affect families. In some cases the issues raised 25 years ago during the White House Conference of Families remain near the top of current political agendas. These include gender equity, gay rights, abortion laws, and the prevention of teen pregnancy. Less visible in 1980, however, but front and center today, are such topics as work and family balance, parenting, fatherhood, and the pressures associated with intergenerational caregiving.

In organizing the collection of articles for presentation in this volume, we recognize at least three large and distinct divisions, within which are several smaller subdivisions. First, one can view family issues from both a micro and macro level. That is, in some cases problems that beset particular families are homegrown, meaning that private decisions can create public burdens. This is certainly true with respect to teen pregnancy, for example. But families are also affected by broader, macro forces, such as economic fluctuations and shifts in political power, that may make them more or less vulnerable to policy initiatives put forth by one political party instead of the other.

Similarly, the articles can also be divided by another category: state vs. family responsibility for solutions to family problems. That is, where, and under what circumstances, should the line be drawn that clearly divides the role of the family from that of the state in providing care to the old and vulnerable? This is particularly true with respect to the care of pre-school children (home vs. child care center) as well as the care of the frail elderly (in-home care vs. the nursing home). Costs are shifted to or from families and taxpayers depending on how the question concerning caregiving responsibilities is answered.

And a third way the articles can be organized is to divide them into U.S. family policy vs. international policy. In a postmodern world in which a dominant force is globalization, it is not surprising that both the challenges and the solutions affecting families know no borders. Although the first group of articles in this collection concerns family issues in the United States, the same or similar issues have surfaced in other nations and some are covered here by international scholars. We learn that family problems are not confined by borders and neither are their solutions.

The first four articles provide a macro perspective on family issues. Ken Root's "Job Loss, the Family, and Public Policy" focuses on the impact job loss has on families and refers to both past and current policies that are designed to address this often unpredictable challenge. Yet, despite a fairly large menu of policies designed to assist dislocated workers, needs still exist for terminated workers, their families, and for the communities in which they reside. Particularly troublesome are scenarios in which both partners are employed by the same company in a single-industry community, when that industry shuts down or re-locates. As Senator Daniel Patrick Moynihan reminded us many years ago, the unemployment rate in the United States is very deceiving because it never includes others, such as family members, who are also affected by job loss. In the United States, unlike most industrial nations, a loss of a job also means the loss of health insurance coverage.

Viewing families in another vein, but still from a macro perspective, Pajarita Charles, Dennis Orthner, Anne Jones, and Deborah Mancini offer us a very provocative article on poor families caught up in a vast and insensitive welfare system. In "Poverty and Couple Relationships: Implications for Welfare Policy," the authors remind us that relationships amidst poverty often depend on economic security, employment support, and the building of interpersonal skills, such as training in parenting and the completion of counseling sessions. Such interventions initiated by government action can help strengthen family bonds during particularly difficult times.

With Teresa Ciabattari's contribution, "Single Mothers and Family Values: The Effects of Welfare, Race, and Marriage on Family Attitudes," we get a glimpse into the consequences of policies that are rooted in false assumptions and stereotypes. We learn, for example, that in the federal government's effort to promote marriage it was assumed by policymakers that poor women, particularly poor women of color, have family attitudes that differ from those of other women. Quite the contrary, contend the authors, as findings reveal that unmarried women of color tend to be more traditional in family attitudes than white women.

Sally Bould expands the discussion about larger forces affecting families in her article, "The Need for International Family Policy: Mothers As Workers and As Carers." Basing her study on United Nations documents on working mothers in developing countries and a case study of a child welfare agency in south Asia, she concludes that globalization, which continues to draw more poor and lower class mothers into the formal labor force, is insensitive to the need for appropriate child care. Consequently, poor children are at risk in the developing world. Bould believes that UN and private foundations need to develop a comprehensive policy and funding mechanisms that take into account women's roles as workers and as carers. Local public funding of quality childcare is not yet possible. To develop "sustainable" services under "local control," funding agencies must also offer local staff requisite training.

But not all family issues revolve around the concept of motherhood. Jocelyn Crowley informs us that a growing number of fathers feel neglected in the ongoing debates about the well-being of children and families and, therefore, seek to address what they perceive to be a serious deficiency. In "Organizational Responses to the Fatherhood Crisis: The Case of Fathers' Rights Groups in the United States," Crowley reports on in-depth interviews with fathers who have been personally affected by child support and custody laws. Contrary to popular perception, argues Crowley, the desire to change public policy is only one of many reasons these men join fathers' rights groups.

Viewing fatherhood from a slightly different angle, Ann-Zofie Duvander and Gunnar Andersson explore the consequences for fertility rates of Sweden's effort to encourage more men to use parental leave with greater frequency. In their article, "Gender Equality and Fertility in Sweden: A Study on the Impact of the Father's Uptake of Parental Leave on Continued Childbearing," the authors report that they expected paternal involvement in leave-taking to be positively associated with continued childbearing, because fathers' leave-taking makes it possible for women to continue their labor force involvement. Using longitudinal data and events-history analysis, they did find a positive effect on childbearing if fathers took a moderately long leave, but it made little if any difference if the leave was much longer. Their results suggest that family policy that encourages fathers to take parental leave may help to increase fertility rates, a major concern in most of European nations, where the birthrates remain under replacement level.

Keeping with the caregiving theme, Carol Harvey and Satomi Yoshino explore the interaction between families and government in the care of elders in Canada, Japan, and Australia. The proportion of elderly is rising in industrialized societies, and there are concerns about the ability of public health and pension programs to fully support elders. In "Social Policy for Family Caregivers of Elderly: A Canadian, Japanese, and Australian Comparison," Harvey and Yoshino conclude that elders in Australia and Canada seek independence from offspring, while in Japan filial responsibility to elders is an ingrained cultural ideal. However, in all three nations families express a growing need for greater societal assistance and government intervention. In all three nations, legislation has been introduced to begin to financially compensate family members who care for frail family members, symbolizing a growing williness on the part of governments to recognize this important form of family work.

Nikki Forry and Elaine Anderson follow a similar path in their research on government support of families who provide care to dependents, be they old or young. In "The Child and Dependent Care Tax Credit: A Policy Analysis," they provide an informative historical overview of the Child and Dependent Care Tax Credit (CDCTC) from its inception in 1954 to the present and reveal a pattern of an inequitable benefit distribution that favors higher income families. Barriers and limitations facing lower income families are identified and policy recommendations designed to improve the distribution pattern of CDCTC are offered.

Clearly, not all caregivers in the U.S. are supported financially, nor do they have access to other benefits that are more common in European and Scandinavian countries. By first identifying the major deficiencies in the Family and Medical Leave Act of 1993, such as only 12 weeks of unpaid leave for those who work for companies of 50 or more employees, Steven Wisensale then provides us with a case study of one state's effort to address America's shortcomings. In "California's Paid Leave Law: A Model for Other States?" we learn that through the expansion of Temporary Disability Insurance, California workers can take time off from work with pay to care for a newborn, provide care to an elderly parent, or to assist a domestic partner who has fallen ill. To date, it remains the only paid family leave bill in the United States.

As we move into the remainder of the articles in this collection, we shift completely into an international mode, as each contribution is either about a particular country or is presented in a comparative format in which several countries are analyzed simultaneously and specific similarities and differences are identified. Topics covered in the remaining seven manuscripts range from the challenges produced by declining fertility rates, to leave policies, to gender issues, and to issues generated by an ongoing conflict between work and family.

In "Birthstrikes? Agency and Capabilities in the Reconciliation of Employment and Family," Barbara Hobson and Livia Sz. Oláh consider women's fertility decisions in the 1990s as influenced by particular policy configurations in twelve welfare states. Policy configurations provide different levels of support for maternal employment and for gender equality in families. They discovered that the most obvious "birthstrikes" occurred in societies with fewer policies designed to help mothers reconcile employment with family life and where few protections existed for families during uncertain economic times. In these societies, the most highly educated women are more likely than less educated women to forego motherhood or to delay having second children.

The research of Marina Adler and April Brayfield runs parallel to the work of Hobson and Sz. Oláh in their focus on maternal employment. In "Gender Regimes and Cultures of Care: Public Support for Maternal Employment in Germany and the United States," the authors explore nationally representative survey data on attitudes toward maternal employment. Their purpose is to examine whether there is increasing convergence of values and policies regarding family life in western societies; in particular, whether there was growing support for maternal employment in the 1990s. They found that public attitudes and policies supporting maternal employment are converging in Germany since reunification, although the former West Germany is still more conservative than the former East Germany. In the U.S., there was little evidence of change within the last decade with respect to attitudes and policies supporting maternal employment.

Continuing the discussion of public policy supporting dual-earner families, Peter Moss and Fred Deven, in "Leave Policies and Research: A Cross-National Overview," explore maternity, paternity and parental leave policies in 19 industrialized societies. They report that Australia and the U.S. remain the only affluent countries to have no universal entitlement to paid leave at or after childbirth. They examine research on the utilization, practice and impact of leave policies, reporting that fathers are more likely to take parental leave when it is a paid individual entitlement. They discuss how divergent leave arrangements appear to reflect the values or norms relating to gender and parenting that permeate national social policy. However, they point out that a supranational governmental organization such as the European Union can effectively push some societies to offer leaves, although these are often unpaid. They conclude by offering scholars and policymakers recommendations for future research and governmental action.

In "Seeking the Balance Between Work and Family After Communism," Steven Saxonberg and Tomáš Sirovátka compare two Central European countries' leave and daycare policies before and after the fall of communism, Poland and the Czech Republic. Focusing on survey data covering individuals' abstract and concrete support for gender equality, the authors conclude that post-communist era policies, that tend to support the male-breadwinner family ideal, are increasingly coming in conflict with demands of the general populace, which continues to view gender equity in a more positive light. Catholicism was found to be relatively unimportant as an explanation for the development of state policies and for individuals' attitudes toward gender equality.

Often running parallel to leave policy and equally important in supporting working families, is childcare. Beginning in 1992, the European Union recognized the importance of childcare and urged some uniformity in its adoption by EU members. In "Trading Well-Being for Economic Efficiency: The 1990 Shift in EU Childcare Policies," researchers Inge Bleijenbergh, Jet Bussemaker, and Jeanne de Bruijn examine the development of childcare policy in three welfare states with a history of strong male breadwinner policy models: Germany, the Netherlands, and the United Kingdom, in the context of the development of child care policy in European Union. At the EU and national levels, arguments prioritizing economic efficiency and women's equal employment opportunities have over time gained ground at the expense of concerns for the well-being of children. The EU still allows nation variability in how EU childcare policy goals will be carried out.

Moving away from a comparative analysis of work and family conflict, Kjersti Melberg offers us a case study devoted exclusively to Norway. In "Family Well-Being Between Work, Care and Welfare Politics: The Case of Norway," Melberg examines gender equality, work load, and family dynamics within a progressive social welfare state. However, despite policies that strongly support gender equity and maternal employment, her analysis of a nationally representative survey indicates that the traditional gender divide still persists, affecting both family well-being at home and worker productivity on the job. There is also divergence in terms of national political goals and individuals' attitudes regarding gender equality, which remain more traditional than policy suggests.

Finally, in our concluding article we are reminded that despite the continuing march of globalization and the blurring of political boundaries, each nation has its own story to tell with respect to family policy. In Gerardo Meil's "The Evolution of Family Policy in Spain" we learn how family policy changed over almost seven decades, in response to political, economic and social transformations. The transition to democracy after dictatorship brought about the most dramatic change in family policies, now designed around the goals of improving the economic well-being of low-income families and helping employed individuals reconcile the demands of work and family life. Concerns about low fertility promise to continue to drive change, as does membership in the European Union.

For those of us who have devoted our careers to studying family issues, this collection of papers will give us a greater appreciation for the strong external social, economic, and political forces that have affected the form and function of families over several decades and around the globe. By comparing countries to each other across selected topics or by carving out informative case studies that offer new perspectives on families and the policies that affect them, we are energized anew to become better researchers, teachers, and practitioners. Hopefully, this collection will not only inform but also inspire all of us to continue seeking new solutions to old problems.

In closing, one cannot complete a body of work such as this without recognizing the enormous amount of help provided by others. Therefore, the co-editors would like to thank in particular the authors who participated in this project. Without their hard work, patience, persistence, and cooperative spirit throughout the review and editing process, we would have surely failed in this endeavor. And, we would also like to thank what once was an invisible force that can now be identified, made visible, and thanked publicly for their contribution to this effort. We are of course referring to the wonderfully gracious reviewers who volunteered so much of their limited free time to read the manuscripts, critique their contents and then instruct all of us on how to improve them. In appreciation of their hard work, we provide an alphabetical listing of the reviewers' names.

Wan-Ning Bao
Linda Bell
Karen Bogenschneider
Pat Boling
Berit Brandth
Preston Britner
Chilla Bulbeck
Jill Bystydienski
Thomas Chibucos
Simon Duncan
Patricia Dyk
Anne Lise Ellingsaeter
Marianne Ferber
Michael Fleming
Joris Ghysals
Tammy Henderson
Sandra Hofferth
Johannes Huinink
Norah Keating
Bethany Lctiecq

Isabel Madruga Torremocha
Ann Orloff
Rene Oscarson
Janneke Plantenga
Phyllis Raabe
Minna Rantalaiho
Tine Rostgaard
Graeme Russell
Pamela Schulze
Leigh Ann Simmons
Denise Skinner
Margaret Strati
Sirin Sung
Maxi Szinovacz
Eileen Trzcinski
Tanja van der Lippe
Liset van Dijk
Karin Wall
Susan Warner
Shirley Zimmerman

Job Loss, the Family, and Public Policy

Kenneth A. Root

SUMMARY. Worker-family units in the U.S. have been impacted by significant work-related changes, including mass layoffs and involuntary job loss through shutdowns. Some post-WWII federal policies have been created to assist displaced workers adapt to job loss, thereby reducing stress in family relations. While these policies assisted dislocated workers to adjust to involuntary joblessness, there are still needs that exist for terminated workers, particularly for those individuals who desire long-term training, those worker-family units that are dramatically impacted–including single parent families and family units where both partners have become jobless–and in communities that are dependent on a single industry or have had multiple workforce reductions. *[Article copies available for a fee from The Haworth Document Delivery Service: 1-800-HAWORTH. E-mail address: <docdelivery@haworthpress.com> Website: <http://www.HaworthPress.com> © 2006 by The Haworth Press, Inc. All rights reserved.]*

KEYWORDS. Displaced workers, family adjustments, job loss

Kenneth A. Root is Professor Emeritus of Sociology, Luther College, Decorah, Iowa. A resident of the Minneapolis metro-area, and founder of Ken Root & Associates, he currently conducts research and consults on job loss.

[Haworth co-indexing entry note]: "Job Loss, the Family, and Public Policy." Root, Kenneth A. Co-published simultaneously in *Marriage & Family Review* (The Haworth Press, Inc.) Vol. 39, No. 1/2, 2006, pp. 11-26; and: *Families and Social Policy: National and International Perspectives* (ed: Linda Haas, and Steven K. Wisensale) The Haworth Press, Inc., 2006, pp. 11-26. Single or multiple copies of this article are available for a fee from The Haworth Document Delivery Service [1-800-HAWORTH, 9:00 a.m. - 5:00 p.m. (EST). E-mail address: docdelivery@haworthpress.com].

http://mfr.haworthpress.com
doi:10.1300/J002v39n01_02

Job loss and job security have garnered a focus in contemporary media outlets (Barnett, 2004; DePass, 2005; Diaz & Haga, 2005; Munk, 1999; Peraino et al., 2001). DePass (2005) described a manufacturer's interest in obtaining a state subsidy to invest in new production technology that would continue employment for over 400 long-term employees, raising the question of whether the state should provide a financial subsidy to companies to maintain existing jobs. Diaz and Haga (2005) focused on the 2005 military base closure roster that threatened 180 installations and thousands of civilian positions nationwide. Often the media presentation of job loss is a scenario with one or two families highlighted, but in reality, both the number of mass layoffs and the number of workers affected are large. For example, the Bureau of Labor Statistics (2005) reports that nationwide, in 2004, there were between 1,178-1,458 mass layoff or shutdown events, impacting 114,000 to 150,000 workers–*each month!* The number of mass layoff events was even higher in 2001-2003, affecting 275,000 workers one month (Bureau of Labor Statistics, 2005).

Job loss issues are major challenges confronting worker-family units today. Root and Park (2005) noted that some of their displaced defense worker sample reported they were relieved to be terminated because job loss brought an end to the stress of worrying about losing their job. They had survived four earlier downsizing decisions, were exposed to numerous rumors, and worried about the plant closing completely. For some of these displaced workers, having an opportunity for an early-out was a relief, a point also made by Milkman (1997) in her study of auto workers.

THE NEED FOR POLICY

Employers utilize plant closings and large-scale layoffs when business conditions change, and under those circumstances, some policy is necessary to both warn and assist the community and those displaced from work. Those who have been terminated through no fault of their own are often angered, hurt, and demoralized. Dislocated workers are frequently penalized in their future earnings, and for those who cannot find work and become long-term unemployed, marital instability is heightened (Bernard, 1966).

While Moen (1980) makes the case that our labor force statistics are based on individual data rather than family data, it is clear that the implications of job loss permeate the family and that dislocated worker families generally bear the brunt of job loss. Families of dislocated workers are both impacted by joblessness and assume important roles in providing a supportive response to the immediate crisis (Gore, 1978). Displaced worker and spouse concerns run the gamut from finances, emotional well-being and physical health for all family members, to a pile-up of multiple stressors.

In addition to displaced worker-family units, communities are also left holding the bag when a major employer leaves town. Although a departing firm is unlikely to provide a transfer option, several displaced worker family units leave the community for employment elsewhere. The loss of the departing firm also impacts the community in other ways. For example, tax revenue is reduced but yet there is often an increased demand for the social/mental health services that need to be funded and provided. According to Rothstein (1986) the ripple effect of the original layoff creates additional job loss among supplier firms and subcontractors at three to five times the direct job loss. In impacted communities, finding replacement work after being declared redundant can be very difficult.

Prior to the early 1960s there were no workforce policies affecting dislocated workers, including a pre-notification requirement. Workers could be–and were–terminated on any given day. Neither an advance notice nor a last-minute job-loss announcement was commonly used. For example, Ehrenberg and Jakubson (1988) found in a 1984 U.S. General Accounting Office survey of companies that terminated 100 or more workers in 1983 or 1984, 31 percent of them provided no advance notice, while another 34 percent provided only 1-14 days notice prior to termination. Job loss announcements have now reached near record highs, with Koeber (2002) describing downsizing as a defining feature of a new capitalism under which all types and classes of workers are at risk of losing their jobs.

Manufacturing Jobs Continue to Decline

A number of research endeavors have focused on the closure of automotive plants, meatpacking facilities, and steel mills, as well as other manufacturing sites (Broman, Hamilton & Hoffman, 2001; Buss & Redburn, 1983; Camp, 1995; Dudley, 1994; Leana & Feldman, 1992; Moore, 1996; Root & Park, 2005; Rosen, 1987). These studies emphasize that job loss results in lower pay and benefits for many workers, limited part-time work for others who desire full-time employment, and for some, periods of long-term unemployment that could culminate in becoming permanently discouraged workers. Other workers retire, or are pushed to take an early exit from the labor force. Sandell and Baldwin (1990) report that dislocated older workers, those who did not complete high school, and those who have been "a factory-based blue-collar worker," are likely to have reemployment difficulty. Osterman (1988) maintains that involuntary job losers face poor reemployment prospects, largely because the labor market fails to absorb terminated workers well. The repercussions of job loss are summarized in *Job Loss–A Psychiatric Perspective*: "The only certainty about losing a job is that it hurts, it threatens everyone, not only the person fired but the family, peers and, to a significant extent, the community" (Group, 1982:4).

Bowman (1988), Moore (1996) and Zinn (1987) focus on the significance of urban manufacturing workforce reductions for minority workers, with this decline altering opportunities for both workforce stability and upward mobility. Bureau of Labor Statistics data (2004a) indicates that 14% of black families, 11% of Hispanic families, and 9% of Asian families had an unemployed family member in an average week in 2003, compared to only 7% of white families.

Job Loss Impacts Workers at All Levels, and Families in All Socio-Economic Classes as Well as All Stages in the Life Cycle

White-collar and blue-collar workers alike confront job loss, not only from plants and firms, but also from schools. Several major U.S. public school systems–Cleveland, Detroit, Chicago, Baltimore, and Minneapolis–recently have experienced a major reduction-in-force for school personnel (Root & Root, 2005). Couch (1998) reports that experienced workers between 55 and 64 years of age are now among the highest cohorts of job losers. In addition to experiencing higher earnings losses than younger workers, these displaced older workers worry about the effect job loss will have on their retirement assets. Among those most commonly exiting the labor market after job loss are women, nonwhites, and older workers (Couch, 1998). Attewell (1999) reports that single parents have higher risks of displacement than their counterparts.

Families with two working adults comprise more than 50 percent of all family units that have at least one working adult (Bureau of Labor Statistics, 2004b), but when both partners have been downsized, the impact on the family is significantly more traumatic. Financial needs hit home literally and figuratively more quickly, exacerbating the stress of job loss. Bakke (1940), Cavan (1959) and Komarovsky (1940) provided early documentation that job loss impacts family dynamics through re-arrangement of family roles and financial management, increasing the potential of strained interpersonal relationships.

The Impact of Job Loss Varies–from Insignificance to Major Difficulties

Zinn (1987:162) summarizes the dominant job loss theme:

> The devastating impact of plant shutdowns, corporate relocations, and displaced workers in abandoned communities is well known. Business in general is being affected; municipal budgets are being drained by the rising demands for social services. The mental and physical health of laid-off workers, their families and friends deteri-orates; rates of divorce, alcoholism, depression, and suicide climb.

Families have differing strengths, allowing some displaced worker-families to respond to negative life events better than others. Those strengths–whether social support, family coping strategies, past experi-ence, or ample financial reserves–act as buffers to modify the impact of job loss for the displaced worker, as well as his/her family. For example, Root (1984), summarizing data from four Midwest closures, found that 18-30 percent of displaced worker-family units sent another family member into the labor force. While several studies have reported that most families weather the storm of job loss, Perrucci and Targ (1988) found that 33 percent of their dislocated sample believed their mar-riages decreased in happiness over the eight-month period for which they have data. In other research, worker-family units have been de-scribed as better off after dislocation because the job loss created new opportunities, growth experiences, or less stress (Little, 1976; Thomas, McCabe & Berry, 1980; Zvonkovic, Guss & Ladd, 1988).

While research on male unemployment and family ramifications has been most typical (Buss & Redburn, 1983; Komarovsky, 1940; Larson, 1984), studies by both Perrucci and Targ (1988) and Gordus and Yamakawa (1988) compare involuntary job loss outcomes between male and female displaced worker-family units. Perrucci and Targ (1988) found that the families of married women experienced similar amounts and kinds of economic strain as those of married men, whereas Gordus and Yamakawa (1988) found that unemployment related losses were greater for displaced women than men. Training for displaced workers and single women in particular is often not practical if the duration of training is longer than the period of unemployment insurance, leading Gordus and Yamakawa to advocate for federally funded living cost stipends for displaced women without other means of support. Rosen's (1987) sample of blue-collar women, who have lived for years with rounds of layoff, unemployment, and reemployment, would benefit significantly from a training program, but their involvement would require a stipend.

Cottle (2001), Laczko (1987) and Rayman (1988) focus on those redundant workers who become the long-term unemployed. Rayman (1988) acknowledges the relationship between the duration of job loss and the severity of family problems, a finding supported by research completed by Broman, Hamilton and Hoffman (2001).

DISLOCATED WORKER POLICY

Since the 1960s there have been a range of federal programs created to help the unemployed obtain work, retrain, or receive job search assistance. These programs are: Manpower Development and Training Act (MDTA), Comprehensive Employment and Training Act (CETA), Job Training Partnership Act (JTPA), Worker Adjustment and Retraining Notification Act (WARN), Economic Dislocation and Worker Adjustment Assistance Act (EDWAA), and Workforce Investment Act (WIA), although most states also have, or have had, supplemental state programs to federal programs.

Those state programs have been important, and necessary, since Leigh (1989) notes that in 1986, JTPA Title III programs assisted only seven percent of the number of eligible displaced workers. While other Federal programs offer assistance to dislocated workers under specialized circumstances, their focus centers on income maintenance rather than providing job search assistance or on-the-job training. For example, Trade Adjustment Assistance (TAA) provides income support to dislocated workers who have lost jobs because of foreign trade and import competition. Under this 1962 program, funds were available for training and an Unemployment Insurance (UI) benefit extension for 52 weeks was provided (Leigh, 1989).

The Manpower Development and Training Act (*MDTA*) was enacted in 1962 to offer retraining to those who were jobless due to automation, as well as those who were economically disadvantaged (Ginsburg, 1983). Training for individuals whose skills had become obsolete consisted of either classroom instruction or on-the-job experience. Classroom or institutional training was often completed at vocational schools to prepare displaced workers for the skilled occupations that the Employment Service determined were needed at the local level. Classroom participants received a stipend, while those in workplace training were paid wages, reimbursed 50 percent to the employer by MDTA.

Although MDTA was a federal program, local program agents acting under grants or contracts with the U.S. Department of Labor delivered the services. While there were numerous positive features of this trial-and-error workforce policy, one disadvantage was that individuals were channeled into existing programs, rather than offering training that met the specific needs of the participants. Another disadvantage was that retraining grants were in specific occupations (i.e., welding), and limited, so only a few dislocated workers were involved in retraining at any given period. Critics of MDTA maintained that most of the training and placement opportunities were given to those who were the most qualified and the least needy. In amendments to MDTA in 1968, on-the-job training projects (OJT) were expanded and states were given more authority to initiate their own programs, paving the way for a more decentralized national workforce program.

The Comprehensive Employment Training Act (*CETA*) replaced MDTA. CETA was created in 1973 to help alleviate a high unemployment rate, and to combine various federal funding sources into block grants to local officials who would be in control and held accountable. CETA gave prime sponsorship to local governmental jurisdictions with populations of at least 100,000, with the prime sponsor determining the mix and employment services to be provided (Leigh, 1989). Overall, CETA's emphasis was on short-term job creation programs in public service employment. Critics were opposed to the "make work" programs in the public sector, as well as the "violation" of the contract terms by renewing public service contracts for the same employees. Reagan administration officials later criticized the program as an income support system rather than a training program. The "training" emphasis, and near abolishment of any stipends became a feature of the next training program, the Job Training Partnership Act.

The Job Training Partnership Act (*JTPA*) enacted in October 1983, contained a separate title for dislocated workers (Title III). JTPA created a partnership among business, local elected officials, and state government in administering federally funded employment and training programs for units of local government with an aggregate population of 200,000 or more. Under the JTPA, individual states were also allowed to be in charge of their own programs. To participate, a worker needed to be a state resident and meet one of three criteria: (a) receive notice of layoff after working with the employer for at least three years and unlikely to return; (b) be laid-off due to a facility closure; or (c) be unemployed for at least 15 weeks after employment with the same employer for three years (U.S. Congress, 1986). No funds were provided for public service employment under JTPA, and income and support services were restricted compared to CETA.

JTPA required states to match federal funds on a dollar-for-dollar basis, but the match was reduced if the state's unemployment rate exceeded the national average (U.S. Congress, 1986). While the state match was relatively unimportant in determining whether the resources would be available or not, Levitan and Gallo (1988) note that the matching requirement had an impact on participant selection. Targeted recipients were those receiving unemployment insurance, and there was a tendency to select community colleges as the service providers.

The Economic Dislocation and Worker Adjustment Assistance Act *(EDWAA)* replaced Title III of JTPA in an attempt to improve services to dislocated workers. EDWAA, which became effective in July 1989, created state-level rapid response assistance to sites after pre-notification was given. Rapid Response Teams met with soon-to-be displaced workers and provided information about job search assistance and retraining. Because workers were not provided an income stipend during training, many were forced to forgo this training opportunity.

The Worker Adjustment and Retraining Notification Act (WARN) was passed in 1988, mandating 60 days advance notice to employees and state government if the company was closing or planning to lay off a large number of workers (LeRoy, 1992). This legislation was prompted by a concern over the loss of several thousand workers in the closure or relocation of manufacturing firms. The Office of Technology Assessment (U.S. Congress, 1986) acknowledges that prior to WARN the typical, but not required, notification of termination was two weeks for white-collar workers and seven days for blue-collar workers, although some unionized workers had a pre-notification clause in their contract that provided six months notification (Perrucci & Targ, 1988). Because job loss in the Northeast and Midwest had been particularly acute, state representatives and local community leaders in these regions discussed potential legislation to regulate closures and relocations. Ohio's Community Readjustment Act was proposed in 1977 (Kelly & Webb, 1979), with similar legislation debated in Massachusetts, Illinois, Wisconsin, Pennsylvania, Maine, and Rhode Island. Between 1980 and 1982, plant closure measures were introduced in several states. Rothstein (1986) notes that several states created inter-agency task forces to provide information and technical assistance to workers and communities that would be impacted by job terminations. The proposed state legislation was a response to a perceived job loss crisis and the failed National Employment Priorities Act of 1974. While never enacted, the National Employment Priorities Act contributed to future federal legislation that requires pre-notification to workers and the state.

The benefit of pre-notification was to help soon-to-be-terminated workers anticipate job loss and obtain reemployment more quickly. WARN applied [1] to employers with 100 or more workers when 50 or more lose work in a 30-day period, [2] if mass unemployment equals at least 33 percent of employees, or [3] if at least 500 employees lose their jobs. The legislation contained in WARN was passed as part of the Omnibus Trade and Competitiveness Act, but vetoed by President Reagan in 1988. WARN was resubmitted and passed in July 1988 (Ehrenberg & Jakubson, 1988). Critics maintained that 60 days was not enough time to accomplish the tasks necessary for either worker-family units to prepare for the transition, nor for communities to recruit new industries to employ those who were dislocated.

The Workforce Investment Act (WIA) was signed into law August 7, 1998. The WIA Dislocated Worker component (Title III) focuses on designing and managing training and employment programs at the local level; providing "customers" access to employment, education, training, and information services they need at a one-stop shop; as well as choices in deciding the training program that best fits their needs (Eberts, O'Leary & DeRango, 2002). This legislation also required linkages with TAA that similarly provided some services to those dislocated workers due to foreign trade. Programs which similarly provided some services to those dislocated workers due to foreign trade. In contrast to the JTPA, the WIA emphasizes returning to work rather than entering a training program (Wandner, 2002).

Local Workforce Investment Boards, partnering with local elected officials, are responsible for planning and overseeing the local WIA program. Critics believe there is too long a delay between the request for, and receipt of, federal funds, thus hampering retraining implementation. Other criticisms include shortages in training funds, which in turn create difficult choices. For example, priority is given to recipients of public assistance and other low-income individuals over dislocated workers. Also, there is concern over high attrition among displaced workers from select community college courses (Jacobson, LaLonde, & Sullivan, 2002).

Implementing WARN was a benefit for many soon-to-be displaced worker-family units because the family units now had some lead-time to respond to job loss. When job loss is not sudden, it becomes more manageable and less stressful and displaced workers return to the job market faster when they are given advance warning (Leigh, 1989; Noble, 1993). Unfortunately, WARN does not cover all workers, so it is still possible for reasonably large numbers of workers to be terminated without any preparation. Additionally, some research documents that companies have not adhered to WARN requirements (Addison & Blackburn, 1994). Compliance with the law is crucial and extends the pre-notification WARN provisions to all who are confronted with involuntary job loss.

WARN was also important in providing Job Center and WorkForce personnel with preparation time. Not only were Job Centers better able to prepare for the terminations, but also through EDWAA they were able to meet with the soon-to-be displaced workers through Rapid Response. The pre-notification process minimized the impact of the congestion effect–the then preferred approach for the company to terminate all workers on a specific day, and in the process create an overload on service providers. While the employer's production schedule continues to control the displacement termination dates in a shutdown or downsizing decision, employers are more commonly using staggered release dates, which are beneficial for workers and their families. A significant improvement for those terminated would be worker selection of the release date that best fits their needs.

With continued WIA funding, Rapid Response Teams are important in initiating an early understanding of what help and services are available to dislocated workers. However, there is no one providing continuous monitoring of individual displaced workers. Many displaced workers have a series of consecutive replacement jobs as they search for a good fit with post-displacement employment, and for this reason alone, the availability of long-term counseling would be beneficial. Other modifications in policy or programming could similarly assist dislocated worker-family units.

There are several areas where existing policy is not sensitive to worker-family needs. Each is discussed below. First, our society appears blind to the special needs of those family units where both members of a two-worker family unit are displaced or the adult in a single-parent household is economically dislocated. Recall that Gordus and Yamakawa (1988) have already proposed that women without means of other support should receive a living-cost stipend while they were involved in training.

Second, Trade Adjustment Assistance is a wonderful aid for those who are able to receive it and want it, but Root and Park (2005) have found that those made redundant who do not qualify for TAA, but would like long-term training, are disgruntled when other dislocated workers qualify. While life options are not equal, there is a need to reconsider support for longer-term training for more displaced workers than just those who receive TAA. A further problem with TAA is the fact that service workers, a growing portion of the U.S. labor force, are not covered by TAA at all.

Third, job loss researchers know that younger employees and their spouses experience higher job loss stress levels than older workers. With thousands of U.S. workers in this "threatened" category (Wilson, Larson & Stone, 1993), we have done little to alleviate the stress of perceived job insecurity and the issue will likely remain with us for a considerable time unless some reform measure is implemented.

Fourth, some social science research has focused on the diminished perceptions of self-worth among underemployed workers (Warr, 1984), yet we seem to have little concern for those dislocated workers whose post-displacement wages are significantly less than their pre termination earnings. Our society has seemingly accepted a lower compensation and benefit bar for re-employed job losers.

Fifth, according to Wandner (2002) targeting is the process by which individuals are selected to participate in job training programs. Selection is necessary because the number of potential program participants exceeds the resource capacity, and receipt of services is not an entitlement. The problem is that even if selected for retraining in any non-TAA supported program, an important kink is the length of time UI benefits will run. Most often, that period is six months. This means that while some direct costs may be covered for a longer period of time, the UI benefits run out, and the displaced worker will either have to have alternative income sources, or will have to drop out of their training program. Either option creates a major negative impact on families.

The problem of job displacement is not uniform across occupations, nor evenly distributed in communities or geographical regions of the country. In towns and cities where the unemployment rate is high, both formal and informal job search methods appear plugged as lay-offs and the rippling of joblessness continues. Sociological research documents that primary groups–whether a nuclear family unity, a work group, or a friendship alliance–are important in the daily life of individuals (Komarovsky, 1967), and provide support to overcome stressful life events (Hanlon, 1982). Zippay (1990) notes that among blue-collar workers, networks are interlocking–family members are neighbors, who are also coworkers. These social networks are important in securing work, but networking with relatives is no longer operational in the job search when relatives and friends are also without work.

Further complicating the situation for those confronting job loss is their reluctance to ask for help. Many confronting joblessness are without work for the first time, and they have been accustomed to being the helper rather than needing help. Typically, displaced workers are unfamiliar with how the system works as well as embarrassed by needing some form of assistance. Rayman and Bluestone (1982) acknowledge that while unemployment is a social condition, displaced worker-family units manage it privately.

CONCLUSIONS

The dislocation of experienced workers has been a serious problem in the United States for many years. Some worker-family units are confronted with an inordinate amount of stress and difficulty when they are made redundant. Among the displaced workers most affected are women, minorities, and older worker-family units. Like some terminated workers, some communities are also affected to a greater degree than others after a mass layoff or shutdown occurs. In those communities that lose their dominant industry or encounter a number of workforce reductions, jobs will be more difficult to obtain and a longer spell of unemployment will be likely for those seeking replacement work. Worker-family tensions may be exacerbated under those circumstances.

Prior to WARN, U.S. workers could be made redundant at the end of a given day without much assistance; often released on the same day, even though there could be hundreds of workers terminated in the same city. Other federal workforce policies have been created which have helped many displaced worker-family units. Under provisions of these federal job loss policies, worker-family units are able to retain their family cohesion and have WorkForce assistance that helps them retrain for, or find, replacement work. Thus, displaced workers have been helped by MDTA and more recent legislation through pre-notification, early comprehension of available options through Rapid Response, job search assistance or retraining, opportunities for participation in on-the-job training programs, or relocation assistance, and for some, a cost-of-living stipend or extended unemployment compensation.

While federal policies have helped dislocated workers adjust to involuntary joblessness, important needs persist for displaced employees, particularly those who are impacted the most and reside in communities that are dependent on a single industry or have had multiple workforce reductions. The benefit of pre-notification is not available for all employees, but in a just society, this should be a given. In addition, quality jobs are in short supply, increased opportunities for retraining are sorely needed, and workers in retraining programs outside of TAA still need stipends and/or extended unemployment compensation. Changes in federal economic dislocation policies that would relieve job security stress and extend the breadth of benefits to all displaced workers would be welcomed. In the process, the well-being of workers and worker-family units would be ensured.

REFERENCES

Addison, J. T., & Blackburn, M. L. (1994). Has WARN warned? The impact of advance-notice legislation on the receipt of advance notice. *Journal of Labor Research, XV,* 83-91.

Attewell, P. (1999). The impact of family on job displacement and recovery. *Annals of the American Academy of Political and Social Science, 562,* 66-83.

Bakke, E. W. (1940). *Citizens without work: A study of the effects of unemployment upon the worker's social relations and practices.* New Haven, CT: Yale University Press.

Barnett, M. (2004, May 31). Starting over. *U.S. News & World Report, 136,* 48-51.

Bernard, J. (1966). Marital stability and patterns of status variables. *Journal of Marriage and the Family, 28,* 421-440.

Bowman, P. J. (1988). Postindustrial displacement and family role strains: Challenges to the black family. In P. Voydanoff & L. C. Majka (Eds.), *Families and economic distress: Coping strategies and social policy* (pp. 75-97). Newbury Park, CA: Sage.

Broman, C. L., Hamilton, V. L., & Hoffman, W. S. (2001). *Stress and distress among the unemployed: Hard times and vulnerable people.* New York: Kluwer Academic/Plenum Publishers.

Bureau of Labor Statistics. (2004a). Employment characteristics of families in 2003. Retrieved March 22, 2005, from http://www.bls.gov/news.release/famee.nr0.htm

Bureau of Labor Statistics. (2004b). Table 2. Families by presence and relationship of employed members and family type, 2002-03 annual averages. Retrieved March 22, 2005, from http://www.bls.gov/news.release/famee.t02.htm

Bureau of Labor Statistics. (2005). Table 1. Mass layoff events and initial claimants for unemployment insurance, March 2001-to February 2005, seasonally adjusted. Retrieved March 22, 2005, from http://stats.bls.gov/news.release/mmls.t01.htm.

Buss, T. F., & Redburn, F. S. (1983). *Shutdown at Youngstown: Public policy for mass unemployment*. Albany: State University of New York Press.

Camp, S. D. (1995). *Worker response to plant closings: Steelworkers in Johnstown and Youngstown*. New York: Garland Publishing.

Cavan, R. S. (1959). Unemployment–Crisis of the common man. *Marriage and Family Living, 21,* 139-146.

Cottle, T. J. (2001). *Hardest times: The trauma of long term unemployment*. Westport, CT: Praeger.

Couch, K. A. (1998). Late life job displacement. *The Gerontologist, 38,* 7-18.

DePass, D. (2005, January 24). Shoemaker's blues. *Minneapolis Star Tribune*, pp. D1, D10.

Diaz, K., & Haga, C. (2005, May 14). Pentagon wants to close 180 military facilities. *Minneapolis Star Tribune*, pp. A1, A20.

Dudley, K. M. (1994). *The end of the line: Lost jobs, new lives in postindustrial America*. Chicago: University of Chicago Press.

Eberts, R. W., O'Leary, C. J., & DeRango, K. J. (2002). A frontline decision support system for one-stop centers. In R. W. Eberts, C. J. O'Leary, & S. A. Wandner (Eds.), *Targeting Employment Services* (pp. 337-381). Kalamazoo, MI: W. E. Upjohn Institute for Employment Research.

Ehrenberg, R. G., & Jakubson, G. H. (1988). *Advance notice provisions in plant closing legislation*. Kalamazoo, MI: W. E. Upjohn Institute for Employment Research.

Ginsburg. H. (1983). *Full employment and public policy: The United States and Sweden*. Lexington, MA: Lexington Books.

Gordus, J. P., & Yamakawa, K. (1988). Incomparable losses: Economic and labor market outcomes for unemployed female versus male autoworkers. In P. Voydanoff & L. C. Majka (Eds.), *Families and economic distress: Coping strategies and social policy* (pp. 38-55). Newbury Park, CA: Sage.

Gore, S. (1978). The effect of social support in moderating the health consequences of unemployment. *Journal of Health and Social Behavior, 19,* 157-166.

Group for the Advancement of Psychiatry. (1982). *Job loss–A psychiatric perspective*. New York: Mental Health Materials Center.

Hanlon, M. D. (1982). Primary group assistance during unemployment. *Human Organization, 41,* 156-162.

Jacobson, L., LaLonde, R., & Sullivan, D. (2002). Measure of program performance and the training choices of displaced workers. In R.W. Eberts, C. J. O'Leary & S. A. Wandner (Eds.), *Targeting Employment Services* (pp. 187-215). Kalamazoo, MI: W. E. Upjohn Institute for Employment Research.

Kelly, E., & Webb, L. (Eds.). (1979). *Plant closings: Resources for public officials, trade unionists and community leaders*. Washington, DC: Conference on Alternative State and Local Policies.

Koeber, C. (2002, April). *His and hers downsizing? Gender differences and reemployment levels of displaced workers in the late 1990s*. Paper presented at the meeting of the Midwest Sociological Society, Milwaukee, WI.

Komarovsky, M. (1940). *The unemployed man and his family*. New York: Dryden Press.

Komarovsky, M. (1967). *Blue-collar marriage*. New York: Random House.

Laczko, F. (1987). Older workers, unemployment, and the discouraged worker effect. In S. di Gregorio (Ed.), *Social gerontology: New directions* (pp. 239-252). Kent, England: Croom Helm.

Larson, J. H. (1984). The effect of husband's unemployment on marital and family relations in blue-collar families. *Family Relations, 33,* 503-513.

Leana, C. R., & Feldman, D. C. (1992). Coping with job loss: How individuals, organizations, and communities respond to layoffs. New York: Lexington.

Leigh, D. E. (1989). Assisting displaced workers: Do the states have a better idea? Kalamazoo, MI: W. E. Upjohn Institute for Employment Research.

LeRoy, G. (1992). WARN and EDWAA: Use 'em or lose 'em. *Labor Research Review, 19,* 99-106.

Levitan, S. A., & Gallo, F. (1988). *A second chance: Training for jobs.* Kalamazoo, MI: W. E. Upjohn Institute for Employment Research.

Little, C. B. (1976). Technical-professional unemployment: Middle-class adaptability to personal crisis. *Sociological Quarterly, 17,* 262-275.

Milkman, R. (1997). *Farewell to the factory: Auto workers in the late Twentieth Century.* Berkeley: University of California Press.

Moen, P. (1980). Measuring unemployment: Family considerations. *Human Relations, 33,* 183-193.

Moore, T. S. (1996). *The disposable work force: Worker displacement and employment instability in America.* New York: Aldine de Gruyter.

Munk, N. (1999, February 1). Finished at forty. *Fortune, 139,* 50-61.

Noble, B. P. (1993, February 25). 60-day notice on layoffs undercut, G.A.O. says. *The New York Times,* p. D6.

Osterman, P. (1988). *Employment futures: Reorganization, dislocation, and public policy.* New York: Oxford University Press.

Peraino, K., Stone, B., Downey, S., Thomas, R., Raymond, J., Irwin, T., et al. (2001, February 5). How safe is your Job? *Newsweek,* 36-44.

Perrucci, C. C., & Targ, D. B. (1988). Effects of a plant closing on marriage and family life. In P. Voydanoff & L. C. Majka (Eds.), *Families and economic distress: Coping strategies and social policy* (pp. 55-72). Newbury Park, CA: Sage.

Rayman, P. (1988). Unemployment and family life: The meaning of children. In P. Voydanoff & L. C. Majka (Eds.), *Families and economic distress: Coping strategies and social policy* (pp. 119-135). Newbury Park, CA: Sage.

Rayman, P. A., & Bluestone, B. (1982). *Out of work: The consequences of unemployment in the Hartford Aircraft industry.* Boston: Boston College, Social Welfare Research Institute.

Root, K. A. (1984). The human response to plant closures. Annals of the American Academy of Political and Social Science, 475, 52-66.

Root, K. A., & Park, R. (2005). Older workers confront job loss: Listen to the men from United Defense. Manuscript submitted for publication.

Root, K. A., & Root, S. (2005, August). *Retire, exit the work force, or find other work: Options for displaced teachers in the current public school budget crunch.* Paper presented at the meeting of the Society for the Study of Social Problems, Philadelphia, PA.

Rosen, E. I. (1987). *Bitter choices: Blue-collar women in and out of work.* Chicago: University of Chicago Press.

Rothstein, L. (1986). *Plant closings: Power, politics, and workers.* Dover, MA: Auburn House Publishing Company.

Sandell, S. H., & Baldwin, S. E. (1990). Older workers and employment shifts: Policy responses to displacement. In I. Bluestone, R. J .V. Montgomery, & J. D. Owen (Eds.), *The aging of the American work force* (pp. 126-149). Detroit: Wayne State University Press.

Thomas, L. E., McCabe, E., & Berry, J. E. (1980). Unemployment and family stress: A reassessment. *Family Relations, 29,* 517-524.

U.S. Congress, Office of Technology Assessment. (1986). *Technology and structural unemployment: Reemploying displaced adults* (OTA-ITE-250). Washington, DC: U.S. Government Printing Office.

Wandner, S. A. (2002). Targeting Employment Services under the Workforce Investment Act. In R. W. Eberts, C. J. O'Leary, & S. A. Wandner (Eds.), *Targeting Employment Services* (pp. 1-26). Kalamazoo, MI: W. E. Upjohn Institute for Employment Research.

Warr, P. (1984). Job loss, unemployment and psychological well-being. In V. L. Allen, & E. van de Vliert (Eds.), *Role transitions: Explorations and explanations* (pp. 263-285). New York: Plenum.

Wilson, S. M., Larson, J. H., & Stone, K. L. (1993). Stress among job insecure workers and their spouses. *Family Relations, 42,* 74-81.

Zinn, M. B. (1987). Structural transformation and minority families. In L. Beneria, & C. R. Stimpson (Eds.), *Women, households, and the economy* (pp. 155-172). New Brunswick, NJ: Rutgers University Press.

Zippay, A. (1990/91). The limits of intimates: Social networks and economic status among displaced industrial workers. *Journal of Applied Social Sciences, 15,* 75-96.

Zvonkovic, A. M., Guss, T., & Ladd, L. (1988). Making the most of job loss: Individual and marital features of underemployment. *Family Relations, 37,* 56-62.

Poverty and Couple Relationships: Implications for Welfare Policy

Pajarita Charles
Dennis K. Orthner
Anne Jones
Deborah Mancini

SUMMARY. Previous welfare policies have discouraged men from assuming active roles with their partners and children, leaving many single-mother families without the relational and financial involvement of men. In an effort to inform social policy, this study explores the impact

---

Pajarita Charles, MSW, MPA, is a doctoral student in the School of Social Work, University of North Carolina at Chapel Hill, 301 Pittsboro St., CB# 3550, Suite 400, Chapel Hill, NC 27599-3550 (E-mail: pcharles@email.unc.edu). Dennis K. Orthner, PhD, is Professor in the School of Social Work and Department of Public Policy and is Associate Director of the Jordan Institute for Families at the University of North Carolina at Chapel Hill, 301 Pittsboro St., CB# 3550, Chapel Hill, NC 27599-3550 (E-mail: orthner@email.unc.edu). Anne Jones, PhD, is Clinical Assistant Professor in the School of Social Work, University of North Carolina at Chapel Hill, 301 Pittsboro St., CB# 3550, Chapel Hill, NC 27599-3550 (E-mail: annejone@email.unc.edu). Deborah Mancini, MS, is a consultant based in Roanoke, Virginia (E-mail: mancinid5@earthlink.net).

This research was funded, in part, by a grant from the Department of Social Services, North Carolina Division of Health and Human Services.

The authors thank Demetrius Semien for his research assistance.

[Haworth co-indexing entry note]: "Poverty and Couple Relationships: Implications for Welfare Policy." Charles, Pajarita et al. Co-published simultaneously in *Marriage & Family Review* (The Haworth Press, Inc.) Vol. 39, No. 1/2, 2006, pp. 27-52; and: *Families and Social Policy: National and International Perspectives* (ed: Linda Haas, and Steven K. Wisensale) The Haworth Press, Inc., 2006, pp. 27-52. Single or multiple copies of this article are available for a fee from The Haworth Document Delivery Service [1-800-HAWORTH, 9:00 a.m. - 5:00 p.m. (EST). E-mail address: docdelivery@haworthpress.com].

of economic, human and relationship capital on couple relationships. Focus groups, conducted with 95 low-income African-American and White adults, revealed that economic security, relationship skills, employment support, fathering classes, and couples counseling are critical to successful couplehood. Based on these findings, we suggest that family policies be designed to strengthen at-risk couple relationships by promoting sustained father-family attachment, bolstering men's employment and educational opportunities, and providing parenting and relationship skills training. *[Article copies available for a fee from The Haworth Document Delivery Service: 1-800-HAWORTH. E-mail address: <docdelivery@haworthpress.com> Website: <http://www.HaworthPress. com> © 2006 by The Haworth Press, Inc. All rights reserved.]*

KEYWORDS. Couple relationships, family formation, family policy, poverty, welfare reform

Although U.S. welfare policies established over the past 70 years were intended to strengthen low-income, vulnerable families, some of these policies have discouraged the formation and continuation of marriage, as well as cohabiting and co-parenting relationships among economically disadvantaged families. Public welfare payments and support have been primarily directed toward single mothers and their children, primarily because public laws often limit benefits, such as cash assistance, food stamps or housing vouchers, when another parent is in the household (Seccombe, 1999). As a result, the presence of men or fathers in U.S. poverty households has been discouraged and typically causes termination or the substantial reduction of benefits to the family if men stay involved with their families (Edin, 1997). Thus, what was once called Aid to "Families" with Dependent Children (or AFDC) evolved into what essentially became Aid to *Mothers* with Dependent Children (Horn & Sawhill, 2001).

Various waves of U.S. welfare reform have attempted to address the issue of economic security by shifting more responsibility to the mother's own economic activity. This has led to a variety of reform initiatives that promoted human capital investments on the part of single mothers, including opportunities to complete their education, get job skills, and move quickly into the labor force (Orthner & Kirk, 1995). These reforms, however, did little to encourage men and fathers to assume productive roles in their families and often discouraged men from sustaining long-term relationships with their partners or their children (Cabrera & Peters, 2000). The only substantial outreach to men came in the form of enhanced Child Support Enforcement rules that attempted to capture the income of men as an offset to welfare checks that the mothers were receiving (McLanahan & Carlson, 2002). States were also given the flexibility to use their Temporary Assistance for Needy Families (TANF) funds to support fatherhood programs and employment assistance, but few states have used these funds to provide significant human capital development types of support (Sonenstein, Malm, & Billing, 2002). Unlike mothers, welfare reform has done little to help fathers gain education or employment skills or direct assistance in finding and sustaining jobs.

It is within this context that the next wave of welfare policy reforms is being shaped. Serious considerations are being given to promoting marriage among low-income families and if not marriage, to sustaining couple and co-parenting relationships on behalf of the children. Under the reauthorization of TANF, current policy includes incentives to strengthen couple relationships and reduce the likelihood that men will leave or abandon their families (Ooms, Bouchet, & Parke, 2004).

This article briefly examines the underlying assumptions that will have to be included in a transformed welfare policy that supports full family (including fathers) involvement. It also examines qualitative data from interviews with low-income fathers, mothers and couples that can help us understand the barriers to implementing such a policy as well as some program strategies that may help overcome these barriers.

BACKGROUND

Policies to support the strengthening of low-income couples are being developed and implemented across many states under TANF reauthorization legislation, but research on low-income, unmarried couples and parents is still in its infancy (Orthner, Jones-Sanpei, & Williamson, 2004). We know much more about the status of single-parenthood and its consequences for children than we know about the sources of resilience and stress among their parents. Nonmarital childbearing is of particular concern because evidence strongly suggests that children who grow up in single-parent families are worse off, on average, than children who grow up in two-parent households (McLanahan & Sandefur, 1994). Even after taking into account important family characteristics such as income, race and socioeconomic status, children from single-parent families are more likely to experience unfavorable physical, cognitive, behavioral, and academic outcomes (Duncan & Brooks-Gunn, 1997). Research shows that these children are more likely to be at high risk for the following outcomes: lower socioeconomic achievement, less education, poorer psychological well-being, lower social integration (Amato & Booth, 1997), lower rates of high school and college completion, teenage childbearing, and idleness in young adulthood (McLanahan & Sandefur, 1994).

Evidence from unmarried parents of these children, however, suggests that many of them begin their parenting with the hope of remaining a couple after their child is born (Waller, 2001). Among the national sample of mostly unwed, low-income families in the longitudinal Fragile Families and Child Wellbeing Study, for example, 82% of the parents were in a romantic and intact relationship at the time of the birth of their child and 51% of these couples were cohabiting at the time (McLanahan et al., 2003). Additionally, 80% of the fathers provided financial and other forms of support during their partner's pregnancy and the majority of mothers and fathers (60% and 75% respectively) reported their chances of marrying one another as "good or almost certain" (McLanahan, 2003). Despite high expectations for marriage, only 9% of the couples actually married within one year of their baby's birth. Another 49% continued to be romantically involved and 42% were no longer together (Bendheim-Thoman Center for Research on Child Wellbeing, 2003). Thus, the dissolution patterns that are well chronicled had begun. The dynamics of complex parenting patterns with multiple births from multiple fathers had been put into motion as well.

Research on the potential benefits of two-parent, low-income families, however, is promising. Conger and Conger (2002) report that children from lower-income families who received affective (warmth and nurturing) and structural (rules and consequences) support made competent transitions to adolescence and young adulthood. McCubbin and McCubbin (1996) found that economically disadvantaged couples often demonstrate high levels of warmth, affection, and emotional support for one another. When optimism and collective efficacy are present in low-income families, children perform much better in school and are more likely to go on to college and increase their opportunities. Even rates of physical and sexual abuse of children are much lower among low-income families when the biological father remains in the household than when that father leaves and other men enter the relationship with the mother and children (Wilson, 2002).

In their study of economic and relational assets among low-income families, Orthner, Jones-Senpai and Williamson (2003) note that low-income families with earnings less than $20,000 per year are often weak on economic assets but their relationship assets are not significantly weaker than families with incomes greater than $40,000. On measures of communication, problem-solving, value congruence, and social support, low-income couples exhibited essentially similar patterns of strengths and weakness. The researchers report, "It appears that lower income families typically struggle with the challenges that come from having fewer financial resources but that this does not strongly influence their overall pattern of relationship strength" (p. 19).

While the potential value of men participating in co-parenting relationships is often recognized, low-income women are not always sure that the father's contribution will be helpful. One in ten low-income fathers are involved with the courts and prison systems (Mumola, 2000). Over half of low-income fathers have not completed high school (Randolph, Rose, Fraser, & Orthner, 2004). Many low-income fathers do not have significant training in job skills and the unemployment rates of these fathers are very high (Blau, Kahn, & Waldfogel, 2000). Their roles as fathers are further complicated by involvement with multiple partners that produce children who reside in different households (Carlson & Furstenberg, 2003). Some of these men also bring with them risks of violence due to poor adult relationship modeling and inadequate skills to manage challenging interpersonal relationships (K. L. Anderson, 1997).

Thus, both fathers and mothers in low-income families recognize the potential vulnerability of their relationships. Opportunities for co-parenting are threatened by inadequate fatherhood role modeling and the sometimes competing demands from other partners and children. This promotes a fragile sense of trust and commitment that must be overcome if these new parenting relationships are to be sustained.

FOCUS OF CURRENT RESEARCH

Research suggests that children benefit from a caring relationship with two parents and that many low-income, new unmarried parents wish to maintain their relationship, but face potential obstacles to building and sustaining long-term commitments. Therefore, the question facing policymakers and program developers is this: How do we help low-income couples build and sustain a long-term committed relationship? That is one of the more significant and new family policy questions and a broader question than how to help couples get married. Marriage, among many couples, is still a confusing, if not remote, concept, particularly among lower income women and men who seek career stability, home ownership, and extended family connections (Edin & Kefalas, 2005). But developing the means to help couples and families get a good start, form sound relational commitments, and build a network of social and economic support to sustain those commitments is one of the new policy frontiers.

In this research, we examine the role of economic, human, and relational assets or relationship capital in the motivation to sustain couple relationships. Theories of economic and human capital consistently hypothesize that when persons or groups exhibit greater assets, such as earnings or job skills, outcomes based on these assets will be greater (Coleman, 1988). Just as having financial capital, such as income, savings and investments, helps us feel more secure in our lives, other forms of "capital" represent assets that can be accumulated and retained as a means of achieving other benefits. Economic capital, which includes financial capital, as well as security in the form of health insurance, household assets and reduced debt, has been consistently linked to family strength outcomes (cf. Orthner et al., 2004). Human capital includes personal assets that can foster economic capital and promote economic and personal security. Education, job skills, work history and personal motivation to succeed are examples of human capital. A third dimension is relationship capital. Similar to social capital (Putnam, 2000), relationship capital is based on the quality of the connections between the people who make up a household, such as having shared values and communication and problem-solving skills (Orthner et al., 2003).

Based on the research findings discussed above, as well as the assumptions of how capital assets may contribute to couple commitments, we expected that men and women in our focus group interviews with low-income couples and parents would report wanting to enter and maintain relationships with partners that offer opportunities for these sources of capital. We also anticipated that they would exit relationships that failed to deliver them. We hoped to learn more about which specific economic and human sources of capital were most pivotal to the sustainability of their relationships and which mechanisms and resources they would endorse as most likely to help increase their potential for long-term partnering and parenting together.

METHODS

Focus group interviews were employed to gather information from single parents and couples about the role of economic, human, and relationship capital in their relationships and to learn about their needs and interests in participating in couple development programs. Feedback from focus groups has been found to be more specific, spontaneous, and meaningful than that obtained from individual surveys and questionnaires (Patton, 2002; Stewart & Shamdasani, 1990). Group interviews may also be particularly advantageous with low-income, vulnerable individuals because of the "safety in numbers" factor (Patton, 2002). In addition to offering a safe environment, the collective nature of focus groups may provide participants with a more empowering and validating experience, especially for historically oppressed individuals (Madriz, 2000).

Sampling Strategy

As is typical for focus groups, a purposeful sampling strategy was utilized in order to ensure that participants possessed characteristics reflecting those of the study population and had experiences relevant to the central purpose of the research (Patton, 2002). Male and female residents of North Carolina were recruited who fit the primary criteria of being economically disadvantaged and able to share information about couple relationships. Additionally, participants were recruited based on the following demographic characteristics: residence (urban and rural); race (African-American and White); and relationship status (single mothers, single fathers, single people without children, married couples, and cohabiting couples). These subcategories were created to produce a range of perspectives on the topics of interest.

Participants were recruited through community organizations such as social service agencies and churches, personal referrals (snowballing), and advertisements posted at local agencies and businesses. In some instances, the group was "piggybacked" on to another event, such as a job training session or parenting group meeting. Incentives in the form of $10 grocery store gift certificates, child care, and transportation (if needed) were provided in order to alleviate obstacles that may have inhibited participation in the study (Morgan & Scannell, 1998). The use of incentives was also intended to convey appreciation for the participants' time and willingness to share their perspectives and experiences.

Group Characteristics and Procedures

Ninety-five men and women, most of whom were parents of young children, participated in twelve focus groups conducted between March and July 2004. The groups ranged in size from 4 to 14 participants, the larger number reflecting a decision to over recruit in anticipation of low attendance rates. Reflecting the higher rate of poverty among African-Americans compared to Whites in North Carolina (U.S. Bureau of the Census, 2000), as well as the out-of-wedlock birth rate (Buescher, 1997), 79% of group participants were African-American and 21% were White. To increase the comfort level and avoid any power differential (Casey & Krueger, 2005), groups were deliberately created to be as homogeneous as possible. For example, separate groups were conducted for men and women (except for couples) and African-Americans and Whites.

Table 1 contains participant characteristics by gender, race, couple status, and parental status for the full sample ($N = 95$). The sample consisted of 47 female participants and 48 male participants. The age of participants ranged from 17 to 52 with an average age of 25. Thirty-three focus group members or 35% of the sample were married, 14 or 15% of the sample were living with a partner, and 48 or 50% of the sample were single. Most of the participants, regardless of current relationship status, had children and hence were recruited to the group because of current or previous relationship experience. The focus groups were conducted in various urban and rural North Carolina community settings, such as recreation and job centers and churches that were both familiar to and convenient for participants. Each group lasted ninety minutes and was audio-taped.

An eight focal question interview guide was used. The interview protocol was based on findings from the Fragile Families and Child Wellbeing Study (McLanahan et al., 2003) and the work of Orthner and his colleagues (2003). As seen in the Appendix, the protocol covered four areas related to couple relationships: (1) barriers to young couples staying together; (2) social and emotional factors that help to stabilize relationships; (3) community services and resources that help couples sustain their relationship; and (4) preferences on potential providers, location of services, and needed supplemental supports and incentives, e.g., child care. Although questions were consistent across groups, the interview protocol was modified slightly to reflect the group composition. Each question was also accompanied by standard probes to encourage specificity and to keep the interviews focused. The groups were

TABLE 1. Focus Group Participant Characteristics by Gender (n = 95)

Sample Characteristics	Women		Men		Total	
	n	%	n	%	n	%
Race						
White	7	14	13	27	20	21
Black	40	85	35	73	75	79
Total	47	100	48	100	95	100
Couple Status						
Married	9	19	24	50	33	35
Cohabiting	6	13	8	17	14	15
Single	32	68	16	33	48	50
Total	47	100	48	100	95	100
Parental Status						
Have children	41	87	35	73	76	80
No children	6	13	3	6	9	9
Total	47	100	38[a]	79[a]	85[a]	89[a]

[a] 10 male participants did not provide information on parenting status. Percents do not add up to 100 because of the missing data.

facilitated by a trained moderator who was selected because of his expertise and experience with focus groups. This leader, a mature doctoral student in sociology, participated in all project planning meetings and assisted in the development of the focus group interview guide and protocol. As moderator, he conducted the group interviews while an assistant moderator took notes, monitored the recording equipment, and ensured that all forms, including an informed consent document, were completed.

Data Analysis

A thematic analytic approach was utilized through a notes-based, question-by-question format. The moderator recorded his own impressions (about content and process) and those of the assistant immediately upon completion of the group session. These notes included process information, such as a description of the setting, the variability of responses, intensity of responses, nonverbal communications, and overall group dynamics. Later, using his notes and listening to the audiotapes, the moderator prepared a summary of the group's responses on a question-by-question basis, supporting his points with illustrative quotes. A second member of the team, utilizing notes, quotes, and tapes, examined the findings across gender groups (Casey & Krueger, 2005; Krueger, 1998) for the purpose of identifying any key differences between male and female informants in the four major areas of interest (relationship barriers, stabilizing factors, needed resources, and preferred service providers). To accomplish this, data tables were created for each focus group question and participant responses were compared across gender groups. Findings were then analyzed for dominant themes within questions and by gender.

Efforts were made also to achieve fidelity in the data analysis. Notes from each group were derived from the observations of both the moderator and the assistant moderator. Their collaborative experiences and impressions were shared with the research team. The opportunity to discuss findings was a reflexive process and one that minimized the effects of researcher bias. The participation of a second person that reviewed the data across groups for gender differences also added another perspective and balance to the analytic process.

Although focus groups afford many advantages over individual interviews, they also have some intrinsic shortcomings which impact these findings and the level of exactness in reporting them. One disadvantage is that focus groups do not typically afford the same level of precision and accuracy as do individual interviews. Frequency, the times a comment is made, is difficult to determine because it may be said multiple times by the same individuals (Casey & Krueger, 2005). Another shortcoming is that extensiveness, the number of times that different people made a comment, is also limited when using notes, transcripts or tapes because it is often unclear who is speaking. Finally, the response time for any one question is limited. Therefore, even when others do have more to say, their perspectives are often cut off in order to ensure time for the remaining questions (Patton, 2002).

FINDINGS

Results from the focus group analysis are presented within the framework of four domains: (1) factors that impede and sustain relationships; (2) factors that help new parents build strong partnerships and co-parenting relationships; (3) programs to sustain relationships; and (4) service delivery strategies to increase program participation. In the words of both men and women, economic and human capital issues present significant challenges to building lasting unions. Relationship factors including unclear expectations, infidelity, and being unprepared for the role changes associated with new parenthood were also identified as obstacles to what are desired but often fragile and unlikely relationships. Participants identified financial competence, employment support, fathering classes, male social support groups, relationship skills, and couples counseling as program areas needed to help men and women do better in relationships and as parents. Focus group members also indicated that community based settings such as churches, as opposed to public agency locations, would provide the most trusted and comfortable environment for classes and services.

Factors that Impede and Promote Couple Development

Human and Economic Capital. Family income and financial problems emerged as the most frequently mentioned impediment to lasting relationships in most focus group discussions (10 out of 12 groups). African-American and White participants, single parents and couples, and both men and women identified economic security as a chief source of contention in many relationships, as well as one of several criteria necessary for a lasting and successful relationship. Women, both married and single, talked about the "burden" they feel when in a relationship with a man who cannot financially contribute to the household. There was agreement that if a man is not helping [with money] a woman can do better on her own. One African-American single mother reflected on her own past experience with her partner.

> I think you can do better by yourself! And like your rent's due and you don't have it all, where are you going to go? You can't go to your partner because he's not working. Then you have to go to DSS [Department of Social Services] for assistance or family members and some family members might say, you've got this [man] living with you and he's not helping and you're coming to me?

Women reported that they are inclined to "show men the door" if they fail to provide economic support to the family. This tendency toward intolerance for financial insufficiency among underemployed and low-skilled men reflects a growing sentiment by women with the same constraints (Edin & Kefalas, 2005; Edin & Reed, 2005). "If I have to act as if I'm by myself, then I might as well be by myself."

Moreover, some women said they viewed men with limited economic and human capital as "children" with dependencies that cannot be easily met. A single mother reported her view about the burden of having a man in the house when there are already other children who command her attention and require resources.

> Financially, you can't do it by yourself. Me, I got three children and I'm a single parent, so that means if you want to have a relationship with me and my children and come into my home, that means that you're going to have to help out with my bills because I'm doing it by myself. And if I'm going to keep doing it by myself that means that you're there like an extra child.

Married and single mothers talked about wanting a partner who can bring home a steady paycheck, can purchase necessities for the family, such as a car and home, and can maintain a full-time job. More conceptually, they also talked about their need to be in a relationship with someone who can be a provider, who has ambition and plans for the future, and wants to share what he has with her and the children. One mother currently in a relationship stated, "I want a man that wants a better life. You know, who wants to make a family and get a good job and like, has plans!" Women's emphasis on economic issues appears to be associated with the idea that a relationship is contingent on a man's willingness and ability to make not only a romantic commitment, but a financial one too. These findings are consistent with other research that shows low-income women hold traditional middle-class values about family and relationships and desire romantic involvement with men who can contribute to the economic well-being of the household in a customary, male-provider role (Edin & Kefalas, 2005; McLoyd, Cauce, Takeuchi, & Wilson, 2000).

There was slightly more variation among men regarding the association between economic issues and relationships. While one father said that money was the most significant stressor in his life, other male focus group members were somewhat less likely to report concerns over economic issues in ways that directly related to criteria for a lasting relationship. Single fathers pointed to the financial burden associated with having children as a reason for relationship difficulties, while other men expressed expectations that a woman should be able to take care of herself and make financial contributions to the household. They recognized their economic support roles but also were more likely to see this as a shared responsibility.

Women also reported concerns about the effect of social welfare programs on relationships. Several programs, including TANF, food stamps, Medicaid, and childcare subsidies contain economic disincentives for marriage through restrictions on the number of wage earning adults that are allowed to be in the family (Hershey, Devaney, Dion, & McConnell, 2003; Horn & Sawhill, 2001). "To the extent that welfare policies or practices favor one-parent families over two-parent families, they discourage marriage and cohabitation and push biological fathers out of the picture" (McLanahan, Garfinkel, & Mincey, 2001, p. 5). Restrictions like these can leave women pretending their partners do not exist and question whether their partners should stay at all. "Relationships are set up to fail by the welfare system," said one African-American mother. Partnership rules in programs like TANF encourage young mothers to choose between the economic security of federal and state public assistance and the economic insecurity of men who may not be able to provide steady income and support to the household.

Women in the focus groups reported that they needed to focus on meeting basic needs, such as assuring that they had adequate food, clothing, and housing, thus leaving them with little time to work on tenuous relationships. Women suggested that punitive welfare policies that can result in sanctions because of an added presence of a man in the house make some of them feel more economically vulnerable, not less. They noted that the subterfuge can leave some women ineligible for food stamps, cause fathers to conceal their existence, and make the sustainability of a two-parent family impossible. As one woman affirmed, "If we weren't stressed with figuring out how to get food, we could focus on family as a unity concept."

Relationship Capital. The second domain of factors related to relationship success and breakdown includes relationship expectations, values, and skills. These played a central role in both men and women's explanation of why couples struggle to maintain long-term bonds and what contributes to successful partnerships. Relational assets such as sharing of values, willingness to commit to a partnership, honesty, emotional security, communication skills, and the ability to work through conflict were raised in focus groups as criteria for supportive, caring, and lasting relationships. However, relationship expectations and fidelity emerged as the two primary themes.

Expectations. Men and women cited misconceptions and unrealistic expectations as reasons for problematic relationships. They discussed, for example, a lack of understanding from their partner about what relationships require in the way of personal sacrifice and commitment. This finding is similar to research from other qualitative studies that examine marriage barriers among low-income couples. For example, the *Time, Love, Cash, Care, and Children (TLC3) Study*, which included interviews with 75 low-to-moderate income couples, found both partners unsure of their emotional capacity to commit to a long-term relationship and some participants doubtful that the relationship was strong enough to endure the demands of marriage (Gibson, Edin, & McLanahan, 2003).

Focus group members identified childbearing as another area in which misconceptions develop. Couples, some suggested, can develop the false notion that having children is romantic and will "fix problems." An African-American married mother said, "Couples have no idea what they're getting into when they have a baby." A White married mother commented that couples, especially when young, "jump into situations too quickly and get married too fast" without being emotionally prepared, without knowledge of who the partner is, and without knowing if they share the same value systems.

Men appeared to hold some similar relationship expectations as women but had additional concerns and desires as well. They identified communication, commitment, and honesty as being foundational to a good relationship. They also, however, made statements about wanting to be with a woman who does not have too many kids, has a good head on her shoulders, can be a good mother, is physically attractive, and is willing to share her sexual history. Men tended to focus on the sacrifices they make and their frustration with the romantic ideals they say women hold.

Trust. Issues of trust and infidelity were strongly visible in a core group of participants' responses. Although both men and women agreed that distrust of one's partner plays a role in many relationship conflicts, this issue was mentioned more often by women, and in particular single mothers. Research by Katherine Edin and Maria Kefalas (2005) with young unmarried mothers reflects the sentiments of the female focus group members who expressed despair about past relationships in which their partners became involved with other women and in some cases fathered children. One mother whose partner had fathered two of her own children and the child of another woman provided insight into the complexities of multiple-partner fertility families.

So that's why it's real hard for me to trust him because he had this baby by this other woman. I know he goes to see his baby and then I'll wonder, is he still messing with her? And I don't mind him taking the baby out, but I don't like him staying over there with the baby. And he's paying child support to her but he's not paying child support for my baby right now.

A father still in a couple relationship said:

A lot of people let things deter them, break their mind down. They let low self-esteem take them where they want to go out and sleep with a lot of women just to add up. I'm a man but that's not a man at all! A real man would take care of his woman.

Women reported difficulties trusting men because they saw them as often less committed to settling down and pursuing stable, monogamous relationships. A mother in a committed partnership said, "He needs to treat me right. You know, don't be going out and doing all this other stuff with other females when I'm here." One low-income, married woman explained that it is important to feel and know that you are emotionally and sexually "the only one." A single woman without children added that she does not "want a man who is dealing with a lot of females."

These complex and quite painful dynamics can leave women with little desire to pursue long-term relationships, let alone marriage. Many of the single-mother participants in the focus groups reported experiencing relief and even happiness when the man was finally gone and the burden of the relationship lifted. One low-income single African-American mother said she "just couldn't keep putting up with him." "He was like the controlling and jealous type. I told him I needed a drama-free life. I'm glad he's gone."

Helping New Parents Sustain a Relationship

Focus group questions directed at participants about the fragility of relationships in the months following the birth of a baby provide another perspective on the complexity of low-income couples' lives. Fathers identified the stress associated with having a new baby as a significant source of tension for young, economically disadvantaged couples. They talked about the difficulties of making the transition to fatherhood, supporting the mother, and maintaining strong cohesion in the relationship. Men shared their experiences about the overwhelming responsibilities that come with newborn babies, girlfriends and wives who suffer from post-partum depression, and the loss of time and attention typically devoted to the couple relationship.

Men and women both provided a wide range of responses when asked to identify strategies to support young couples with babies. Women with children talked about needing more couple preparation with an emphasis on the new values that children bring, parenting strategies, and the need to share childcare responsibilities more equitably with the father. Some men and women pointed out that a couple's relationship must remain a priority despite the additional obligations that come with having a baby. While several focus group couples proposed that women need to learn how to be less neglectful of their partner and that couples should take time out for themselves, one woman reported how difficult it is to meet all the demands of new motherhood:

> Sometimes it's jealousy. Some men get jealous when you spend too much time with the baby. It's like some men want you to give all your attention to them. And that's a big problem and that's why some couples get separated.

Married couples also shared their perspective on "life after baby." They emphasized that couples, particularly young men and women with little life experience, are generally unaware of the changes that will ensue. Several single men and women without children talked about their discomfort with the parenting role and suggested that young couples who are thinking about pregnancy seek counseling because of the "need for understanding and being able to voice feelings since parenting is an unfamiliar situation."

Programs to Sustain Relationships

The focus group participants were also asked questions about what they thought men and women needed to learn in order to have stronger relationships and be more effective as parents. What kind of programs would work, for them and others like them? These questions were exploratory but helped provide an understanding of intervention models that might be effective in supporting and strengthening low-income couple relationships. These questions were designed to probe for their perspectives on the types of programs and classes that they would use or recommend to others.

The skill areas mentioned most frequently by focus group members were financial competence, communication skills, anger management, and parenting techniques. Additional topics they thought should be considered in the design of services included overall relationship skills, coping with complex family systems, personal development to increase self-esteem, conflict resolution, stress management, domestic violence prevention, divorce prevention, and resource development including budgeting, managing money, and making savings and spending decisions. As one young man explained:

> If you get a girl pregnant and you don't know if you want to be around or not, you need to go talk to someone, a minister, a counselor, just for the long run, talk to somebody to think of the best way . . . basically, you have to handle your responsibilities.

Programs targeted to specific population groups were also discussed. A number of men and women indicated that young, disadvantaged couples should have access to premarital programs, individual and couples counseling, couples groups (both for support and socialization), and support services tied to parenting skills. An African-American father talked about what happens when supports are lacking:

> I think there needs to be support systems for young people today; telephone numbers to talk about their problems or whatever. With a pregnancy, that man is supposed to be her support system and vice-versa. If he ain't got no support, from the moment that bubble pops there's going to be problems and confusion.

Some women suggested that new fathers in particular could use support after a baby's birth and need assistance in acquiring parenting skills. For example, mothers recommended that men learn how to care for a baby and how to best support them as mothers as important first steps in establishing a good co-parenting relationship. Women also made specific program suggestions for men that included "father for a day" workshops and watching educational videos; male focus group participants on the other hand recommended that men attend fatherhood seminars and be provided with semi-structured social opportunities to talk with other fathers.

Child care also emerged as a particularly important program area for married couples, even though they often focused their comments on affordability issues. They commented that parents should be able to "write off child care in taxes" or have the "first five years [of care] free or provided on a sliding scale fee." Other recommendations for programs included mediation services, job training and career development, family shelters, and telephone referral systems specifically geared toward "spreading the word about what is already out there."

In a number of focus groups, men and women recommended that programs be developed with the goal of primary prevention among adolescents to thwart problematic behaviors and poor decisions that often lead to unstable relationship patterns in early adulthood. They recommended that children, adolescents, and young adults be prepared for sexuality and parenting. Parents suggested that middle school children be taught more about sex education and the real demands of caring for a baby at a young age. Adolescents, they felt, should learn about healthy ways to communicate in relationships as well as basic money management skills. One African-American single father worried that more needs to be done to "target African-Americans who are 14-21 years who are having a lot of sex and not thinking about it."

Service Delivery Strategies to Increase Program Participation

Feedback was also solicited from focus group participants about ways that new and existing services could be made more attractive to persons like them. Men and women were asked who should offer classes, where they should be held, and what would engage couples in programs and reduce dropout. By far, the most frequently cited answer regarding location and provider preference was the church. Participants also pointed out, however, that some individuals, especially men, may not be comfortable in church settings for various reasons, not the least of which is confidentiality. Despite these concerns, both men and women seemed to prefer a church environment for delivery of couple and parenting support services. Schools and community colleges were other places proposed by a number of men and women. Additional locations that several members suggested were social service agencies, community centers, public health care settings, recreation centers, and libraries. The settings most often mentioned, however, were organizations with services delivered by trusted people known to community members.

Focus group participants overwhelmingly agreed that incentives are needed to increase involvement. Both men and women reported that this is especially pertinent to men since their participation in family and couple oriented services has traditionally been weak. Specific suggestions from men and women for incentives included money, sports tickets, food vouchers, course credit, coupons, gift certificates, child care, and toys for children. Women commented that on-site free child care is often an issue for many programs and would need to be available for both partners to attend.

For many participants "feeling comfortable" was cited as an important criteria for engaging couples in services. Strategies to encourage participation include "personalized outreach so people understand what kind of help they'd be getting," invitations for services by someone who is known and trusted, and having speakers and program staff be "someone they can relate to" or "someone with recent and relevant experience." Women participants also noted that offering food is an effective technique because it provides a social atmosphere and is something often used at a variety of events by different race and ethnic groups.

Some differences were found among men and women's responses to questions about particular program characteristics. Women stated that they would prefer their male counterparts be present in classes and would like to see a focus on couple-specific activities. Men on the other hand were more likely to report preferences for all male programs so they could "hear the perspective of other men" and "be free to talk . . . [and thereby] avoid couple sessions that will lead to arguments." Both men and women acknowledged the difficulty in successfully engaging men in these programs. Some women thought that while men might be unwilling to go to "classes," some might be open to attending "community college courses." In several focus groups, fathers raised the issue of men's general discomfort with counseling environments and said that some men are opposed to counseling because relationship problems should be worked out by couples privately.

CONCLUSION

The findings from this focus group study of low-income couples, singles and single parents indicate that there is both promise and challenge before us in developing policies and programs that can strengthen relationships. If new policies supporting low-income couple relationships are to be successful, significant obstacles in personal and relationship development have to be overcome and programs and services must be redesigned to promote successful couple engagement and sustain couple commitments. This includes addressing the obstacles that these individuals face.

The obstacles to relationship development reported in this study appear to corroborate our theoretical assumptions. Individuals and couples who demonstrate inadequate economic, human, and relationship capital and assets have a difficult time building a foundation for long-term commitments, both to the partnership and to co-parenting. The aspect of the relationship that is easiest for both men and women to describe and highlight is the economic one. Sustaining a long-term relationship appears to be most contingent on each person, but particularly the father, bringing in a steady income that can be relied on for financial security. Mothers do not appear to be willing to sustain a relationship, and replace government economic assistance, without the assurance that their partners are a reliable economic resource. In some ways this emphasis on economic factors is the easiest test for a new relationship and both mothers and fathers gauge the other's adequacy by this simple measure. They admit that this is only a partial picture of adequacy but it is fundamental to security and trust. Therefore, early relationship success appears to hinge on this factor. Seccombe (1999), in her interviews with economically fragile women, found a similar pattern in which the mothers actively weighed the financial contribution of fathers as a primary gauge for whether the relationship might continue.

Directly linked to this economic capital is the human capital that the partners bring into the relationship. This type of asset is somewhat more abstract but it supports the emphasis the respondents gave to economic capital. In a sense, human capital attributes such as having an education or job skill or motivation to succeed in life, were mentioned but not emphasized as much as economic support, a more tangible byproduct of human capital. Focus group participants acknowledged that a partner's attractiveness increased when they "wanted a better life" and were willing to get the job skills and experience that would make that happen. But like economic capital, this attribute was more likely to be mentioned by women and linked to men's capacity to be a good provider or co-provider. The perceived inadequacy of men's human capital was a major stumbling block to women considering their partner as a long-term investment. And the reality of men's higher rates of school dropout and weaker labor force attachment may continue as a crisis for low-income women for some years to come (Orthner & Randolph, 1999).

The importance of relationship capital to the men and women in this study is particularly noteworthy. Both genders recognized that relationship success requires commitment, trust and good communication. The importance of this attribute paralleled the focus on economic issues in the words of the focus group participants. A good relationship is not just one that has economic security but one in which priority in time and effort is given to the partner and each is able to talk and manage conflicts well with the other. In other words, the quality of the relationship is important to these low-income couples and, as other research has shown, they value the same characteristics in their family as others with more income (Orthner et al., 2004). Their perspectives also echo research on impoverished African-American, young men who have been found to have images of what family life should be like that are very similar to other, more economically advantaged, young men. Unfortunately, when these dreams of partnership, stability, respect, and status go unrealized, anger and domestic violence often ensue (E. Anderson, 2005).

IMPLICATIONS FOR POLICY AND PRACTICE

Information from the focus group participants indicates that any successful strategy for engaging and sustaining low-income couples will require a comprehensive family support approach. Simply focusing on one aspect of family well-being, whether it is financial security, human capital development, or relationship skills, will not be sufficient to adequately promote couple and co-parenting relationships. Policies to strengthen these couples will have to be built around new assumptions. Informed by our study findings, we suggest (1) supporting and encouraging father presence in the household unless indicators of violence are evident or incidents occur; (2) providing fathers public assistance to help them gain employment skills, placements, and support; (3) offering parenting and relationship skills training and support to both men and women; (4) providing counseling for couples that are experiencing relationship challenges; and (5) offering mentors or support groups that encourage new relationship and parenting values.

These policy assumptions sometimes represent a significant change from current policies. In every case, men are considered potentially valuable allies in the economic support for their families as well as a relationship resource for their female partners and for their children. Our data indicate that these assumptions are not easy to make, and that without substantial and early family support, the probabilities of success may be low. Once men have left the relationship, and have not engaged with their children, they are less likely to come back or be welcomed back by their former partners. Thus, low-income couples who want to sustain their relationship will be viewed as pioneers in their communities and among their peers. These couples will need competent assistance, support, and on-going encouragement as they face numerous challenges to building and sustaining their relationships.

One policy challenge that must be overcome is that of different agencies implementing policies differently. Right now, responsibilities for economic assistance, education and training, employment support, mental health and substance abuse issues, health care, and parent and family development skills training are lodged in different federal and state departments, divisions, and agencies. This makes it difficult for families to receive integrated support and assistance when the funding, policy support, and accountability cross multiple boundaries. A successful strategy would integrate these different streams into a comprehensive family support agency with all the tools and resources to foster couple and family well-being from pregnancy through parenting.

This is the service delivery model that is currently being supported by the U.S. Administration for Children and Families through the Building Strong Families (BSF) initiative (Dion & Devaney, 2003; Dion et al., 2003). A somewhat parallel comprehensive strategy is encouraged by the Center for Law and Social Policy in their "marriage-plus" program and policy model (Parke, 2004). Both of these program models, especially BSF, recommend that services be directed toward couples during their pregnancy who seek to establish a successful relationship. The reasoning is in large part based on data from the Fragile Families and Child Wellbeing Study which showed that new parents are more likely to have positive thoughts and feelings about their relationship and hope for their future (Dion & Devaney, 2003). These couples would have the support of a "family coordinator" to help them access services, couple and parenting education, job skills and placement assistance, a couple support network, and fathering support groups. Assistance would be provided as long as the couple needs it but at least for the first three years after the birth of their child.

This type of program model, we suspect, would be supported by the men and women in our focus groups. When asked what kind of support they felt would help couples make their relationships a long-term success, they gave priority to economic and employment support, parenting, relationship classes, or mentoring, and support that is not conditioned by the man leaving the household. One issue the couples raised was where and by whom this support might best be provided. Here they offered the recommendation that a community-based, perhaps faith-based location, would be most trusted as a safe and convenient place for these services. They also recommended that the provider be a trusted agent that can offer confidential or private support, while helping them through what are likely to be major challenges they will face. These observations make it likely that services for low-income couples and parents may need to be contracted to faith-based or other non-profit services that can coordinate and link programs across the myriad networks that now provide these various program elements.

In conclusion, the current policy and program environment for families in poverty will need substantial adjustment if priority is given to encouraging two-parent families to rear their own children. The lack of support for men and fathers will need to be substantially revised and replaced with new services that seek to engage men during pregnancy and continue to provide economic, human capital, and relationship development assistance throughout the early years of parenting. There is substantial skepticism that this assistance will indeed be enough to change the life-course trajectories of these families, even from the men and women involved, but there is also hope that this support will make it possible for a growing number of what are now fragile families to become successful models for the future.

REFERENCES

Amato, P. R., & Booth, A. (1997). *A generation at risk: Growing up in an era of family upheaval*. Cambridge, MA: Harvard University Press.

Anderson, E. (2005). *Inner city men who have babies but seldom marry*. Paper presented at the Sociology Colloquium, Department of Sociology, University of North Carolina at Chapel Hill.

Anderson, K. L. (1997). Gender, status and domestic violence: An integration of feminist and family violence approaches. *Journal of Marriage and the Family, 59*, 655-669.

Bendheim-Thoman Center for Research on Child Wellbeing. (2003). *Union formation and dissolution in fragile families* (No. 14). Princeton, NJ: Author.

Blau, F. D., Kahn, L. W., & Waldfogel, J. (2000). Understanding young women's marriage decisions: The role labor and marriage market conditions. *Industrial and Labor Relations Review, 53*, 524-548.

Buescher, P. A. (1997). *Trends in births to unmarried women in North Carolina, 1940-1995* (Statistical Brief Number 8). North Carolina Department of Environment, Health, and Natural Resources.

Cabrera, N., & Peters, H. E. (2000). Public policies and father involvement. *Marriage & Family Review, 29*, 295-314.

Carlson, M., & Furstenberg, F. (2003). *Complex families: Documenting the prevalence and correlates of multi-partnered fertility in the United States*. (Working Paper #03-14-FF). Princeton: Bendheim-Thoman Center for Research on Child Wellbeing.

Casey, M. A., & Krueger, R. (2005). An overview of focus group interviewing. In A. R. Roberts & K. R. Yeager (Eds.), *Evidence-based practice manual: Research and outcome measures in health and human services*. Oxford: Oxford University Press.

Coleman, J. S. (1988). Social capital in the creation of human capital. *American Journal of Sociology, 94* (Supplement: Organizations and Institutions: Sociological and Economic Approaches to the Analysis of Social Structure), S95-S120.

Conger, R. D., & Conger, K. J. (2002). Resilience in Midwestern families: Selected findings from the first decade of a prospective, longitudinal study. *Journal of Marriage and Family, 64*, 361-373.

Dion, M. R., & Devaney, B. (2003). *Strengthening relationships and supporting healthy marriage among unwed parents* (BSF In Brief, No. 1). Princeton, NJ: Mathematica Policy Research, Inc.

Dion, M. R., Devaney, B., McConnell, S., Ford, M., Hill, H., & Winston, P. (2003). *Helping unwed parents build strong and healthy marriages: A conceptual framework for interventions*. Washington, DC: Mathematica Policy Research, Inc.

Duncan, G., & Brooks-Gunn, J. (1997). The effects of poverty on children. *The Future of Children, 7*, 55-71.

Edin, K. (1997). *Making ends meet: How single mothers survive welfare and low-wage work*. New York: Russell Sage Foundation.

Edin, K., & Kefalas, M. (2005). *Promises I can keep: Why poor women put motherhood before marriage*. Berkeley: University of California Press.

Edin, K., & Reed, J. M. (2005). Why don't they just get married? Barriers to marriage among the disadvantaged. *The Future of Children, 15*, 117-137.

Gibson, C., Edin, K., & McLanahan, S. (2003). *High hopes but even higher expectations: The retreat from marriage among low-income couples.* (Working Paper #03-06-FF). Princeton, NJ: Bendheim-Thoman Center for Research on Child Wellbeing.

Hershey, A. M., Devaney, B., Dion, R., & McConnell, S. (2003). *Building strong families: Guidelines for developing programs.* Washington, DC: Mathematica Policy Reseach, Inc.

Horn, W. F., & Sawhill, I. V. (2001). Fathers, marriage, and welfare reform. In R. Blank & R. Haskins (Eds.), *The new world of welfare* (pp. 421-441). Washington, DC: The Brookings Institution.

Krueger, R. A. (1998). Analyzing and reporting focus group reports. In *The focus group kit, Vol. 6.* Thousand Oaks, CA: Sage.

Madriz, E. (2000). Focus groups in feminist research. In N. K. Denzin & Y. S. Lincoln (Eds.), *Handbook of qualitative research* (2nd ed.). Thousand Oaks, CA: Sage.

McCubbin, M., & McCubbin, H. (1996). Resiliency in families: A conceptual model of family adjustment and adaptation in response to stress and crisis. In H. McCubbin, A. Thompson & M. McCubbin (Eds.), *Family assessment: Resiliency, coping and adaptation–Inventories for research and practice* (pp. 1-64). Madison, WI: University of Wisconsin System.

McLanahan, S. (2003). *Fragile families and the marriage agenda.* (Working Paper #03-16-FF). Princeton, NJ: Bendheim-Thoman Center for Research on Child Wellbeing.

McLanahan, S., & Carlson, M. (2002). Welfare reform, fertility, and father involvement. *The Future of Children, 12,* 147-163.

McLanahan, S., Garfinkel, I., & Mincey, R. B. (2001). *Fragile families, welfare reform, and marriage* (No. 10, Policy Brief). Washington, DC: The Brookings Institution.

McLanahan, S., Garfinkel, I., Reichman, N., Teitler, J., Carlson, M., & Audigier, C. N. (2003). *The fragile families and child wellbeing study: Baseline national report.* Princeton, NJ: Bendheim-Thoman Center for Research on Child Wellbeing.

McLanahan, S., & Sandefur, G. (1994). *Growing up with a single parent: What hurts, what helps.* Cambridge, MA: Harvard University Press.

McLoyd, V. C., Cauce, A. M., Takeuchi, D., & Wilson, L. (2000). Marital processes and parental socialization in families of color: A decade of review of research. *Journal of Marriage and the Family, 62,* 1070-1093.

Morgan, D. L., & Scannell, A. U. (1998). *Planning focus groups (The focus group kit, Vol. 2).* Thousand Oaks: Sage Publications.

Mumola, C. J. (2000). *Incarcerated parents and their children.* Washington, DC: Bureau of Justice Statistics, U.S. Department of Justice.

Ooms, T., Bouchet, S., & Parke, M. (2004). *Beyond marriage licenses: Efforts in states to strengthen marriage and two-parent families.* Washington, DC: Center for Law and Social Policy.

Orthner, D. K., Jones-Sanpei, H., & Williamson, S. (2003). Family strength and income in households with children. *Journal of Family Social Work, 7,* 5-23.

Orthner, D. K., Jones-Sanpei, H., & Williamson, S. (2004). The resilience and strengths of low-income families. *Family Relations, 53,* 159-167.

Orthner, D. K., & Kirk, R. (1995). Evaluation of welfare employment programs. In R. Edwards (Ed.), *Encyclopedia of Social Work* (19th ed.). Washington, DC: National Association of Social Workers.

Orthner, D. K., & Randolph, K. A. (1999). Welfare reform and high school dropout patterns for children. *Children and Youth Services Review, 21,* 785-804.

Parke, M. (2004). *Who are "Fragile Families" and what do we know about them?* (Couples and Marriage Series, Brief No. 4). Washington, DC: Center for Law and Social Policy.

Patton, M. Q. (2002). *Qualitative research & evaluation methods* (3rd ed.). Thousand Oaks, CA: Sage.

Putnam, R. D. (2000). *Bowling alone: The collapse and revival of American community.* New York: Simon & Schuster.

Randolph, K. A., Rose, R., Fraser, M., & Orthner, D. K. (2004). Examining the impact of changes in maternal employment on high school completion among low-income youth. *Journal of Family and Economic Issues, 25,* 279-299.

Seccombe, K. (1999). *So you think I drive a Cadillac? Welfare recipients' perspectives on the system and its reforms.* Boston: Allyn & Bacon.

Sonenstein, F., Malm, K., & Billing, A. (2002). *Study of fathers' involvement in permanency planning and child welfare casework.* Washington, DC: Urban Institute.

Stewart, D. W., & Shamdasani, P. N. (1990). *Focus groups: Theory and practice.* London: Sage.

U.S. Bureau of the Census. (2000). Census Summary File 3, Tables P6, P159A-P159B. Washington, DC: U.S. Bureau of the Census.

Waller, M. R. (2001). High hopes: Unwed parents' expectations about marriage. *Children and Youth Services Review, 23,* 457-484.

Wilson, R. F. (2002). Fractured families, fragile children–the sexual vulnerability of girls in the aftermath of divorce. *Child and Family Law Quarterly, 14,* 1-23.

APPENDIX

Interview Guide Used with Single Mothers

1. From what I understand, lots of young women like you say they want to stay together with the fathers of their children but seem to have a hard time making it today. Why do you think that is true?
2. What kinds of things need to be in place for young couple relationships to be successful today? (i.e., what do women and men look for in a partner who they want to have a long-term relationship with?)
3. Tell me more about what you think women are looking for in a partner?
4. Now tell me more about what you think men are looking for in a partner?
5. We have learned that lots of couples say they want to stay together but often break up after their child is born. What kinds of things could be done to help more of those couples stay together?
6. What kinds of programs or classes or activities would you be willing to attend or participate in that might help you with your own relationships?
7. Who could offer those kinds of programs that you would be willing to attend?
8. If the types of programs you just mentioned actually existed, would you and people you know actually go? What would it take to get you to go?

Single Mothers and Family Values:
The Effects of Welfare, Race,
and Marriage on Family Attitudes

Teresa Ciabattari

SUMMARY. In recent years the federal government has made marriage promotion a central part of its welfare reform initiatives. These promotion efforts are based on the assumption that poor women, particularly women of color, have family attitudes that differ from those of other women. This article tests that assumption using the Fragile Families and Child Wellbeing Study, a nationally representative sample of births to single mothers in urban areas. Results show significant differences in family attitudes between married and unmarried White women, but few differences for women of color. In fact, unmarried women of color tend to be more traditional than White women. In addition, welfare recipients are similar to non-recipients in gender traditionalism and attitudes towards marriage, and low-income women often express the most support for traditional gender roles. Implications for marriage promotion policies are discussed. *[Article copies available for a fee from The Haworth Document Delivery Service: 1-800-HAWORTH. E-mail address: <docdelivery@ haworthpress.com> Website: <http://www.HaworthPress.com> © 2006 by The Haworth Press, Inc. All rights reserved.]*

KEYWORDS. Low-income women, marriage, single mothers, welfare reform

Teresa Ciabattari, PhD, is Assistant Professor in the Department of Sociology at Sonoma State University (E-mail: teresa.ciabattari@sonoma.edu).

[Haworth co-indexing entry note]: "Single Mothers and Family Values: The Effects of Welfare, Race, and Marriage on Family Attitudes." Ciabattari, Teresa. Co-published simultaneously in *Marriage & Family Review* (The Haworth Press, Inc.) Vol. 39, No. 1/2, 2006, pp. 53-73; and: *Families and Social Policy: National and International Perspectives* (ed: Linda Haas, and Steven K. Wisensale) The Haworth Press, Inc., 2006, pp. 53-73. Single or multiple copies of this article are available for a fee from The Haworth Document Delivery Service [1-800-HAWORTH, 9:00 a.m. - 5:00 p.m. (EST). E-mail address: docdelivery@haworthpress.com].

The federal government has made marriage promotion a central component of its welfare reform efforts. The proposed initiatives seek to increase marriage rates, reduce divorce, and decrease non-marital childbearing by using welfare funds for education, counseling, and media campaigns that emphasize the value of marriage. These programs are the latest examples of an ideology that has long infused U.S. welfare policies, what Abramovitz (1996) calls the *family ethic*, "a dominant social norm" which mandates that "proper women marry and have children while being supported by and subordinate to a male breadwinner" (p. 3). Current marriage promotion programs are meant to encourage poor women to live up to this family and gender ideal.

Part of the rationale for marriage promotion is the perception "that low income women are reluctant to marry and that their family values are out of step with mainstream America (i.e., White and middle-class families)" (Lichter, Batson, & Brown, 2004, p. 4), a perception that is applied especially to African American single mothers (Jones & Luo, 1999; Thomas, 1994). But what is the empirical basis for these assumptions? Do women who are welfare recipients have different family values than other women? By analyzing national data on single mothers, this article will address this question and explore the linkages between welfare receipt, marital status, race/ethnicity, and attitudes about marriage and family.

This study makes several contributions. First, I use an important new dataset, the Fragile Families and Child Wellbeing Study. This is a national sample of urban single mothers that includes a comparison group of married mothers. The respondents are mainly women with low incomes and over half of the sample are women of color, including African American women and both native- and foreign-born Latinas. Second, this analysis addresses an important empirical need. In the controversy surrounding marriage promotion and welfare reauthorization, there were many calls for more empirical data on welfare recipients' family attitudes, behaviors, and needs (Lichter et al., 2004; National Council on Family Relations [NCFR], 2003). This article attempts to fill that gap and help us understand if and how poor single mothers differ from married mothers in family attitudes. By subjecting the ideological assumptions of marriage promotion policies to empirical scrutiny, this article will inform ongoing policy debates about recent federal and state efforts to promote marriage.

MARRIAGE PROMOTION POLICIES
AND THE FAMILY ETHIC

Policymakers and much of the American public express concern about the values of welfare recipients and other low-income families (Aaron, Mann, & Taylor, 1994). They believe that welfare recipients lack a work ethic, have little respect for the institution of marriage, and go on to teach these problematic attitudes and behaviors to their children in an ongoing culture of poverty (Bullock, 1999; Gilens, 1999; Jones & Luo, 1999; Ricketts & Sawhill, 1988; Thomas, 1994). This perception that welfare recipients have different values than the general public may explain why most Americans distrust the welfare system and those who use it (Gilens, 1999).

In fact, the 1996 welfare reform bill–the Personal Responsibility and Work Opportunity Reconciliation Act (PRWORA)–was designed specifically to address these value concerns. Its key components are embeed with ideological currents that reflect dominant values and ideals: "Public policies represent standards, or rules, for conduct. . . . They reflect what we [society] value, what we believe, and what we think is in our best interests" (Lerner, Sparks, & McCubbin, 2000, p. 380). For example, the work requirements and "work-first" strategy intended to address the perceived lack of work ethic among welfare recipients. Similarly, the bill explicitly promoted marriage as an anti-poverty strategy, and marriage was mentioned in three of the four stated goals of the TANF program: (1) to end the dependence of needy parents on government benefits by promoting job preparation, work, and marriage; (2) to prevent and reduce the incidence of out-of-wedlock pregnancies; and (3) to encourage the formation and maintenance of two-parent families.[1]

Although the new work requirements and time limits received the most attention at the time PRWORA was passed and in the first few years of its implementation, marriage promotion is now becoming a more prominent, and well-funded, strategy. President Bush has made marriage promotion a focal point of his welfare reform proposals, and Congress has responded favorably to his suggestions. The version of the TANF reauthorization bill that passed the House in 2003 provides $1.8 billion over five years to promote marriage under the Healthy Marriage Initiative (Parke, 2004). Activities allowed under this initiative include advertising campaigns on the value of marriage, high school education programs to teach the value of marriage and marriage skills, pre-marital education programs, marriage mentoring, and divorce reduction strategies.[2]

Implicit in these programs is the assumption that welfare recipients and other low-income women (and men) need to be taught the value of marriage. This is consistent with what Susan Thomas (1994) calls the "myth of the culture of single motherhood," which locates the causes of poverty in the individual behavioral and moral pathology of single mothers. For example, this myth blames single mothers' poverty on inappropriate sexual behavior, mistimed childbearing, a lack of work ethic, and a disregard for the institution of marriage. This myth has direct implications for poverty reduction. If moral weakness and poor decisions are seen as causes of poverty, moral education and behavioral reforms become solutions to poverty. It focuses on reforming individuals rather than redesigning social and economic structures.

SINGLE MOTHERS, WELFARE, AND FAMILY ATTITUDES

But do welfare recipients and other poor women have different family attitudes than other women? The assumption is that differences in marriage and childbearing behaviors between poor and non-poor women, and among White, Black, and Latina women, reflect underlying differences in values and attitudes. However, research using national-level data to explore low-income women's marital and family attitudes is scarce (Lichter et al., 2004).

That research which does exist shows a complex picture in which poor women aspire to, and think very highly of, marriage, even as they experience significant barriers to achieving and maintaining it. Ironically, it is poor women's high regard for marriage that may contribute to low marriage rates (Edin & Kefalas, 2005). They tend to view marriage as a culmination of personal, financial, and relational success, a success that is very difficult to achieve, given limited resources and opportunities (Cherlin, 2004).

Recent research has documented women's desire for marriage. Waller (2001), for example, found that unmarried parents in the Fragile Families study, especially those who are cohabiting, have high expectations for marriage. More than half of the whole sample and 75% of cohabitors report a pretty good or almost certain chance of marriage. Similarly, Lichter et al. (2004) found that single mothers desire marriage as much as childless single women, yet they also express lower expectations for actually getting married. Employment, income, and receipt of public assistance have no effect on women's desires for marriage (Bulcroft & Bulcroft, 1993; South, 1993), although South (1993) found that more highly educated women did express a slightly stronger desire to marry. He also documented no racial/ethnic differences in marital desires. Similarly, Sassler and Schoen (1999) found that attitudes cannot explain Black/White differences in marital behaviors.

Several recent studies demonstrate the complex relationships between race/ethnicity and marital attitudes. Using the National Survey of Families and Households, Bulcroft and Bulcroft (1993) found that Black women perceived more economic, social, and emotional benefits from marriage than White women, yet also expressed lower expectations for marriage. Black women were also less willing to marry men with fewer resources. In addition, Jones and Luo (1999) found that African Americans, both poor and nonpoor, are more approving of single motherhood than Whites. In studies of the marital attitudes of Latinos, Oropesa (1996) found that both Mexican Americans and Puerto Ricans, especially those who are foreign-born, are more pro-nuptial than Whites, although Puerto Ricans are also more likely to approve of cohabitation. South (1993) found that Hispanic men had higher desire for marriage than White men, but there were no differences between White and Hispanic women in their desires for marriage.

Welfare recipients and low-income single mothers have not been the focus of studies using national data, although they have been the focus of several important ethnographic analyses (Coley, 2002; Edin, 2000; Edin & Kefalas, 2005; Gibson-Davis, Edin, & McLanahan, 2005). These analyses have emphasized not only women's desire for marriage, but also the multiple barriers to successful relationship building that they face, including the need to reach financial and relationship stability *before* entering into marriage (Edin, 2000; Gibson-Davis et al., 2004). Gender mistrust and violence are also real concerns for many women that inhibit their ability to transfer marital desires into marriage (Coley, 2002; Edin, 2000).

In sum, the existing literature shows that poor women have strong desires to marry, but also express reservations about, and face obstacles to, achieving this goal. This analysis builds on previous research by exploring low-income single mothers' attitudes on a variety of marriage and family items and by examining specifically the effects of welfare receipt and race/ethnicity on these attitudes.

DATA AND METHODS

This article analyzes the Fragile Families and Child Wellbeing Study,[3] a nationally representative sample of nonmarital births in U.S. cities with populations over 200,000 that also includes a comparison group of married mothers. The baseline data were collected from a sample of families in 20 U.S. cities between February 1998 and September 2000, immediately after the birth of the focal child. This sample is ideally suited to this analysis because it comprises women who have been the object of most of the attention surrounding welfare reform: primarily poor, single mothers living in urban areas. Respondents with missing data on any dependent or independent variable were excluded, and all analyses used weighted data ($N = 2299$).

Dependent Variables

The Fragile Families study includes twelve items measuring attitudes towards families, marriage, and gender. For each item, respondents were asked to strongly agree, agree, disagree, or strongly disagree. The items are listed in Table 1. Correlation matrices were examined and factor analysis was conducted to explore whether these items could be combined into one or several scales (analyses not shown). Analyses of the 12 items showed that 60 of the 66 inter-item correlations (91%) were less than .30 and only one was greater than .50.[4] Factor analysis of the 12 items showed factors with limited face validity, and the resultant alphas for potential scales were moderate (less than .68). As a result, I decided not to combine the items into scales. In addition, because of the large number of items, I have collapsed the categories so that respondents who answered strongly agree or agree are coded 1 and those who answered disagree or strongly disagree are coded 0.[5]

Independent Variables

The focal independent variables are marital status, race/ethnicity, welfare receipt, and income. Although about half of unmarried mothers are cohabiting with a partner (Sigle-Rushton & McLanahan, 2002), the rhetoric and ideology of welfare and marriage promotion emphasizes the differences between married and unmarried women. Thus, the analysis makes only this more basic distinction. Additional analyses differentiating married, cohabiting, and non-cohabiting women show results consistent with those reported here, and are available from the author by request. To capture interactions, I used a combined measure of marital status and race/ethnicity. Women were placed into one of eight categories: married White, unmarried White, married Black, unmarried Black, married native-born Latina, unmarried native-born Latina, married for-

TABLE 1. Dependent Variable Items

	Percentage agreeing or strongly agreeing		
	Unmarried	Married	Total
Marital Attitudes:			
The main advantage of marriage is financial security.	41.9	26.6*	37.8
All in all, there are more advantages to being single than being married.	34.0	10.5*	27.8
It is better for a couple to get married than to just live together.	51.7	70.2*	56.6
Living together is just the same as being married.	45.7	17.4*	38.2
Marriage and Child Well-being:			
A mother living alone can bring up her child as well as a married couple.	83.3	56.4*	76.2
It is better for children if their parents are married.	63.9	82.1*	68.8
When there are children in the family, parents should stay together even if they don't get along.	8.5	14.6*	10.1
Gender Traditionalism:			
The important decisions in the family should be made by the man of the house.	12.3	19.0*	14.1
It is much better for everyone if the man earns the main living and the woman takes care of the home and family.	24.9	32.0*	26.8
It is more important for a man to spend time with his family than to work as many hours as he can.	63.3	80.3*	67.8
Gender Mistrust:			
In a dating relationship, a man is largely out to take advantage of a woman.	15.6	7.5*	13.5
Men cannot be trusted to be faithful.	19.7	6.7*	16.3
N	1,689	610	2,299

* Significantly different than unmarried mothers at *p* <= .05

eign-born Latina, and unmarried foreign-born Latina. Latinas were differentiated by nativity because foreign-born women tend to have more traditional attitudes than native-born (Oropesa, 1996; Oropesa & Gorman, 2000).

The survey asked women if they have received welfare or food stamps in the 12 months prior to birth; those who responded yes were coded 1 on the welfare receipt variable and those who have not were coded 0. Finally, the variable measuring income divides women into three categories, based on household income in the previous 12 months: $0-14,999, $15,000-34,999, and $35,000 or more.

Several additional control variables were also included in the models. First, I controlled for education, identifying women as having less than a high school degree, a high school degree, or some college or a college degree, including vocational training and associate degrees. Because religiosity is highly correlated with attitudes towards family and marriage, I also controlled for whether the respondent is a frequent church attendee, defined as attending religious service at least several times per month. Also, previous research has shown that one's family of origin affects familial attitudes, so I included controls for whether the mother was living with both of her biological parents at age 15. Finally, I included controls for the parity of the focal birth and the mother's age at birth.

Analytical Strategy

Analysis proceeded in several steps. First, I examined descriptive statistics on all independent and dependent variables. Next, I ran multivariate logistic regression models where the dependent variable measures 1 if the respondent strongly agrees or agrees with the statement and 0 if she disagrees or strongly disagrees with the statement (tables available from the author). I then used the coefficients (log odds) from the logistic regression equations to calculate predicted probabilities for women in each category of the focal independent variables, with other variables set at their modes or means. This technique allows for a more detailed comparison of the estimated effects of the variables of interest. Because of the large number of models that were run, I present the predicted probabilities only for the variables that show significant effects in the multivariate logistic regression models.

RESULTS

Descriptives

Table 2 shows descriptive statistics for the independent variables. A plurality of the sample (37%) are unmarried Black women. Unmarried native-born Latinas are the second largest group (17%), and married and unmarried White women each make up about 14% of the sample. The rest of the sample are married Black women (6%), married native-born Latinas (4%), married foreign-born Latinas (3%), and unmarried foreign-born Latinas (4%). Only 20% of the unmarried mothers are White, compared to 54% of the married mothers. Consistent with the sample design, about 73% of the respondents are unmarried. Thirty-five percent of the respondents report receiving welfare or food stamps in the 12 months prior to the interview, 44% of unmarried

TABLE 2. Descriptive Statistics for Independent Variables

| | Percentage / Mean | | |
	Unmarried Mothers	Married Mothers	Total
Race/Marital Status:			
Married White	—	53.9	14.3
Unmarried White	20.2	—	14.8
Married Black	—	21.8	5.8
Unmarried Black	50.6	—	37.2
Married native-born Latina	—	14.3	3.8
Unmarried native-born Latina	23.2	—	17.1
Married foreign-born Latina	—	10.0	2.7
Unmarried foreign-born Latina	6.0	—	4.4
Received welfare or food stamps	44.2	11.0*	35.4
Education:			
Less than high school	34.4	10.8	28.1
High school degree	34.7	20.2	30.8
Some college or college degree	30.9	69.0	41.0
Household Income:			
$0 - 14,999	46.4	11.2	37.0
$15,000 - 34,999	32.5	23.6	30.1
$35,000 +	21.2	65.3	32.9
Living with both parents at age 15	35.8	62.6*	42.9
Attends religious service regularly	33.1	48.7*	37.2
Parity *(Mean)*	2.0	2.0	2.0
Age *(Mean)*	24.0	29.3*	25.4
N	1,689	610	2,299

* Significantly different than unmarried mothers at $p <= .05$

women and 11% of married women. Unmarried mothers are about evenly distributed by education level, with about one-third of the respondents in each of the three education categories. However, over two-thirds (69%) of the married mothers have some college or a college degree. Similarly, the unmarried mothers report much lower household incomes: 46% report household incomes less than $15,000 per year and only 21% have incomes greater that $35,000. Among married women, 65% are in the highest income group and only 11% have incomes less than $15,000. Unmarried mothers are also less likely than married mothers to have lived with both parents at age 15 (36% vs. 63%, respectively) and to attend religious services regularly (33% vs. 49%, respectively). The mean parity for both groups of mothers is 2.0, and the mean age of unmarried mothers is 24.0, compared to 29.3 for married mothers.

Table 1 shows the percentage of respondents agreeing or strongly agreeing with each dependent variable statement, by marital status. The results show that married women are more traditional than unmarried women. They are more likely to agree that it is better to get married than to live together, more likely to agree it is better for children if their parents are married, less likely to agree that a single mother can raise a child as well as a married couple, and are more gender traditional. Unmarried women are more likely than married women to mistrust men.

Multivariate Analysis

To test whether these differences in attitudes can be explained by compositional differences in the samples, I ran logistic regression models to predict the os of agreeing with each statement controlling for the independent variables listed in Table 2 (tables available from author). I then used significant results from these models to compute the estimated effects of marital status, welfare, and income on select dependent variables. These effects are shown in Tables 3 to 5, respectively.

Table 3 shows the estimated effects of marital status on the 12 attitude items by race/ethnicity. The probabilities are computed based on the full multivariate logistic regression models, with all covariates held constant. T-tests for significant differences in the probabilities test for differences between marital status categories within each racial/ethnic group and between each racial/ethnic category within the marital status group. For example, I test whether the estimated probability for unmarried White women is significantly different than the probability for married White women, unmarried Black women, and both groups of unmarried Latinas.

The results show that marital status affects White women's attitudes more than it affects the attitudes of women of color, with significant differences for White mothers on 8 of the 12 items. Unmarried White mothers are more likely than married mothers to agree that there are more advantages to being single than being married ($Pr = .29$ & $Pr = .11$, respectively), that living together is equivalent to marriage ($Pr = .50$ & $Pr = .18$), and that a single mother can raise her child as well as a married couple ($Pr = .81$ & $Pr = .68$). They are less likely to agree that it is better to get married than to live together ($Pr = .40$ & $Pr = .69$), that it is better for children if their parents are married ($Pr = .63$ & $Pr = .77$), that parents should stay together for the children ($Pr = .02$ & $Pr = .12$), that important decisions should be made by men ($Pr = .05$ & $Pr = .13$), and that it is better for men to work and women to care for the home ($Pr = .24$ &

TABLE 3. Estimated Effects of Marital Status on Family Attitudes, by Race/Ethnicity

	White Unmarried	White Married	Black Unmarried	Black Married	Native-born Latina Unmarried	Native-born Latina Married	Foreign-born Latina Unmarried	Foreign-born Latina Married
Marital Attitudes:								
The main advantage of marriage is financial security.	0.400	0.315[c]	0.626	0.534	0.474	0.496[c]	0.524	0.325
All in all, there are more advantages to being single than being married.	0.290[abcd]	0.112[abcd]	0.432[b]	0.342[b]	0.424[ac]	0.243[ac]	0.509[ad]	0.298[ad]
It is better for a couple to get married than to just live together.	0.397[ab]	0.689[ac]	0.566[abe]	0.698[ae]	0.420[e]	0.536[ceg]	0.562	0.752[g]
Living together is just the same as being married.	0.503[ac]	0.176[ac]	0.412[ef]	0.282[e]	0.673[ace]	0.459[ace]	0.614[af]	0.313[a]
Marriage and Child Well-being:								
A mother living alone can bring up her child as well as a married couple.	0.813[abc]	0.676[abc]	0.913[bf]	0.864[bf]	0.912[cg]	0.859[c]	0.743[fg]	0.741[f]
It is better for children if their parents are married.	0.627[ad]	0.769[a]	0.568[f]	0.690	0.571[g]	0.678	0.909[dfg]	0.792
When there are children in the family, parents should stay together even if they don't get along.	0.021[abd]	0.120[a]	0.069[be]	0.078	0.031[ae]	0.107[a]	0.072[d]	0.074

TABLE 3 (continued)

	White Unmarried	White Married	Black Unmarried	Black Married	Native-born Latina Unmarried	Native-born Latina Married	Foreign-born Latina Unmarried	Foreign-born Latina Married
Gender Traditionalism:								
The important decisions in the family should be made by the man of the house.	0.052[acd]	0.125[a]	0.092	0.145	0.113[c]	0.163	0.144[d]	0.195
It is much better for everyone if the man earns the main living and the woman takes care of the home and family.	0.239[abd]	0.381[abd]	0.149[bef]	0.231[bf]	0.227[aeg]	0.367[ag]	0.579[dfg]	0.608[dfg]
It is more important for a man to spend time with his family than to work as many hours as he can.	0.800[bd]	0.829[b]	0.626[be]	0.534[bef]	0.721[e]	0.766[e]	0.647[d]	0.744[f]
Gender Mistrust:								
In a dating relationship, a man is largely out to take take advantage of a woman.	0.068[cd]	0.053[cd]	0.103[ef]	0.066[e]	0.169[ce]	0.193[ce]	0.265[df]	0.178[d]
Men cannot be trusted to be faithful.	0.086[bcd]	0.054[cd]	0.220[bf]	0.131	0.253[cg]	0.247[c]	0.420[dfg]	0.273[d]
N	341	329	855	133	392	87	101	61

Notes: Based on logistic regression models in Table 3. Probabilities are for mothers with a high school degree, with household income $0 - 14,999, who did not receive welfare, who did not live with both biological parents at age 15, who do not attend religious services regularly, who have 2 children, and are 25 years old.

a. Within race difference in probability is significant at p <= .05.
b. Within marital status, White vs. Black difference is significant at p <= .05.
c. Within marital status, White vs. native-born Latina difference is significant at p <= .05.
d. Within marital status, White vs. foreign-born Latina difference is significant at p <= .05.
e. Within marital status, Black vs. native-born Latina difference is significant at p <= .05.
f. Within marital status, Black vs. foreign-born Latina difference is significant at p <= .05.
g. Within marital status, native-born vs. foreign-born Latina difference is significant at p <= .05.

Pr = .38). Thus, the results for White women show consistent and significant differences in the attitudes of married and unmarried women.

The results for women of color, however, are much different. For Black women, only one difference by marital status is significant: unmarried Black women are less likely to agree that it is better to get married than to live together (Pr = .57 & Pr = .70), and this difference is much smaller than it is for Whites (Δ Pr = .13 for Blacks and Δ Pr = .29 for Whites). On all other items, there are no differences in the attitudes of married and unmarried Black women. Unmarried and married Latinas also hold similar attitudes. Both native- and foreign-born Latinas who are not married are more likely than married Latinas to agree that there are more advantages to being single and that living together is the same as being married. In addition, unmarried native-born Latinas are also less likely than married women to agree that parents should stay together for the children (Pr = .03 & Pr = .11, respectively). In sum, the effects of marital status on family attitudes are strong and consistent for White women, but few significant effects emerge for women of color.

Several other racial/ethnic patterns in attitudes are evident in Table 3. Foreign-born Latinas are more likely than all other women to support separate spheres, and women of color are more likely than Whites to see the advantages of being single. In addition, most women agree that single mothers can raise good children, but within each marital status, White women and foreign-born Latinas are least likely to agree. Similarly, few women agree that men should make the important decisions, but all Latinas and married White and Black women are more likely to agree. Black women and unmarried foreign-born Latinas are least likely to agree that men should spend time with their families rather than work. Finally, Latinas are most mistrustful of men.

Tables 4 and 5 focus specifically on unmarried women and examine more closely the effects of welfare receipt and income on their attitudes. Only attitude items that are significantly affected by these variables in the full multivariate models are examined (results not shown). For welfare, the logistic regression models show that women who have received welfare are no different from those who have not, except on one item: welfare recipients are less likely to agree that men should spend time with family rather than work as many hours as possible. There are no significant differences between welfare recipients and non-recipients on the other 11 attitude items. The estimated effect of welfare receipt on this item is shown in Table 4 for unmarried mothers. For all racial/ethnic groups, recipients are more likely than non-recipients to

TABLE 4. Estimated Effects of Welfare Receipt on the Probability of Agreeing that "It is more important for a man to spend time with this family than to work as many hours as he can," Unmarried Mothers by Race/Ethnicity

	White	Black	Native-born Latina	Foreign-born Latina
Received welfare	0.684[abc]	0.476[ab]	0.584[a]	0.498[ac]
Did not receive welfare	0.800[bc]	0.626[b]	0.721	0.647[c]
N	341	855	392	101

Notes: Based on logistic regression models in Table 3. Probabilities are for unmarried mothers with a high school degree, with household income $0 - 14,999, who did not live with both biological parents at age 15, who do not attend religious services regularly, who have 2 children, and are 25 years old.
a. Significantly different than probability for non-recipients at $p <= .05$.
b. White vs. Black difference is significant at $p <= .05$.
c. White vs. foreign-born Latina difference is significant at $p <= .05$.

agree. For example, the difference in probability for Whites is .12, for Blacks is .15, for native-born Latinas is .14, and for foreign-born Latinas is .15. In addition, Black women and foreign-born Latinas are least likely to agree with this statement.

Table 5 shows the estimated effects of income on select attitudes for unmarried women. On the first three marital attitude items, the highest income women in all racial/ethnic groups are less likely to agree than the lowest income women. Specifically, higher income women are less likely to agree that there are more advantages to being single than being married (Pr = .19 & Pr = .29, respectively), that it is better to get married than to live together (Pr = .30 & Pr = .40), and that the main advantage of marriage is financial security (Pr = .26 & Pr = .40). Interestingly, high-income women are less likely to recognize the advantages of being single, but also less likely to value marriage over cohabitation.

Table 5 also shows that low-income women are more likely to agree in separate spheres–that it is better for men to work and women to care for the home. For all four racial/ethnic groups, women in households earning $15,000-$34,999 and more than $35,000 are less likely than the lowest income women to agree with this statement. In addition, higher income women of color are less likely to agree that men cannot be trusted to be faithful. Income has no effect on the attitudes of White women on this item. Finally, Black women whose income is more than $35,000 are less likely than women whose income is less than $15,000

TABLE 5. Estimated Effects of Income on Select Family Attitude Items for Unmarried Mothers, by Race/Ethnicity

	(1)	(2)	(3)	(4)	(5)	(6)	N
White Women							
$0 to 14,999 (ref.)	0.400	0.290	0.397	0.239	0.021	0.086	102
$15,000 to 34,999	0.376	0.216	0.342	0.158*	0.012	0.050	131
$35,000 or more	0.261*	0.186*	0.295*	0.108*	0.007	0.046	108
Black Women							
$0 to 14,999 (ref.)	0.455	0.432	0.566	0.149	0.069	0.220	443
$15,000 to 34,999	0.430	0.338	0.507	0.095*	0.040	0.137*	254
$35,000 or more	0.307*	0.298*	0.453*	0.064*	0.024*	0.127*	158
Native-born Latinas							
$0 to 14,999 (ref.)	0.474	0.424	0.420	0.227	0.031	0.253	186
$15,000 to 34,999	0.449	0.332	0.363	0.149*	0.018	0.160*	128
$35,000 or more	0.324*	0.291*	0.315*	0.102*	0.011	0.148*	78
Foreign-born Latinas							
$0 to 14,999 (ref.)	0.524	0.509	0.562	0.579	0.072	0.420	52
$15,000 to 34,999	0.499	0.411	0.503	0.452*	0.042	0.289*	35
$35,000 or more	0.368*	0.366*	0.450*	0.348*	0.026	0.271*	14

* $p <= .05$.

Notes: Based on logistic regression models in Table 3. Probabilities are for unmarried mothers with a high school degree, who did not receive welfare, who did not live with both biological parents at age 15, who do not attend religious services regularly, who have 2 children, and are 25 years old.
(1) The main advantage of marriage is financial security.
(2) All in all, there are more advantages to being single than being married.
(3) It is better for a couple to get married than to just live together.
(4) It is much better for everyone if the man earns the main living and the woman takes care of the home and family.
(5) When there are children in the family, parents should stay together even if they don't get along.
(6) Men cannot be trusted to be faithful.

to agree that parents should stay together for the children. In sum, the results in Table 5 show that although differences by income are not widespread, when they do occur, low-income women tend to be more traditional than higher income women: they think it is better to get married than to live together, that it is better for men to work and women to care for the home, and, for Black women, that parents should stay together for the children.

In addition to marital status, welfare receipt, and income, several other independent variables in the multivariate models have important effects on women's attitudes (results not shown). For example, less educated women are more likely to think that marriage is better for children, more likely to recognize the financial advantages of marriage, more mistrustful of men, and more supportive of separate spheres. Women who are more religiously active are also more gender traditional, more pro-nuptial, and less supportive of cohabitation.

DISCUSSION AND CONCLUSIONS

This article tests the ideological assumptions underlying current federal efforts to promote marriage, in particular, the assumption that welfare recipients and other poor women have different family values than other women. Not surprisingly, the attitudes of the women in this sample mirror the attitudes present in the larger culture (Axinn & Thornton, 2000). Most approve of single motherhood, even if they recognize it is not ideal, most approve of cohabitation, and few advocate that parents should stay together for the sake of the children.

Results also show that, in general, welfare recipients do not differ from other women in their family and marital attitudes. On only one variable are their attitudes significantly different: welfare recipients are less likely to agree that a man should spend time with family rather than work as many hours as possible. This difference is likely attributable to women's need for the additional earnings from men's work hours, rather than a disregard for men's time with their families. In addition, it is consistent with low-income women's strong support of separate spheres, where men are expected to be the primary breadwinner.

Although there are no widespread differences by welfare receipt, there are some differences by marital status, but primarily for White women. Married White women are more conservative than unmarried women: they are more likely to agree that children are better off with married parents and that separate spheres is preferable, and less likely to agree that being single has more advantages than being married. In addition, unmarried White women are often less traditional than unmarried women of color. For example, they are least likely to agree that important decisions should be made by men and that it is better to get married than to live together. Similarly, unmarried Black women and foreign-born Latinas are often most conservative; they are most likely to agree that parents should stay together for the children and that it is better to get married than to live together.

In fact, one of the most consistent findings is the conservatism of foreign-born Latinas, likely reflecting the more conservative cultural attitudes of their countries of origin (Oropesa, 1996). Although, even here, there is variation. For example, Latinas are most likely to view cohabitation as equivalent to marriage. This may reflect the history of long-term cohabitation in many Latin American countries, including Puerto Rico (Manning & Landale, 1996). In addition, foreign-born Latinas are most likely to express gender mistrust and to see more advantages to being single than being married.

On only half of the items does income have a significant effect, and on the pair of these items that most reflect "traditional family values"–approving of marriage over cohabitation and support of separate spheres–low-income women are more traditional than higher income women. Yet, at the same time, low-income women see advantages to being single, see financial advantage to marriage, and for women of color, mistrust men.

A primary limitation of this study is its inability to address issues of causality. It is possible that women's attitudes affect their behavior, for example, that more traditional White women are more likely to marry, but it is also possible that behaviors change one's attitudes. This latter pattern is consistent with research on divorce and attitudes, which shows that behavioral change often precedes attitudinal change. For example, Cherlin (1992) found that the overall rise in divorce rates in the 1970s preceded the large shift in attitudes towards divorce. Similarly, Thornton (1985) analyzed longitudinal data and found no effect of women's attitudes towards divorce on the likelihood of divorce, but he did find that women who divorced became more accepting of divorce in later years. In a later study, Axinn and Thornton (1992) also found that young people entering into cohabiting unions were no more approving of divorce, but became so over the course of their cohabitation. This reciprocal relationship between attitudes and behaviors is especially relevant in this study for the items regarding single motherhood. Few unmarried women who have just given birth will say that single motherhood is bad for children, even if they would have also agreed that marriage is ideal.

Together, these results show real complexity and ambiguity in women's attitudes. It is difficult, if not impossible, to find clear patterns of groups having more or less "family values" than others. Public discourse and public policies need to acknowledge and reflect this complexity. For example, the absence of difference in welfare recipients' attitudes suggests that it is unjustified to target welfare recipients with marriage promotion efforts to change marital attitudes. Welfare recipients do not differ from other women in their attitudes, and policies should not treat them as if they do.

However, it is also clear that women do not view non-marriage as a deterrent to childrearing, nor do they think that children will suffer if they are raised by a single mother. Improving well-being for all children, regardless of parental marital status, necessitates policies that ease the burdens of single parenthood by improving access to financial, educational, and child care resources. Marriage itself may not improve child well-being if it does not also increase familial and financial stability.

Finally, this analysis calls into question the "common wisdom" that low marriage rates among poor women, especially African American women, can be explained by their values. Rather, it is the obstacles to relationship and marital stability, including lack of financial resources, gender mistrust, and high expectations about companionate marriage (Cherlin, 2004; Edin, 2000; Edin & Kefalas, 2005; Gibson-Davis et al., 2004) that make marriage difficult to achieve. If policymakers want to increase marriage rates, policies should focus on reducing these barriers. Although the ability of policies to reduce gender mistrust or to improve relationship quality is limited and/or untested (NCFR, 2003), policies can focus on improving couples' financial stability so that they feel more secure to enter into this lifelong commitment.

NOTES

1. A proposed change to the wording of this final goal was included in recent reauthorization bills and makes marriage even more explicit: "to encourage the formation and maintenance of healthy, two-parent married families" (H.R. 4737, 2002).

2. A complete list of allowable activities is available at http://www.acf.hhs. gov/healthymarriage/about/mission.html.

3. The Fragile Families Study was funded by a grant from NICHD (#R01HD36916) and a consortium of private foundations. A full list of funders can be found at http://crcw.princeton.edu/fragilefamilies/funders.asp.

4. Pearson's $r = .55$ for it is better for a couple to get married and it is better for children if parents are married.

5. Ordinal logistic regression equations using the full range of responses were also run. The results are very similar to those reported here. For simplicity of presentation, given the large number of items, I report the logistic regression results here.

REFERENCES

Aaron, H. J., Mann, T. E., & Taylor, T. (Eds.) (1994). *Values and public policy*. Washington, D.C.: The Brookings Institution.

Abramovitz, M. (1996). *Regulating the lives of women: Social welfare policy from colonial times to the present*. Boston, MA: South End Press.

Axinn, W. G. and Thornton, A. (1992). The relationship between cohabitation and divorce: Selectivity or causal influence? *Demography, 29*, 357-374.

Axinn, W. G. and Thornton, A. (2000). Transformation in the meaning of marriage. In L. J. Waite (Ed.), *Ties that bind: Perspectives on marriage and cohabitation* (pp. 147-165). New York: Aldine de Gruyter.

Bulcroft, R. A., & Bulcroft, K. A. (1993). Race differences in attitudinal and motivational factors in the decision to marry. *Journal of Marriage and Family, 55*, 338-355.

Bullock, H. E. (1999). Attributions for poverty: A comparison of mile-class and welfare recipient attitudes. *Journal of Applied Social Psychology, 29*, 2059-2082.

Cherlin, A. J. (1992). *Marriage, divorce, remarriage*. Cambridge, MA: Harvard University Press.

Cherlin, A. J. (2004). The deinstitutionalization of American marriage. *Journal of Marriage and Family, 66*, 848-861.

Coley, R. L. (2002). What mothers teach, what daughters learn: Gender mistrust and self-sufficiency among low-income women. In A. Booth & A. C. Crouter (Eds.), *Just living together: Implications of cohabitation on families, children, and social policy* (pp. 97-105). Mahwah, NJ: Lawrence Erlbaum Associates.

Edin, K. (2000). What do low-income single mothers say about marriage? *Social Problems, 47*, 112-133.

Edin, K., & Kefalas, M. (2005). *Promises I can keep: Why poor women put motherhood before marriage*. Berkeley, CA: University of California Press.

Gibson-Davis, C. M., Edin K., & McLanahan, S. (2005). High hopes but even higher expectations: The retreat from marriage among low-income couples. *Journal of Marriage and Family, 67*, 1301-1312.

Gilens, M. (1999). *Why Americans hate welfare: Race, media, and the politics of antipoverty policy*. Chicago: University of Chicago Press.

Jones, R. K., & Luo, Y. (1999). The culture of poverty and African-American culture: An empirical assessment. *Sociological Perspectives, 42*, 439-458.

Lerner, R. M., Sparks, E. E., & McCubbin, L. D. (2000). Family diversity and family policy. In D. H. Demo, K. R. Allen & M. A. Fine (Eds.), *Handbook of family diversity* (pp. 380-401). New York: Oxford University Press.

Lichter, D. T., Batson, C. D., & Brown, J. B. (2004). Welfare reform and marriage promotion: The marital expectations and desires of single and cohabiting mothers. *Social Service Review, 78*, 2-25.

Manning, W. D., & Landale, N. S. (1996). Racial and ethnic differences in the role of cohabitation in premarital childbearing. *Journal of Marriage and Family, 58*, 63-77.

National Council on Family Relations. (2003). *Marriage promotion in low-income families*. Retrieved December 13, 2004, from National Council on Family Relations Web site: http://www.ncfr.org/pdf/Marriage_Promotion_Fact_Sheet.pdf.

Oropesa, R. S. (1996). Normative beliefs about marriage and cohabitation: A comparison of non-Latino Whites, Mexican Americans, and Puerto Ricans. *Journal of Marriage and Family, 58*, 49-62.

Oropesa, R. S., & Gorman, B. K. (2000). Ethnicity, immigration, and beliefs about marriage as a 'tie that binds'. In L. J. Waite (Ed.), *Ties that bind: Perspectives on marriage and cohabitation* (pp. 188-211). New York: Aldine de Gruyter.

Parke, M. (2004). Marriage-related provisions in welfare reauthorization proposals: A summary. Retrieved January 19, 2005, from Center for Law and Social Policy Web site: http://www.clasp.org/publications/marr_prov_upd.pdf.

Ricketts, E. R., & Sawhill, I. V. (1988). Defining and measuring the underclass. *Journal of Policy Analysis and Management, 7*, 316-325.

Sassler, S., & Schoen, R. (1999). The effect of attitudes and economic activity on marriage. *Journal of Marriage and Family, 61*, 147-159.

Sigle-Rushton, W., & McLanahan, S. S. (2002). The living arrangements of new unmarried mothers. *Demography, 39*, 415-433.

South, S. J. (1993). Racial and ethnic differences in the desire to marry. *Journal of Marriage and Family, 55*, 357-370.

Thomas, S. L. (1994). From the culture of poverty to the culture of single motherhood: The new poverty paradigm. *Women & Politics, 14*, 65-97.

Thornton, A. (1985). Changing attitudes toward separation and divorce: Causes and consequences. *American Journal of Sociology, 90*, 856-872.

Personal Responsibility, Work, and Family Promotion Act of 2002, H.R. 4737, 107th Cong. (2002).

Waller, M. R. (2001). High hopes: Unwed parents' expectations about marriage. *Children and Youth Services Review, 23*, 457-484.

The Need for International Family Policy: Mothers As Workers and As Carers

Sally Bould

SUMMARY. This article reviews the policies of the United Nations with regard to families where mothers are working in developing countries. The focus is child care, which is being passed over in United Nations' efforts on gender mainstreaming and empowering women as well as ignored in United Nations' statements on poor children. This is especially problematic because globalization is now drawing poor and working class mothers into the formal labor force where combining child care with productive activity is no longer possible. The history of Care, Health and Education for Children in Poverty, an organization located in South Asia, provides a grassroots example. Popular goals of privatization, sustainability and local control are putting poor children at risk in the developing world. *[Article copies available for a fee from The Haworth Document Delivery Service: 1-800-HAWORTH. E-mail address: <docdelivery@*

Sally Bould is Professor Emerita, Department of Sociology, University of Delaware.

Address correspondence to: Sally Bould, Department of Sociology, University of Delaware, Newark, DE 19716 (E-mail: salbould@udel.edu).

Support for this research was from the Center for International Studies at the University of Delaware, Newark, Delaware. The author would like to thank her research assistants, Julissa Gutierrez, Stella Ilel, Leigh Snyder and Milena Mladenovich. An earlier version of this paper was presented at Cornell University's conference, 75 Years of Development Research, May 7-9, 2004.

[Haworth co-indexing entry note]: "The Need for International Family Policy: Mothers As Workers and As Carers." Bould, Sally. Co-published simultaneously in *Marriage & Family Review* (The Haworth Press, Inc.) Vol. 39, No. 1/2, 2006, pp. 75-98; and: *Families and Social Policy: National and International Perspectives* (ed: Linda Haas, and Steven K. Wisensale) The Haworth Press, Inc., 2006, pp. 75-98. Single or multiple copies of this article are available for a fee from The Haworth Document Delivery Service [1-800-HAWORTH, 9:00 a.m. - 5:00 p.m. (EST). E-mail address: docdelivery@haworthpress.com].

KEYWORDS. Child care, family policy, United Nations policy, work and family

INTRODUCTION

This article reviews the history of international policies of the United Nations (UN) with respect to women as workers and women as carers for young children. These international policies of the UN are critical because, directly or indirectly, they impact funding of development programs focused on women and children. Developing countries generally lack the resources to fund child care and are dependent on international donors for such programs. Yet, the need for child care for working mothers is glossed over in the current discussions of Gender and Development (GAD). This article follows the history of one child care organization in a South Asian country,[1] but it will argue that the issue of child care is world wide. Globalization has separated the home from the place of work for mothers throughout the developing world and for poor and working class women the urgent need for child care has often been overlooked by the United Nations and other development organizations.

Much of family policy in the developed world has revolved around the provision of child care for working mothers. Children are dependent on the care of others, and this burden falls predominantly on mothers (Fineman, 2002; Folbre, 1994; Kittay, 1999; Kittay & Feder, 2002; Windebank, 2001). More importantly, child care advocates such as Barbara Bergmann (1996a) have pointed out that adequate child care can alleviate poverty. Inadequate child care, as in the United States under the Personal Responsibility and Work Opportunity Reconciliation Act 1996, creates a child care crisis for poor single mothers who are now expected to work (Chaudry, 2004). The UN's 1995 Human Development Report, *Gender and Human Development,* focused upon the very high rates of women's poverty, but in the following 10 years there has been no discussion of the role of child care in promoting the reduction of poverty among women in developing countries. In this 1995 Human Development Report, women were estimated to be 70% of the 1.3 billion poor in the world. Women are disproportionately represented in poverty in developing countries (UNDP, 1995), because they have more limited access to income generating opportunities and have responsibilities for children. Furthermore, women and children may not have a right to support from the men in their family (Blumberg, 1991; Tinker, 1976), or the men are unable to support them because of underemployment, alcohol abuse, absence or death (Narayan et al., 2000). Poverty rates are very high in the South Asian region with 83% in Bangladesh, 80% in India, 66% in Pakistan and 51% in Sri Lanka living on less than $2 a day (UNDP, 2005b).

Active policy discussions and debates concerning public responsibility for the care of children, especially poor children, are generally focused on the situation in developed countries and deal with the extent the state should subsidize child care, especially for poor families (Bergmann 1996b; Helburn & Bergmann, 2003). In low-income developing countries, few discussions are underway as national policy and limited resources are focused on child health and schooling. Middle-income developing countries that do have a policy of child care in place, such as Mexico and Argentina, are cutting back those programs due to budget shortfalls.[2] International donor agencies and the UN are similarly focused elsewhere. Since UN policy is especially critical in obtaining the outside financing necessary for such programs, this article focuses on international policy as reflected in UN publications. For the UN, the issue is now "gender mainstreaming," the discussion and practice of which does not include child care (Cf. UN, 2002; UN, 2003).

Reports discussing the "promotion of equity between women and men" and better access for women to the labor market (Daeren, 2001, p. 15) as goals have not included discussions of child care. In the four case studies of family and work produced by the Division for Social Policy and Development Family Unit (UN, 2000), only the developed country, The Netherlands, reports at length on child care as an important factor. The most recent publication under the auspices of the UN, *Gender Equality* (UNRISD, 2005), devotes a section to the issue of "Women, work and social policy" (pp. 65-140), but there is no discussion of child care except in the brief discussion of "women's employment in OECD countries," where there is a vague reference to "institutions" and to nannies (pp. 69-71) available to women in Western Europe. In the rest of this section there are detailed discussions of women's increasing participation in the paid work force, especially in Asia, but no reference to the issues of child care. In an earlier section on "Trends in gender differences in access to opportunities and resources" (UNRISD, 2005, pp. 52-54), there is no reference to child care as a necessary resource. Another recent UN publication on the situation in Latin America refers to a need for a more equitable distribution and "greater compatibility between paid work and family responsibilities" (Daeren, 2001, p. 17), again without any reference to the child care needed by poor and working class women. In Staudt's (1998) broad discussion of gender issues, *Policy, Politics and Gender*, there is also a lack of discussion of issues of child care (see also Kasente, Lockwood, Vivian & Whitehead, 2002). Part of the explanation for this lack of attention to child care issues in developing countries may be the widespread availability of cheap labor so that middle class women in developing countries do not have the same problem as middle class women in developed countries; many can afford live-in help when they have young children.

This article proposes a new family policy that could direct international funding organizations toward important gaps in the programs for gender equality and poverty alleviation. These funding organizations have the resources to allocate funds to the important issues raised by mothers as carers and as workers in the developing world. A specific case in the South Asian region in the town of "Sangupur" is examined as an example where international funding policies are putting poor children and their families at risk.

MYTHS INHIBITING AN INTERNATIONAL FAMILY CHILD CARE POLICY

Two myths have been pervasive and have limited an active push for an international family policy that focuses on mothers as workers and as care providers in development policy since World War II. The first, derived from traditional family expectations, is that mothers in developing countries are engaged in full-time child care at home. The second, that developed as criticism of the first, argues that women in developing countries typically combine child care and productive activity; since these women have managed without help, there is no need for child care. The corollary to the second myth is that if the working mother does need help, there are other female family members who can take care of the children.

The first myth was predominant during the UN's early development (1961-1970). It was perpetuated by western economists who dominated development activity. Policymakers assumed that family organization and traditional family expectations found in middle class families in Canada, the United States and Western Europe in the 1950s existed also in developing countries. Women's role was to raise children and to take care of the home (Cf. Staudt, 1998, p. 101). For example, W. W. Rostow in his book, *The Stages of Economic Growth* (1961, p. 91), referred to women only once in a parenthetical remark about their full-time duties in child care. As the UN summarized the situation during this period:

> Development projects concentrated on literacy courses, home economic programs, child care [at home] and family planning activities. However, welfare and family oriented programmes, though no doubt valuable, nonetheless had the effect of reinforcing women's traditional role with the family. (UN, 1999, p. ix)

Development activities for women had been focused on family planning and health, and especially children's health and well-being. This focus fits with the overall emphasis on traditional home economics, or "domestic science," as it developed during the 1950s and 1960s (Rogers, 1980: 85ff). These activities were criticized by feminists who saw the programs as narrowly conceiving of women as care providers and ignoring women as workers. Women's projects had been focused on how to help women be better homemakers in what Rogers called *The Domestication of Women* (1980). This emphasis was found in national and multinational foreign assistance programs. Professional women in international development work in the UN or the U.S. Agency for International Development (AID) were typically concentrated in departments of health and family planning. And family planning was narrowly conceived as reducing the number of children per family, not on planning for work combined with child care. Even Ulla Olin, a professional woman at the UN, and Principal Officer at the UN's Development Program, envisioned women's most important role as home managers; in 1976, she emphasized the "biological basis of human behavior" (Olin, 1976, p. 127). Similarly, private funding of development activities was dominated by charitable organizations whose goal was to help poor children; sometimes these programs included mothers, especially in their responsibility for child health.

This first myth, that women don't "work," was roundly criticized by Irene Tinker in her article, "The adverse impact of development on women" (1976; see also Blumberg, 1976; Boserup, 1970). Furthermore, she points out that every member of poor families must work and contribute to family income. In the mid-1970s, development planners were still assuming that women generally had "leisure" time to focus on child care.

Problems in developing adequate data on labor force participation for women in developing countries contributed to this first myth. A general lack of recognition of women's economic activity was hampered by cultural expectations in which women were not expected to work in the same way as men. In South Asia, these cultural norms were partly the result of British colonial rule (Cf. Rogers, 1980: 36ff). Reporting on data around 1980, the U.S. Agency for International Development outlined the problem:

> As in other developing regions, norms in Asian countries often do not promote the reporting of women's work as constituting a formal part of the labor force and the resulting statistics show a large discrepancy between female and male participation rates. These rates are especially low for women in Middle South Asia. (U.S. Bureau of the Census, 1985: 33)

For example, in 1981 in Bangladesh, only 5% of women were reported as participating in the labor force, ignoring the extensive participation of women as unpaid family workers in this predominantly rural population (U.S. Bureau of the Census, 1985, p. 33).

The second myth was based on an overgeneralization of Boserup's (1970) forceful argument for recognition of women as workers, not just child carers. She focused upon women's agricultural work as "own account" (self-employed) workers or unpaid family workers. Women combined their work as providers of child carers with economic activity; the first myth had allowed development planners to ignore this work. The issue was the "invisibility" of women's productive activity. Typically this form of women's traditional agricultural work was integrated with their carework; small children were carried on their mothers' backs in the fields, while older children were part of the unpaid family labor force. Much of women's labor was centered around home production in kitchen gardens and small livestock. Agricultural development experts, typically men, did not "see" these activities (Rogers, 1980, pp. 54-56). In these situations, however, the dependence of children and their need for care was not an overwhelming issue since the home was also the place of work.

Today, there is a strong emphasis on women's productive roles in developing countries; for example, in the case of Bangladesh, the reported labor force participation rate for women is 56% in 2000 (UN Statistics Division, 2004) up from only 5% in 1981. This dramatic increase in the labor force participation over a short time of 20 years no doubt reflects better reporting in the rural regions. Seventy-three percent of economically active women in Bangladesh are reported as working as contributing (unpaid) family members in family enterprises in 2000 (UN Statistics Division, 2004). This economic activity in Bangladesh still reflects women's place of work in and near their homes so that child care can be combined with market work. But in countries like Sri Lanka, 60% of economically active women in 2003 are wage and salaried workers outside the home (UN Statistics Division, 2004). This economic activity generally precludes the combination of work and child care at the place of work. Clearly the economic activity of women is now more widely reported and recognized but important observers have failed to acknowledge the dependency of children and the need for support for child care, especially among poor women.

The Mexico City conference where the UN set forth the first Decade for Women (1976 to 1985) highlighted the need for women to be included in development, but ignored child care. This conference brought women's issues to the attention of everyone involved in development activities and created "international 'networks' among female elite" (Charlton, 1984, p. 206). Pressure was put on international organizations to hire women in positions that were not directly related to family planning and child health (Himmelstrand, 1997). Opportunities became available for the first time for women from developing countries to achieve professional positions in international organizations (Charlton, 1984). The women's movement in international development opened up important opportunities for educated women to become integrated into the developing economies of their own countries. Internationally, women's issues have followed the pattern of the U.S. women's movement. The first priority was enabling educated women to compete successfully in economic structures that had once excluded them. Their role as mothers of young children was not central to this effort. This was true in large part because the women who were going out to work had the financial means to hire help for child care. This was even more the case for educated third world women who had a very large pool of poor women who could be hired at extremely low wages, even as live-in nannies. Thus, women's issues became issues that focused on the needs of middle class women as individuals and their right to work. There was no need for a "family policy" as these women had the resources to manage in the private market; poor women's potential need for child care was overlooked, although a maid was often allowed to bring her young child with her when she cared for her employer's children.

With globalization, poor women have entered the paid labor force as agricultural workers or as factory workers, a move that has separated the home from the place of work, a place where children are not welcome. Traditional approaches to child care, such as bringing the child to the fields for agricultural work, or combining child care with an at-home business, are simply not appropriate when the workplace is separated from the home and the mothers are employed for eight or more hours a day. Once women were acknowledged as economically productive, economists changed their labor supply models so that women and men workers were assumed to have identical labor supply functions. (See Barnum & Squire, 1978.) This assumption ignores women's responsibilities for dependent children. The participation of women in the paid labor force in South Asia is now broadly recognized and a recent publication of the Asian Development Bank on poverty reduction notes that women "are the primary caregivers in the home" and often "major contributors to the market as well" (Thukral, 2002, p. 243). But Thukral (2002) does not mention any issues about mothers combining market work with child care; neither do other authors in this volume devoted to issues of poverty reduction.

A corollary to the second myth is that other family members will be available to provide child care while the mother is away at work. The "grandmother solution" is one that is widely assumed by development economists.[3] The availability of grandmothers for child care, however, is scarce among poor families since the life expectancy among the poor is still quite low in developing countries. If alive, the grandmother is very likely to be disabled and if the grandmother is able, she is likely to be employed for pay, also. The same is true for other female relatives as poverty or near poverty means that every able-bodied adult in the family will try to generate income for the family (Tinker, 1976). Aunts and other adult women family members are likely to be working mothers themselves. Unlike the situation during the industrial revolution in the west, globalization in developing countries is drawing mothers into full-time paid jobs away from home.

With the success in reducing fertility, there are fewer older children to care for younger children, but even where there are older children they should be in school and not doing child care (Kahn, 1993). Egypt has high levels of child labor and there is a "high rate of [school] dropouts because of family responsibilities [of girls]" (UN, 2000, p. 15). India also has high levels of child labor (UN, 2000). A survey in the rural Tamhur district of India revealed that the need for child care often resulted in older girls dropping out of school; Tara (1985, p. 114) recommends child care centers so that older girls can continue their education. Even in Sri Lanka where women have high literacy rates, a survey of three communities indicated that child care needs of families were often met by restricting the education of girls (Rice & Wilber as discussed in Kahn, 2002: 217). In Argentina, cutbacks in publicly funded day care and the recourse to private solutions have resulted in lower school attendance: "School drop out rates started to climb in 1996 as low-income families started to take their children out of school at an early age" (UN, 2000, p. 4).

Ironically the success of women's organizations and feminist organizations to get women included in the development process as producers and not just caregivers has shifted the focus from poor children to adult women in their economically active roles. In both situations, however, the need for a family policy has been overlooked. In the first development decades poor children were the focus. Their mothers were only involved in carrying out instructions for better child health even if the emphasis, e.g., nutrition, was not attainable due to poverty (Rogers, 1980). In the later development decades, adult women are conceptualized as "individuals" and their care for dependents is ignored (Nussbaum, 2002). It is time to develop an international family policy where the focus is on poor families with young children where the mother works in the paid labor market.

The lack of attention to child care in discussions of globalization is, in part, the result of a narrow focus on young childless women factory workers (Ahmed & Bould, 2004). Salzinger (2003) for example, mentions child care only once, even though she estimates that a significant minority of the maquila factory workers are mothers (with 20% being single mothers) and labor shortages will no doubt draw more mothers into this labor force. In the context of globalization, family policy in developing countries needs to focus on issues raised by mothers who are both carers and workers. Globalization has drawn mothers into the paid workforce throughout the developing world and consequently has created a child care crisis. Nevertheless much of the discussion about women and globalization does not acknowledge that this full-time workforce participation requires full-time child care. (See Kelly & Sassen, 1995.) Even though Salzinger (2003) lives with a single mother working in the maquila factories, she does not mention her host's child care arrangements.

How many women working as wage and salary workers cannot rely on existing forms of child care? Data on this question are inadequate in the U.S. (Chaudry, 2004; Helburn & Bergmann, 2003) and are practically nonexistent for developing countries. The most critical variable here is the social class of the family. Higher class families in the town of "Sangupur," the site of the fieldwork, rely on hiring low wage workers for in-home care. But, here, as elsewhere, the supply of low wage women for child care is being reduced by the opportunity for higher wages in other low skilled jobs such as in garment factories. This is true even where working as a nanny pays more than beginning wages in factory work. The traditional status of the nanny in developing countries is generally one of a servant, a very low status occupation that brings shame on the woman. Now that she has other forms of paid work as an option, she seeks to have a higher status job with opportunity, even if the initial pay is lower (Ahmed & Bould, 2004).

In the town of "Sangupur," there is a child care center for infants and preschoolers. It is located near the municipal buildings where many middle class women have white collar government jobs. It is available for mothers to stop by on their lunch time, and provides access before and after work; it is also quickly reachable in the case of an emergency. The mothers pay the full cost of this care. Of course, better-off families may also have a non-working adult female family member who can provide child care. None of these alternatives are available for poor families. Furthermore, the vast majority of jobs that these poor women hold are "wage employment in informal jobs (that is without secure contracts, worker benefits or legal protection)" (UNRISD, 2005, p. 76). The mother has to go to work even if she cannot find adequate child care, even if she has to leave her children alone; if she does not go to work, she is likely to lose her job and therefore will be unable to feed her family. Self-employed women, however, can still combine work with child care. During our fieldwork research, we visited one mother with two small children. She had a successful sewing business making wedding dresses. Her sewing machine was in the bedroom next to the double bed. While she sewed, she kept the children on the bed next to her.

The error of ignoring women's child care needs under myth two discussed earlier results in a negative impact similar to the ignoring of women's productive activity in myth one. Under myth one, women had the most to lose when seen only in terms of their care providing role. Ignoring the importance of women's productive labor, this myth made it more difficult for women to carry out their economic responsibilities in providing for their families (Staudt, 1998). Ignoring women's labor and productivity had the most negative impact on poor women whose labor was essential to feeding the family. According to Rao:

Most development policies and projects have, in fact, had severe negative impacts on the survival chances of *poor women and their families*. Moreover, such policies and large-scale projects often fail to meet their goals when women's labor contributions at the household and project levels are overlooked, their need for economic incentives are not understood and resources relevant to their productive work are misdirected to men. (Rao, 1991, p. 2, italics added)

Two decades later, it is possible to rewrite the preceding statement such that development planners have now moved to "gender mainstreaming" and are including women's labor as critical to the development process; the emphasis is on providing equal access to the paid labor market for men and women (UNRISD 2005, pp. 63ff). Nevertheless, a critical resource for women's full economic participation, child care, is overlooked. The most severe negative impact of this is on *poor and working class women and their families*.

There is another reason why poor women and their children stand to lose the most from lack of adequate child care. Adequate child care also provides for preschool education; for example, this is recognized in France where all children 3 years of age and over can enroll in an *école maternelle* financed by the Ministry of Education. Bergmann (1996a) notes that these programs in France are especially effective for poor and minority children. Children of poor families in the developing world face severe difficulties in succeeding in school without adequate preparation. And poor parents in the South Asian region rarely have the literacy skills necessary to help their children prepare for primary schooling. Difficulties at school most often result in leaving school for poor children whose parents often could use the child's labor (Cf. Tara, 1985). While the UN has established the right of a child to schooling, it has not yet recognized that this right for poor children needs to be supported by preschool activities.

CARE, HEALTH, AND EDUCATION FOR CHILDREN IN POVERTY (CHECP)

The inadequacy of development policy with respect to poor women's economic opportunities is reflected in the history of the non-governmental organization (NGO), Care, Health and Education for Children in Poverty (CHECP), located in the town of "Sangupur" in a South Asian country. Fieldwork was conducted in the summer of 2003 by the author and three students. There was a meeting with the mothers at the center, as well as observation of the activities of the center. Newsletters of the center were reviewed and are referred to below. Key informants were critical in providing the history of the organization as well as in describing its current situation. Key informants consisted of two board members, one of whom was a founding member, as well as the current director of the organization, who also worked in setting up the organization. Interviews were done by telephone with two funding officers from different funding agencies. Clarifications and additional information have been obtained through telephone and e-mail correspondence.[4]

Reflecting myth one, the policy of the early development decades, the initiative to establish development assistance in "Sangupur" was prompted by publicity involving the dire need of children. A BBC broadcast in the early seventies showed the horrific situation of the children of the Delit Hindus, the lowest Hindu status. The Terre des Hommes Foundation, from Lausanne, Switzerland, carried out a survey in 1974 that showed that children were suffering from malnutrition and neglect. There was a high level of child mortality and morbidity. "Diseases like scabies and worms were prevalent."[5] Moreover, these poor children were often excluded from government schools.

The donor agency, Terre des Hommes, focused on children rather than families. This child focus was implemented, in part, by the building of an orphanage at CHECP in 1978. As was the case in the West during the industrial revolution, an orphanage typically served children who had a living parent(s) who was unable to care for them. Poor parents left their children at the orphanage in order to assure that their children received food and shelter.

According to one of the founders of CHECP, Terre des Hommes' main focus was "consistently on the children; to fight malnutrition, several feeding centers were opened in 1977. This was for needy children, breast-feeding mothers and pregnant women to receive medical, nutritional and general care."[6] In 1978, a day nursery was added with the goal of improving children's health and mitigating neglect. The goal was to help vulnerable children who come from "single parent households, orphans, malnourished, lacking care because both parents are working . . ." (CHECP, 1997, p. 7). Even in 2000, one funding proposal describes the target children as "neglected" children, implicitly blaming poor mothers, describing the "need to care for children who are neglected and left alone while parents are at work" (CHECP, 2000, p. 3). The mothers were provided education in "health, nutrition, agriculture, handicrafts." Nowhere in these documents is there a mention of the need for employment for these poor mothers or that poor nutrition was the result of the mothers' severe lack of income.

The provision of "day care" has remained last on the list of purposes of CHECP. A bulletin (CHECP, 1996, p. 1) lists the purposes of the organization as dealing with "problems with malnutrition among the very young children, education and training for the older children who have had no schooling, women's health and child care for young women." This approach to day care reflects the initial policy of Head Start in the U.S. in the sixties; the policy focuses on the child and the child's need for preschool education and health care. There is limited conceptualization of the mother as a "working mother" who needs child care and pre-school activities for her children while she pursues employment to help feed her family. The assumption is, rather, that poor mothers were providing "an inadequate home environment" (Vinovskis, 2005, p. 70). Lady Bird Johnson reported in her diary, "It will include a medical examination, one good free meal a day and the simplest rudimentary teaching in manners and vocabulary improvement" (quoted in Vinovskis, 2005, p. 74). This all sounds like the program at CHECP that now serves about 100 children.

The importance of parents' employment was acknowledged but not the working mother; the effort was focused on "adult persons"; the goal was to get one parent a job, not both parents. But the low level of wages would require both parents to work in order to provide a minimal standard of living. The future employment of young people was the impetus for vocational training programs. But these programs fit the old style gender division of labor, with an afternoon sewing school for girls and carpentry for boys (CHECP, 2000, p. 4). The training did not take into account labor market opportunities. The vocational training was not likely to lead to income-generating activity where there was no market analysis and no business skills were taught. The feminist critiques of these types of programs were well-founded (Rogers, 1980).

In spite of the early focus on traditional women's roles, this organization made significant progress in child health and education of children. The school no longer exists because the children are now able to go to government schools; the orphanage is in disuse because the children are now with their families. But the imminent collapse of the current day care center could result in the need to rebuild the orphanage for children whose parents can no longer afford to care for them.

GENDER AT THE CENTER?

The first successful pressure from women's organizations to include women in the international development process took effect in the U.S. in the 1973 "Percy Amendment" to the 1961 Foreign Assistance Act. This amendment, Section 113, required "particular attention to those programs, projects and activities which tend to integrate women into the national economies of foreign countries, thus improving their status and assisting the total development effort." The emphasis was on the status of women and their productive role in the development process. Subsequently the U.S. Agency for International Development (USAID) created an office of Women in Development. In Canada, the Canadian International Development Agency appointed the first coordinator for women in development in 1976 (Charlton, 1984). This new direction in development policy was highly critical of the narrow focus on women as carers, a focus that ignored women's economic activity. But there was still no move to integrate women's economic activity with the needs of children's health and family planning. An example of this lack of integration was found in the structure of the Centre for Development and Population Activities. Before 1982, this organization had one branch for "family planning and health" and another branch for "women-and-development activities" (Charlton, 1984, p. 209).

The new Women in Development (WID) focus of the late 1970s and 1980s shifted the focus away from children and toward the economic activity of women. Yet another shift occurred from WID, with its emphasis on women's access to economic benefits, to Gender and Development (GAD), where equality of the genders was the focus. By 1999, this shift is pronounced a success: "Today, gender is finally at the center of development policies, after three decades of struggle" (UN, 1999, p. vii). But this research suggests that children have been moved to the periphery with gender mainstreaming as central: "Mainstreaming a gender perspective is the process of assessing the implications for men and women of any planned action, including legislations, policies and programmes" (UN, 1999, p. ix). Again it is only men and women that are at center stage, not boys and girls, and definitely not families. "All that a gender-transformative policy can hope to do is to provide women with enabling resources which will allow them to take greater control of their own lives" (Kabeer as quoted in UN, 1999, p. x). This approach ignores the fact that in developing countries the majority of poor women are mothers; they can only take greater control of their own lives if they have options for the care of their children when they are young. And for girls, their education will be limited by their families' need for child care services. Unfortunately, the UN's "enabling resources" do not include child care. In the discussion of the UN Millennium Development Goal Number 3, "promote gender equity and empower women," Kabeer (2003) makes no mention of child care.

Empowerment is an empty term unless it enables poor women to both work and assure care for their very young children and provide educational opportunities for their preschool children. The current focus on "empowerment" has even resulted in downplaying the role of income. For example, Rowlands (1999, p. 146) stresses that "an exclusive focus on economic activities does not automatically create a space for women to look at their own role as women," and she emphasizes confidence and self-esteem. Endeley (2001) sees income as necessary but not sufficient for empowerment. In the report by the Women and Development Unit, entitled "Understanding Poverty from a Gender Perspective," there is a caution against a focus on material deprivation measures of poverty because

> policy makers risked ending up with poverty reduction strategies which were designed to impact on the situation of women, but neglected to alter gender conditions. This would lead the State to prioritize the satisfaction of women's practical and immediate needs, while ignoring their strategic interests and thus reinforcing the cultural patterns and objective conditions that perpetuated gender inequality. (UN, 2004, p. 57)

Providing child care for working mothers does "reinforce" cultural patterns of female caregiving but it is necessary also to confront issues of poverty and inequality for poor and working class women. Among the UN publications, Chant is one of the few commentators who recognizes that there needs to be a "greater recognition of women's disproportionate responsibility for raising children through public-sponsored provision of child care . . ." (2003, p. 36), but her voice seems lost.

Wage income can empower poor women if they have adequate child care (Ahmed & Bould, 2004). The "new analysis of poverty" assumes that, for poor women, power and status are the key; but that has never been the case; low status and powerlessness have always been the result of poverty for women as well as men. In the long run, higher economic resources result in higher status and power (Weber, 1963). This "new" analysis ignores the dimension of economic resources by focusing on needs of power and status that are urgent for middle class women. Income plus child care including preschool education is the only way poor mothers can hope to empower themselves and their children. This is especially true if these mothers also face ethnic, racial or caste discrimination.

PRIVATIZATION, SUSTAINABILITY AND LOCAL CONTROL

For more than 20 years, Care, Health and Education of Children in Poverty (CHECP), enabled by consistent funding from the Terre des Hommes Foundation, in Lausanne, Switzerland, made effective strides in promoting poor children's health, education and welfare with an integrated approach of infant and child health together with child care and preschool and after school education. These programs enabled mothers to enter the paid workforce knowing that their children were not only cared for but prepared for school (CHECP, 2000). But the continued success of the CHECP program requires a family policy approach which can deal with the long-term funding issues involved in providing child care for poor working mothers. No such family policy has been developed; instead, development policy has focused upon privatization, sustainability and local control. None of these fashionable approaches are effective in providing child care for poor and working class mothers.

Privatization is the buzzword of development agencies and is likely to become the only acceptable philosophy with the appointment of Wolfowitz as head of the World Bank. According to its supporters, privatization is the key to development and is the best way to help the world's poor. Although many feel that privatization is a long run solution, few actually believe that it will help the poor in the short run (Phillips, 2003). Privatization of child care, of course, has been the goal of neo-liberal policies in those few cases where there were some efforts at publicly supported child care such as was the case in Argentina (UN, 2000, p. 3ff). But for low-income developing countries, the possibilities of publicly funded day care are limited. This leaves the international funding agencies as the only possible sources of funds for assisting organizations like CHECP.

International funding agencies, however, are similarly constrained by "sustainability," a popular concept of the 1990s. Projects were to be sustainable, that is, after a certain point in their development they could be sustained without the donor's continued funding. Donors would no longer have to continue funding forever. The projects need only be funded for a few years, and subsequently they could manage to sustain themselves. The new philosophy is that "no grantmaker wants to adopt" a program (Kiritz & Mundell, l988, p. 10). Terre des Hommes wanted to move on to other projects involving other, more severely disadvantaged children. While there are certainly possibilities of creative self-financing that might work in some cases, the charitable donor organizations helping children have little experience in guiding NGOs in the fundraising process that is now necessary. Much more attention needs to be paid to how to enable poor mothers to provide good quality care for their children using all the means available. But with day care off the agenda it is hard to see how this could be accomplished, even where it might be possible.

Another popular idea now for donor organizations is that of "local control." Local control was established for CHECP; it was registered as an NGO with the legal status of a non-profit organization. In l994, CHECP took over full management and responsibility of all former Terre des Hommes activities (CHECP, 1997). This reflects the shift in philosophy of donor agencies from continued charitable support for a worthy cause, the children, to the new approach which gets the donor agency out from under the responsibility of running and financing an organization. With outside control comes the external imposition of management. Terre des Hommes had strict central administrative control during the years it funded and managed CHECP. This approach has the drawback of being paternalistic and neo-colonial in that Europeans or North Americans controlled the organization. If the funding organization does not like what the local staff members are doing, it can simply fire the staff and hire replacements. But once local control is established, the funding agency only provides the money with no control over how it is spent. If it does not like how the management handles the program or the money, it can simply withdraw funds. Under local control, children in poverty are put at risk when the funding becomes less secure and less available and/or if management is not effective in securing and managing funds. Organizations under local control have to compete for funding and under the current emphasis on competition, it is expected that the "best" program will be funded. The result is that if the day care/preschool program is not judged the best, it will simply have to close its doors and leave the children outside.

In the shift to "local control," moreover, there is often scant effort to retrain the old style managers. These are individuals who typically have been trained in child health care and preschool education. They have had no training in fundraising or in the politics necessary for securing funds from charitable sources. Their job definition has changed dramatically but they have little opportunity to learn their new jobs. Besides, people who have devoted their life to child health and care may not want to reorient themselves away from their area of training. In any case, this lack of training and support for necessary fundraising puts the children and their mothers at risk. This is the situation of the NGO, CHECP. The program was begun and funded for years by the Terre des Hommes Foundation. In a radical change of policy in the early 1990s, the management of CHECP was given over to the control of a local board of directors. This "local control," however, ended the ongoing funding of the donor agency, Terre des Hommes. Fortunately, similar funding was available from a North American donor agency for a few more years. But that funding is now threatened with the "new" goals of women's empowerment. This is ironic because with globalization, poor women can find jobs, but they are likely to be left without safe child care, let alone help with keeping their children healthy and preparing their children for the education which is required in the modern world. Care, Health and Education for Children in Poverty (CHECP) is now at risk of sinking without a trace. The only funding left is for the feeding programs from Hope for Children, a charitable funding organization in the United Kingdom.

CONCLUSION

Why has the gender in development emphasis shifted away from the earlier focus on child care, health and schooling? The swing of the pendulum has gone to the other extreme. The process began with a narrow focus on children. Given the perceptions of women's role in the West during the first development decade as primarily carers of young children, this was a logical outcome. But now projects have moved to the other extreme, seeing women as primarily workers and ignoring their caregiving roles. The report of the UN Millennium Project Task Force on Education Gender Equality (2005) prepared by a group of 27 leading experts devotes only one page out of 257 pages (2005, p. 97) to the issue of child care. Moreover, there is no discussion of child care in the section on "making it happen." Instead the report proposes to study women's poverty, do a gender analysis, and develop a system for gender-aware public spending documentation as well as a public sector management strategy. Meanwhile it is clear that poor women need child care and poor children need preschool education. Ignoring these immediate needs, while studying and planning, leaves these women and their children at risk.

The women's movement, especially in the U.S., pushed for a recognition of women as following the decade of the fifties when women were only to be carers of children; the trends in international development thinking have taken a similar shift. In view of the importance of women's roles in development, this shift was effective in reorienting the focus to women's productive roles. In the process, however, women's caregiving roles have been ignored. The lack of full recognition of women's caregiving roles is now being addressed by feminist scholars in the developed world (Gerstel & Gallager, 1994; Kittay, 1999; Kittay & Felder, 2002). There is a danger in the "citizen as worker model," because it treats everyone as "individuals" and does not recognize the importance of family roles and the dependency needs of children. The real danger of the citizen as worker model in the developing world is that poor mothers will be unable to combine work and care responsibilities in ways that promote their children's health and education. This is a practical and immediate need of poor women and their children that should not be ignored by the state. Where the state cannot manage, this critical need should be met by international donor organizations, including the UN.

A coherent international family policy that focuses on mothers in both their provider roles and their caregiver roles would be a first step. It is not possible to "alter gender conditions" without explicit attention to the immediate dependency needs of children, especially poor children. To wait until men are equal participants in child care is to sacrifice poor children and their mothers to an ideal of gender equality which will take many decades to achieve even in the developed countries (Acker, 1998). Although critics of the emphasis on low-income women stress the importance of status and power, they do not understand that the low status and low power of poor women can be changed only if their material situation improves. Donor organizations as well as international organizations need a clear family policy so that they are not blown about by the winds of fashionable ideas. If there had been such a family policy, perhaps less money would have been spent to "empower women" and more money would have been spent to deal with the issues of families where globalization has drawn poor mothers into the work force. Unfortunately, the history of international assistance is one of bifurcation into "children's needs" and "women's needs," as if these two population groups were separate and not intimately linked in their families. As the Communitarian Network position paper on the family states,

"Government [or donor organizations] cannot intervene to promote child welfare while remaining neutral about the family" (1991, p. 2).

The focus on needy children is still the subject of UN initiatives under the auspices of UNICEF. But this focus still is not based on a clear, coherent family policy. The needs of children, as outlined on the UNICEF Web site (UNICEF, 2005), do not include the need for day care and/or preschool education. The UN should set an example by bringing together "women" and "children," rather than maintain the current organization whereby UNICEF discusses needs of poor children but not daycare, and Gender and Development (in the Executive Summary), discusses supporting women without mention of day care (UNDP, 2005a). It is time for a strong emphasis on women as workers *and* as carers in developing a family policy that is viable for all families.

Organizations that provide child care for poor mothers should be developed so the staff have the skills and training necessary for both sustainability and local control. These organizations need the approach outlined by Oxfam called "capacity-building" (Eade, 1997). Issues of child care are not just issues of developed countries. The UN Millennium Development Goals of gender equality, education for girls, and poverty alleviation are achievable only with a family policy approach that includes child care and preschool programs.

NOTES

1. The South Asian region identified by the United Nations includes Afghanistan, Bangladesh, Bhutan, India, Iran, Maldives, Nepal, Pakistan and Sri Lanka. The USAID publication (U.S. Bureau of the Census, 1985) uses the term "Middle South Asia" to refer to all of the countries above except Bhutan, Iran and the Maldives. A more specific location is not presented in order to protect the privacy of the key informants and the NGO.

2. Exceptions are found in higher per capita developing countries in Latin America. Mexico has established Centros de Asistencia Infantil Comunitarios to provide care, education, health for vulnerable preschool children–www.dif.gob.mx/grups/menores/centroscaic.html (Systema Nacional para el Desarrollo Integral de la Familia of the government of Mexico, Mexico D.F.). The situation in Chile is presented at a government Web site, Gobierno de Chile, Ministerio de Educacion, Junta Nacional de Jardines Infantiles–www.Junji.cl (Chilean Ministry of Education, National Organization of Child Care Centers. Argentina is described in a UN publication (UN, 2000).

3. The "grandmother solution" was proposed by many economists when an earlier version of this article was presented at the Cornell University conference "75 Years of Development Research." Sponsored by the Program on Comparative Economic Development, Department of Economics, May 7-9, 2004.

4. A detailed history of the organization was provided by one of the current board members who was involved in the founding of CHECP. Information on the situation of the children in those early years was provided by the current director who also worked for the organization at its inception. This information was corroborated by telephone and e-mail correspondence with a funding officer at Terre des Hommes. Once CHECP was established as an independent NGO, a newsletter, *News and Views*, was occasionally produced. After 2000, when funds became tight, this newsletter project was abandoned.

5. This is from private correspondence with one of the current board members, who was also a founding member.

6. This is from private correspondence with one of the current board members, who was also a founding member.

REFERENCES

Acker, J. (1998). Women, families, and public policy in Sweden. In S. J. Ferguson (Ed.), *Shifting the center* (pp. 681-695). Mountain View, CA: Mayfield.

Ahmed, S. S. and Bould, S. (2004). One able daughter is worth 10 illiterate sons. *Journal of Marriage and Family, 66*, 1332-1341.

Barnum, H. and Squire, L. (1978). An economic application of the theory of the farm household. *Journal of Development Economics, 6*, 79-102.

Bergmann, B. R. (1996a). *Saving our children from poverty: What the United States can learn from France.* New York, NY: Russell Sage Foundation.

Bergmann, B. R. (1996b). Child care: The key to ending child poverty. In I. Garfinkel, J. L. Hochschild & S. S. McLanahan (Eds.), *Social policies for children* (pp. 112-135). Washington D. C.: Brookings Institution.

Blumberg, R. L. (1976). Fairy tales and facts: Economy family, fertility and the female. In I. Tinker, B. B. Bramsen & M. Buvinic (Eds.), *Women and world development* (pp. 12-21). New York, NY: Praeger.

Blumberg, R. L. (1991). Income under female versus male control. In R. L. Blumberg (Ed.), *Gender, family and economy: The triple overlap* (pp. 97-127). Newbury Park, CA: Sage Publications.

Boserup, E., (1970). *Women's role in economic development.* New York, NY: St. Martin's Press.

Chant, S. (2003). *New contributions to the analysis of poverty: Methodological and conceptual challenges to understanding poverty from a gender perspective.* Santiago, Chile: United Nations.

Charlton, S. E. M. (1984). *Women in third world development.* Boulder, CO: Westview Press.

Chaudry, A. (2004). *Putting children first: How low-wage working mothers manage child care.* New York, NY: Russell Sage Foundation.

CHECP (Care, Health and Education for Children in Poverty) (1996). *News and Views.* No. 4 (July-December).

CHECP (1997). *News and views.* No. 6 (December).

CHECP (2000). *News and views.* No. 6 (December).

Communitarian Network (1991). *A Communitarian position paper on the family.* Washington, D.C.: Author.

Daeren, L. (2001). *The gender perspective in economic and labour policies.* Santiago, Chile: United Nations.

Eade, D. (1997). *Capacity-building: An approach to people-centered development.* Oxford, England: Oxfam.

Endeley, J. B. (2001). Conceptualizing women's empowerment in societies in Cameroon: How does money fit in? In C. Sweetman (Ed.) *Gender, development, and money* (pp. 34-41). Oxford, England: Oxfam.

Fineman, M. L. A. (2002). Masking dependency: The political role of family rhetoric. In E. F. Kittay and E. K. Feder (Eds.), *The subject of care: Feminist perspectives on dependency* (pp. 215-244). New York, NY: Rowan and Littlefield.

Folbre, N. (1994). *Who pays for the kids?* London, UK: Routledge.

Gerstel, N. & Gallagher, S. (1994). Caring for kith and kin: Gender, employment and the privatization of care. *Social Problems, 41,* 519-539.

Helburn, S. W. & Bergmann, B. R. (2003). *America's child care problem.* New York: NY: Palgrave Macmillan.

Himmelstrand, K. (1997). Can an AID bureaucracy empower women? In K. Staudt, (Ed.), *Women, international development, and politics* (pp. 123-135). Philadelphia, PA: Temple University Press.

Kabeer, N. (2003). Gender equality and women's empowerment. (An edited version of *Gender mainstreaming in poverty eradication.*) London, UK: Commonwealth Secretariat.

Kahn, S. R. (1993). South Asia. In E. M. King & M. A. Hill (Eds.), *Women's education in developing countries* (pp. 211-246). Baltimore, MD: The Johns Hopkins University Press.

Kasente, D., Lockwood, M., Vivian, J. & Whitehead, A. (2002). Gender and the expansion of nontraditional agricultural exports in Uganda. In S. Razavi (Ed.), *Shifting burdens* (pp. 35-65). Bloomfield, CT: Kumarian Press.

Kelly, M. P. F. & Sassen, S. (1995). Recasting women in the global economy. In C. E. Bose & E. Acosta-Belen (Eds.), *Women in the Latin American Development Process* (pp. 99-124). Philadelphia, PA: Temple University Press.

Kiritz, N. J. & Mundell, H. (1988). *Program planning & proposal writing: Introductory version.* Los Angeles, CA: The Grantsmanship Center.

Kittay, E. F. (1999). *Love's labor.* New York, NY: Routledge.

Kittay, E. F. & Feder, E. K. (Eds.). (2002). *The subject of care: Feminist perspectives on dependency.* New York, NY: Rowan and Littlefield.

Narayan, D., Patel, R., Schafft, K., Rademacher, A., & Koch-Schulte, S. 2000. *Voices of the poor.* New York, NY: Oxford University Press.

Nussbaum, M. C. (2002). The future of feminist liberalism. In E. F. Kittay & E. K. Feder (Eds.), *The subject of care: Feminist perspectives on dependency* (pp. 186-214). New York, NY: Rowan and Littlefield.

Olin, U. (1976). A case for women as co-managers. In I. Tinker, B.B. Bramsen & M. Buvinic (Eds.), *Women and world development* (pp. 105-128). New York, NY: Praeger.

Phillips, M. M. (2003). The World Bank as privatization agnostic. *The Wall Street Journal* (July 21, p. A2).

Rao, A. (1991). Introduction. In A. Rao, M. B. Anderson & C. A. Overholt (Eds.), *Gender analysis in development planning* (pp. 1-8). W. Hartford, CT: Kumarian Press.

Rogers, B. (1980). *The domestication of women.* London, UK: Tavistock.

Rostow, W. W. (1961). *The stages of economic growth.* London, UK: Cambridge University Press.

Rowlands, J. (1999). Empowerment examined. In D. Eade (Ed.) *Development with women* (pp. 141-150). London, UK: Oxfam.

Salzinger, L. (2003). *Genders in production.* Berkeley, CA: University of California Press.

Staudt, K. (1998). *Policy, politics and gender.* West Hartford, CT: Kumarian Press.

Tara, S. N. (1985). *Education in a rural environment.* New Delhi, India: Ashish Publishing House.

Thukral, E. G. (2002). Poverty and gender in India. In C. Edmonds & S. Medina (Eds.), *Defining an agenda for poverty reduction, Volume 1* (pp. 233-253). Manila, Philippines: Asian Development Bank.

Tinker, I. (1976). The adverse impact of development on women. In I. Tinker, M. B. Bramson & M. Buvinic (Eds.), *Women and world development* (pp. 22-34), New York, NY: Praeger.

United Nations (1999). *1999 world survey on the role of women in development.* New York, NY: United Nations.

United Nations (2000). *Families and the world of work.* New York, NY: United Nations.

United Nations (2002). *Gender mainstreaming: An overview.* New York, NY: United Nations.

United Nations (2003). *Putting gender mainstreaming into practice.* New York, NY: United Nations.

United Nations (2004). *Understanding poverty from a gender perspective.* Santiago, Chile: United Nations.

United Nations Development Programme (1995). *Human development reports.* Oxford, UK: Oxford University Press.

United Nations Development Program (2005a). *Taskforce on education and gender equality.* Executive Summary, pp. 10-25. Retrieved September 6, 2005 from http://www.mdgender.net/upload/monographs/Task_Force_3

United Nations Development Program (2005b). *Human development report, 2005.* Table 3: Human and income poverty. Retrieved September 7, 2005 from http://hdr.undp.org/statistics/data/indicators.cfm?x=24&y=1&z=1

UNICEF (2005). *The state of the world's children, official summary.* Retrieved September 6, 2005 from http://www.unicef.org/publications/index_24433.html.

United Nations Millennium Project (2005). *Taking action: Achieving gender equality and empowering women.* London, U.K.: Earthscan.

United Nations Research Institute for Social Development (UNRISD) (2005). *Gender equality.* Geneva, Switzerland: UNRISD.

United Nations Statistics Division (2004). *Statistics and indicators on men and women.* Retrieved September 9, 2005 from http://unstats.un.org/unsd/demographic/products/indwm/indwm2.htm

U.S. Bureau of the Census (1985). *Women of the world: A chartbook for developing regions*. Washington, D.C.: U.S. Government Printing Office.

Weber, M. (1963). Class, status, party. In S. M. Miller (Ed.), *Max Weber* (pp. 42-58). New York, NY: Thomas Y. Crowell.

Windebank, J. (2002). Dual-earner couples in Britain and France. *Work, Employment and Society, 15*, 269-290.

Vinovskis, M. A. (2005). *The birth of Head Start*. Chicago, IL: University of Chicago Press.

Organizational Responses
to the Fatherhood Crisis:
The Case of Fathers' Rights Groups
in the United States

Jocelyn Elise Crowley

SUMMARY. The emergence of fathers' rights groups, predominantly composed of men who have been personally affected by child support and custody laws, have been understudied up until this point. This article, based on 158 in-depth interviews, identifies individual motivations of members who join these groups, as well as their impressions on overcoming obstacles to further growth. Contrary to popular perception, the desire to change public policy is only one of the many reasons these men choose to join; equally, if not more important, are their needs for legal and emotional assistance. While acknowledging barriers to attracting new members, most are optimistic that their network of grassroots groups will soon become a strong, national social movement working on

---

Jocelyn Elise Crowley, PhD, is Associate Professor of Public Policy in the Edward J. Bloustein School of Planning and Public Policy at Rutgers, the State University of New Jersey.

The author gratefully thanks Margaret Watson for her exceptional research and editorial assistance. In addition, the author sincerely thanks M. B. Crowley and the anonymous referees who significantly improved the quality of the manuscript.

[Haworth co-indexing entry note]: "Organizational Responses to the Fatherhood Crisis: The Case of Fathers' Rights Groups in the United States." Crowley, Jocelyn Elise. Co-published simultaneously in *Marriage & Family Review* (The Haworth Press, Inc.) Vol. 39, No. 1/2, 2006, pp. 99-120; and: *Families and Social Policy: National and International Perspectives* (ed: Linda Haas, and Steven K. Wisensale) The Haworth Press, Inc., 2006, pp. 99-120. Single or multiple copies of this article are available for a fee from The Haworth Document Delivery Service [1-800-HAWORTH, 9:00 a.m. - 5:00 p.m. (EST). E-mail address: docdelivery@haworthpress.com].

behalf of fatherhood issues. The article concludes with several recommendations for policymakers to consider these groups' claims. *[Article copies available for a fee from The Haworth Document Delivery Service: 1-800-HAWORTH. E-mail address: <docdelivery@haworthpress.com> Website: <http://www.HaworthPress.com> © 2006 by The Haworth Press, Inc. All rights reserved.]*

KEYWORDS. Child custody, child support, father's rights groups

In recent years, policymakers have grown increasingly concerned about fatherless families in the United States. The statistics related to children living with only one parent suggest the need for such urgency. From 1970-2000, the percentage of children living with a sole parent grew from 12% to 28%.[1] More often than not, this sole parent is the mother. Divorce, separation, and never-married parents are the central drivers behind this trend which leave increasing numbers of children with only one primary caregiver in their critical developing years (McLanahan, 1998). Although there are differences across racial, ethnic, and class lines, most fathers are simply parenting less than mothers, if they are parenting at all (Dowd, 2000).

The consequences of growing up in single-parent families are now well known. Researchers have demonstrated that children from these non-traditional families are more likely to engage in criminal activity than their counterparts in two-parent families (Conamor & Phillips, 2002; Popenoe, 1996). They are also more likely to drop out of high school, lag academically if they stay in school, experience a teenage pregnancy, and undergo long periods of unemployment (Krein & Beller, 1988; Painter & Levine, 2004; Kiernan, 1992). Children living in single-parent families are also exposed to higher risks for sexual abuse by non-relatives (Lauritsen, 2003). Still other scholars have pointed to the reduction in income and quality adult interaction as the most central deleterious outcomes associated with growing up in a single-parent home (McLanahan, 1985; Simons, 1996).

While most observers agree that fatherlessness is a problem, there is much less consensus on what needs to be done to turn this negative trend around. As a result, a variety of organizations have sprung up to address what they view as the key "causal factors" behind the fatherlessness phenomenon. Most of these organizations are "top-down" in nature; that is, they are composed of a core set of paid or unpaid professionals that attempt to shape the fatherhood debate. Membership is either not possible for the mass public, or is defined simply through a financial contribution. Some, however, are "bottom-up" organizations; that is, they are composed of actual members who physically meet and work together on a more grassroots level to address some particular aspect of fatherlessness.

One of the most understudied of these "bottom-up" groups are fathers' rights organizations located across the United States (Messner, 1997). These are grassroots organizations made up of mostly men who are predominantly interested in how the child support and child custody systems, including visitation enforcement, affect fathers. Their existence is not without controversy. Women's groups, for example, have responded to them with alarm, arguing that fathers' groups aim to restructure both child support and custody policy in ways that disadvantage mothers (Crowley, 2003). More specifically, they maintain that the sole purpose of fathers' rights groups is to overturn all of the economic and social progress that they have earned over the past several decades, especially when it comes to women's roles as mothers. Beyond these broad characterizations and accusations, however, little is known about these groups' actual membership composition and goals. What do the men who join hope to achieve from these groups? Are they really interested in a fundamental shift in public policy with respect to their responsibilities when their families break down as some women's groups argue, or do other factors motivate their participation? What about the future? Are they confident in their ability to bring more men into their ranks?

This article aims to answer exactly these questions by first beginning with an overview of recent organizational responses to the fatherhood crisis. Second, in order to present the concerns of fathers' rights groups more specifically, I describe my research methodology which involves 158 in-depth interviews with leaders and members located across the United States. Third, I present the results from this membership study, and fourth, I conclude with several recommendations for policymakers as they consider these groups' primary concerns.

RECENT ORGANIZATIONAL RESPONSES TO THE FATHERHOOD CRISIS

A variety of organizations now operate within the current political landscape to address the epidemic of fatherlessness across the United

States. While they each argue that fatherlessness is a problem which needs to be remedied, they disagree as to its causes. Generally speaking, these groups can be categorized according to the one particular cure for the fatherhood crisis they promote: pro-marriage, economic empowerment, spiritual leadership, or fathers' rights.

Pro-Marriage Groups

Individuals involved in pro-marriage groups begin with the premise that the modern American family has recently undergone a massive, negative transformation (Gavanas, 2004; Popenoe, 1996; Blankenhorn, 1995). Over the past several decades, these groups claim, feminists and other liberals have advocated new family forms that wrongly assert a moral equivalence between two-parent and female-headed households. In this new social order espoused by these "progressives," men and women have interchangeable roles in the family. Pro-marriage groups disagree. In stark contrast to these interchangeability claims, pro-marriage adherents argue that men and women perform worthy, necessary, and unique tasks within the American family (Coltrane, 2001). These differences are both natural and valuable; other family types are simply inferior. Pro-marriage groups, therefore, seek to restore monogamous, lifelong marriage as the central institution that forms the foundation of all societies. Only with this restoration, they maintain, will fathers be able to reclaim a sense of their own importance in their children's lives.

The National Fatherhood Initiative (NFI), founded in 1994 by Dr. Wade Horn and Don Eberly, is, perhaps, the most influential of the pro-marriage groups operating in the United States today. It promotes media campaigns on the significance of marriage and family, and also produces educational programs for targeted groups of families who might be experiencing higher levels of stress than usual, such as those with fathers in the military or in jail. Another influential group is the Institute for American Values, formed in 1987 by David Blankenhorn. This organization generates research on the topic of fatherlessness in the United States, and has published numerous books and reports on the importance of marriage in American culture. Other pro-marriage groups include the Institute for Responsible Fatherhood and Family Revitalization (IRFFR), begun by Charles Ballard in 1982, and the National Center for Fathering (NCF), started by Ken Canfield in 1990. IRFFR has engaged in innovative policymaking by actively sending married couples to live in low income communities as role models. NCF provides tips on how men can be better fathers and offers training seminars on the topic of strong father and mother partnerships in raising children. Public affiliation in each of these organizations is simply by donation; only NFI calls its donors "members," and even here, membership is defined chiefly by financial contributions.

Economic Empowerment Groups

In contrast to pro-marriage groups which view traditional partnerships between men and women as central in revitalizing fatherhood, economic empowerment organizations look to jobs, particularly for low income, African-American men, as the panacea for fatherlessness (Mincy & Pouncy, 1997, 1999; Gavanas, 2004; Doolittle & Lynn, 1998; Doolittle et al., 1998). These groups focus on deficits in the educational and labor markets as the primary causes of problems for these men in the "relationship market." In this view, the severe lack of employment for a substantial percentage of the male population creates a situation in which family responsibilities become almost impossible to assume and then manage (Wilson, 1996). As a result, men may father children, but then fail to adequately raise them (Sorenson & Zibman, 2001). These organizations thus look to economic opportunity as the principle way to advance men's interest in creating strong bonds with their children. Marriage to their children's mother might be one option for these men in establishing more robust family ties, but it clearly is not the most significant pathway to becoming strong fathers.

Economic empowerment groups, also known as fragile family organizations, take on a variety of forms all across the United States. The National Partnership for Community Leadership (NPCL), for example, began in 1996 as a vehicle to distribute grants to community-based organizations to run a variety of programs for low-income fathers. One of its most important projects is the Partnership for Fragile Families initiative which encourages parents to establish legal paternity, remain involved with their children after birth, and find gainful, long-lasting employment. NPCL often collaborates with the National Practitioners Network for Fathers and Families (NPNFF), founded in 1995. This group provides conferences, training, and technical support for those interested in improving the lives of fathers in fragile families. In the same vein, the Center for Family Policy and Practice (CFPP), established in 1995, advocates for families in economically tenuous circumstances, including situations where fathers have had their parental rights terminated. This group also offers legal assistance and workshops on the topics of custody and child support enforcement, with a specific focus on those fathers who are currently incarcerated. The public cannot join NPCL at all and can only affiliate with CFPP by donation. Membership in NPNFF is defined chiefly by financial contribution, but is aimed at academics and practitioners working in the field rather than the general public.

Spiritual Leadership Groups

Like pro-marriage and economic empowerment organizations, groups that emphasize spiritual leadership remain highly concerned with the loss of familial leadership power among contemporary men. However, instead of pointing to the demise of marriage or declining employment opportunities as the causes of this deficiency, spiritually based groups place the blame for these changes on the increasing secularization of contemporary society–through such factors as movies, television, and popular music–that move men and women away from their true, God-given family roles. According to these groups, men and women are biologically different, leading them to occupy unique roles in the social structure. In this view, men are the natural heads of households, with women assuming secondary positions of support.

Unfortunately, according to these groups, the turbulent social activism of the 1960s, which included the women's movement, toppled this order in the name of "progress." In order for societies to function most healthfully, then, men must take back these leadership roles in their families. More directly, spiritually oriented groups aim to change men's hearts into stronger, authority-motivated forces over their families and advance the idea that all men should live their lives in accordance with certain religious principles. In doing such, proponents hope to bring American society back into a purer, God-centered form of social order.

One of the most influential groups with this philosophy is the Christian Promise Keepers (Coltrane, 2001). From its beginnings in 1990 with only 72 followers, leader Bill McCartney built a transformative movement of men across the United States that seeks to put Jesus Christ first in all of his followers' lives. By 1995, the organization was able to fill several football stadiums across a multitude of American cities with devoted adherents (Quicke & Robinson, 2000; Messner, 1997). By 2003, the Promise Keepers continued to show strength by holding 18 arena conferences that attracted more than 170,000 men who responded to the charismatic character of these meetings (Johnson, 2000). While Christian belief systems tend to dominate these spiritually oriented organizations, other belief systems are represented as well. For example, the Million Man March took place in 1995 under the guidance of Minister Louis Farrakhan and the Nation of Islam. Although the March had many goals, a chief tenet of those who attended was to restore male responsibility in their key roles as husbands and fathers (Baker-Fletcher, 1998; Gabbidon, 2000). Public "membership" in groups like these is usually through the attendance of large-scale rallies or conferences at which there might be a price for admission.

Fathers' Rights Groups

Finally, others see the problem of fatherlessness through the lens of individual rights (Williams & Williams, 1995; Coltrane & Hickman, 1992; Fineman, 1991). Fathers' rights groups, located throughout the country, take on a variety of forms, including national offices with state-level chapters, freestanding national or state units, or state-level groups with local chapters. In stark contrast to many of the groups described above, public membership is available; it is also usually through yearly paid dues instead of sporadic monetary contributions. More importantly, these groups actually meet *in-person on a regular basis*. Like their counterparts in other countries, the majority of fathers' rights groups in the United States claim that men are victims of discrimination in the area of family law, especially with respect to child support and custody issues (Bertoia & Drakich, 1993). Sympathizers argue that current family law is corrupt; only when fathers achieve "equal rights" with mothers will their significant value to families be properly acknowledged and restored (Baskerville, 2002). However, beyond these broad claims, little else is known about the motivations of the men who join these groups and their perceptions of what is holding them back from constituting a larger social movement. It is to these questions that this analysis now turns.

METHODOLOGY

My primary methodological aim in this project was to conduct one-hour telephone interviews with both leaders and rank-and-file members of fathers' rights groups across the United States. Similar to the work of Arendell (1995) and Waller (2002), this intensive interview strategy represented the best way to capture the complexity of these men's lives and how their organizational affiliation fits into their every day existence. Because no centralized list of "fathers' rights" groups exists, I first searched the Internet and non-profit directories for possible groups. This was difficult in that organizations that are involved in these issues describe themselves in many ways. Some prefer the term "fathers' rights" group. Others identify themselves as "children's rights" groups and adamantly deny that they are interested in "fathers' rights." Still others qualify themselves as "family rights" groups. Further complicating matters is the fact that many of these groups are highly ephemeral in nature. Intra-group in-fighting is common, leading to the rapid birth and demise of these types of organizations over short periods of time. It is therefore nearly impossible to compile a comprehensive list of such groups that remains consistently stable. As a first step, then, I attempted to identify at least 3-4 viable groups per state.

In deciding which of these groups to include in this analysis, I examined their array of activities, mission statements, and goals. If child support and child custody issues were primary, then they were in the pool of potentially sampled groups. They also had to meet two other criteria. First, all selected groups had to be active within their particular jurisdiction on family issues; that is, they could not simply be post office boxes without members. More specifically, all groups had to meet a certain threshold of regularly scheduled activities, including monthly or quarterly in-person meetings. Second, I also chose groups to provide the research project with maximum geographic and thus membership diversity. In the end, I had a potential sampling pool of 50 groups.

Next, I attempted to make contact with each group's leader. Four leaders declined participation on behalf of their group and two leaders declined because their groups were no longer active. Fourteen group leaders did not respond to my request for information, and four group leaders' contact information was no longer in service at the time of my request for access. This left me with a final sample of 26 groups,[2] including seven from the northeast, eight from the mid-west, nine from the south, and two from the west.

Once the group's leader agreed to be interviewed, I requested permission to publicize my study to group members. This is the typical "snowball sampling" technique, a procedure that is necessary when group members are difficult to reach. While most leaders were helpful and forthcoming during the interview process, a small minority was not willing to provide additional assistance in reaching members. These diverse reactions translated into varied levels of success in recruiting potential members to the study. The maximum number of interviews I obtained from one group was 20, while the minimum was only one. In the end, I secured a total of 158 interviews and conducted them during the summer of 2003. I asked all of my respondents questions on six topics, of which the second is the focus of this article: (1) Demographics, (2) Group Patterns of Recruitment and Goals, (3) Relationships with Past Partners, (4) Relationships with Their Children, (5) Political Behavior, and (6) Challenges Related to Leadership (asked of leaders only).

As the final part of this first methodological strategy, the taped interviews were transcribed. I then analyzed the written transcriptions of this work using grounded theory methods with the help of the qualitative software analysis program, Atlas.ti. By using this method, I was able to draw upon the words of each of my respondents to create categories of meaning across the interviews (Strauss & Corbin, 1990). These categories were constantly compared, developed, and refined in order to produce the theoretical understandings of membership behavior presented here. It is also important to note that throughout this article, I illustrate my most important arguments with quotes taken from my research participants. All quotes that are used here are verbatim, and all names have been changed to protect the confidentiality of my respondents.[3]

FATHERS' RIGHTS MEMBERS: WHO THEY ARE

Fathers' rights groups in the United States are not monolithic by any means; rather, they attract a wide variety of individuals with diverse backgrounds and experiences. Out of the 158 individuals sampled for this study, 85% were male and 15% were female. Women involved in the groups tended to be second wives and mothers of men with outstanding custody and child support decisions. In this article, however, I focus only on male membership patterns since they constitute the core group of activists. Overall, the majority of members in the groups were in their thirties and forties, while the mean age of the sample was 46, the range of ages represented was between 23 to 76.[4]

There is one important difference between the fathers' rights members that I interviewed and fathers that have been the focus of other studies related to child support and custody issues; this difference relates to socio-demographic advantage. The majority of research in this area has focused on profiling low-income fathers who tend to come from minority backgrounds, possess low levels of education, and are either underemployed or are unemployed (Sorensen & Zibman, 2001). In contrast, my fathers' rights sample was 87% white, while only 8% were Black, 2% were Hispanic, and 1% were Asian. Less than 1% characterized themselves as being of multiple races or an unspecified race, and 1% of all respondents refused to disclose their race.

In addition, while my respondents were not asked directly about their incomes, they did report their level of educational achievement as well as their occupation. Overall, the sample was highly educated. Those who had a high school diploma or a GED composed 9% of the sample, while those who had an associate's degree, some college credits, or some other type of post-high school vocational training made up 31% of all respondents in the study. In addition, 30% of the respondents held a bachelor's degree or a bachelor's degree plus some other graduate training, while the remaining 30% held doctorates, master's degrees, or professional degrees (law, medical, or dental degrees). Corresponding to these high levels of educational achievement, fully 78% of all respondents occupied traditionally white-collar jobs, while only 13% occupied blue-collar jobs. About 6% were retired, and the remainder were either unemployed, students, or volunteers.

In terms of their living situations at the time of the interviews, about 51% of the respondents were divorced or separated, 41% were married, and the remaining 8% were either single or widowed. Over the course of their lives, however, a full 79% had experienced a divorce. Most were divorced once or twice; the maximum number of divorces received by one respondent was six. These divorces took place as recently as 2003 and as early as 1973. There was also wide variation in the number of children reported by these respondents. The average number of biological children in this study was two, although one respondent reported having 12 children. Interestingly, some members of fathers' rights groups were simply activists; they did not have any children of their own.

Members came together in these groups mostly through monthly meetings that lasted from 1-2 hours in length in an individual member's or leader's home, or they were conducted in spaces that were donated either by a local church, library, or business organization. Sometimes the group gathered in a local cafe or restaurant. The content of meetings varied from group to group, but most included the leader following a simple agenda covering a variety of issues currently facing individual members or the organization as a whole. The key questions thus remain: What motivates individuals to join these groups? What do they hope to achieve through their organizational affiliations?

Personal Case Management

By far, the most common answer to the question of why individuals joined their local fathers' rights groups was not the desire to transform public policy, but rather the need for help with their own personal child support and custody issues. In fact, 49% of all respondents in the sample declared that personal case management was a central reason for joining.[5] Most fathers' groups studied here spent a significant amount of time during each meeting providing individual consultations to members. Usually any member who was having a personal family problem—most often related to child support and custody—had an opportunity to speak at the meeting. As these organizations are not licensed to practice law, leaders were careful to insist that they were only offering general information and not legal advice. In addition to the leaders offering options regarding legal tactics, other group members often provided their opinion as to the most effective strategies for handling a particular type of problem, especially if they experienced a similar challenge in their own lives. Sometimes local attorneys also attended these meetings with the dual aim of both offering information about the court system, as well as recruiting new clients for their legal practices.

Members turned to the group after feeling a sense of shock when they initially faced the court system. They did not know what to expect, and the group offered help in understanding the processes under which they would now need to operate in order to secure the most favorable child support and custody decisions. In short, the group gave them the resources that they needed to move forward with their cases.

> What I found through the court system was (that) they ignore the parental input and desires of fathers. My kids' mom asked for the divorce, I didn't want it; there was no infidelity, she up and said one day she wanted a divorce. It shocked me. I was the one who bathed the kids every night, I put them to bed, (and) I read them stories. I was always the first one up and fed them breakfast. I was a very involved father, very involved parent. . . . I immediately filed (I learned pretty quick what joint custody or shared custody was) for shared custody, but they gave me some temporary custody because the mother for the first couple of weeks wouldn't let me see the kids. It was every other weekend, Wednesday nights for 2-1/2 hours, which is what I have now. It took a year to get the trial and the trial was a joke, it was like 15 minutes. . . . The more I went to the court, the more I saw (that) they were missing reality and

there was nowhere to help that, there was nothing. Then I contacted (my local fathers' group) and thought long and I thought if there is nothing around there, I am going to start something. So I did and the more I got involved, the more it helped me. –Tito

Other fathers at first tried to get information themselves about the court system through a local library or through other online reference tools. However, they frequently found themselves so overwhelmed by the sheer quantity of complex family laws that they turned to the group for aid in sorting through it all.

I was doing so many things on my own like joining a law library at the city-county building, researching (and) reading hundreds of cases of law and trying to do my own work. I said, there has to be a better way, maybe to get to the point a lot quicker instead of my working in circles and, you know, feeling so alone and depressed, down and out about it. I (was) talking to a friend of mine who went through a divorce and actually knew (the local fathers' group leader) who started the local chapter of (a national fathers' group) and he said, give him a call. . . . When I finally hooked up with him, it was like a light bulb lit for both of us. He is like, boy, you've already done a lot of things that we would have already recommended and you are already up to speed with most of the things I need to explain to you, but I can help you, (if you) join. That's what happened. –Reed

Still others turned to the group when their financial resources no longer permitted them to continue paying attorneys to fight on their behalf. For these fathers, the group provided them with the information that they needed to continue pressing their claims for more favorable child support and custody arrangements without the assistance of a lawyer.

(I joined) because after 6 1/2 years, now it's 7 1/2 years, of not seeing my children and litigating against a brick wall, I've gone through 5 lawyers and over $20,000 at that point, now it's over $25,000 . . . I wasn't getting anywhere and I wanted to first see if there was some more information that I could find out, even though my case is out of state. –Tristan

In each of the examples cited above, fathers found elements of their personal child support and child custody cases to be too overwhelming to experience alone. They therefore turned to their local fathers' rights group to provide them with the nuts and bolts of case management.

Emotional Support

Approximately one in five (17%) of respondents in this study declared that emotional support was a motivating factor behind their joining their local fathers' group. Numerous respondents reported feeling isolated in the period immediately following their family's breakdown. To these respondents, women have an advantage over men in that they have strong networks of friendship upon which to rely during stressful periods of their lives. Men tend to lack these networks, and thus the group became the only place where they could encounter solace during a difficult time.

> When I was going through my divorce and the issues that were raised and what we perceived as the unfairness (of the situation), I felt I was alone. . . . I discovered when (the group) contacted me that I wasn't (alone) and there were many, many, many men in (a) similar situation. All of us (were) out in the wilderness with no place to go, and this (group) was a place that brought us all together where we could share feelings and emotions and come up with strategies on how to proceed with our cases. –Juan

Others looked to the group for emotional benefits after they settled their divorce cases, when they were seeking a new beginning for their lives.

> I was looking for, at that point, more just social support, social connections. As far as my situation was concerned it was pretty much a done deal, there was not a whole lot I could do about it. I wasn't in a great deal of economic or emotional pain at that point . . . I was more in the process of putting my own life together and so for me it was just very therapeutic to take my anger about the situation and use it in a very constructive manner by being part of an organized group. –Ryan

Fathers, then, used the groups as places where they could share their experiences with others, and, as such, draw upon the emotional sustenance offered by men in similar circumstances. Once they became more stable emotionally themselves, they could then return the favor by offering their assistance to all newcomers to the group.

Changing Public Policy

Interestingly, only one in five respondents (17%) stated that a desire to affect federal and state level public policy was central in their decision to join fathers' rights groups. At the federal level, the Personal Responsibility and Work Opportunity Reconciliation Act (PRWORA) of 1996 continued the several decade-long trend of strengthening child support enforcement efforts in the United States against non-paying parents. More specifically, among many measures, PRWORA introduced a directory of new hires in order to track down delinquents, improved interstate collection mechanisms, and mandated the creation of strong procedures to revoke drivers' and professional licenses when parents fall behind in their payments. States followed suit with hard-line enforcement policies of their own, such as tough, new arrearage penalties, including jail time. Also at the state level, most fathers continued to face judges that used the "best interest of the child" standard for making custody determinations. Although on its face gender-neutral, this best interest standard still resulted in mothers receiving custody in the overwhelming majority of cases.

Fathers who sought to change laws such as these quickly discovered the power of numbers in affecting the political process. More specifically, they learned that when acting in isolation, most policymakers would not listen or respond to their calls for change. However, when they aggregated their claims and interests, policymakers were much more likely to at least provide them with a hearing.

> (I joined) because I have been very frustrated with the public policies towards noncustodial parents in our state . . . I had spent, oh, since my divorce, I have spent five to six years writing letters and talking to state senators and doing many things by myself, and I eventually realized that as a single voice, I wasn't getting very far. So I felt it was best to lend my voice to an organization. –Lawrence

Still others cited the need to change public policy in order to create a better world for their children in the areas of child support and custody.

> I've always been active. I did not like being told how much time I could spend with my kids. If I wanted more time, it was (only) at the grace of the other parent. If I didn't do something (like join the group), what is going to change for my son and daughter? –Gerard

Others echoed this view of wanting to improve the future for others, but expressed a desire to do so not just for their offspring, but for fathers everywhere.

> Every holiday, especially after separating from the kids, it (is not only) hell on the father but everyone around you. It affects you at work and every aspect of your life and who is around (you). It is so wrong. I am a strong Catholic. My faith has grown over the last years and this is so wrong that if I can help other men from going through this, I'm going to. –Pablo

Interestingly, even though their reason for affiliating was not dominant, those who joined with the aim of changing policy tended to express a stronger desire than other respondents to continue their activities with the group for an indefinite time into the future. Only when they reached their goal of "true equality" in terms of family policy would they end their struggle for fathers' rights.

BARRIERS TO ENCOURAGING OTHER MEN TO JOIN

While many men have been motivated to join fathers' groups, most members acknowledge that there is a vast, untapped constituency that shares their plight. These untapped potential participants are mostly men, who, for a variety of reasons, have not yet been mobilized to fight on behalf of fathers' rights. Their explanations for others "not joining" are important in that they indicate the capacity of these groups to grow in the future. Interestingly, while 23 respondents discussed this theme in their interviews, no one dominant explanation emerged for the lack of mobilization; approximately 20% of this group mentioned each of the following barriers to participation: new life priorities, a lack of group exposure, men's ineffective "natural" organizing skills, and a general dearth of personal resources.

New Life Priorities

One reason cited by fathers' rights group members as to why more men do not join their organizations is the existence of new priorities in their lives. The family separation process takes an extreme toll on these men, and most want to look forward, not backward.

> I think people are basically selfish–maybe that's not the best word–self-interested which is a little less harsh and judgmental. But if you, through the horrors of divorce, take the emotional and financial beating you are going to take, whoever you are, man or woman, mother or father, grandparent or whatever, you take all the beatings and you (want to just) pack up all that emotional baggage and tuck it away in the back of your head and get on with your life. –Gerald

Moreover, if a man has started to put his family's break-up behind him, he may also have a new love interest who does not necessarily want him to become involved in a group that deals with "problems from the past."

> (Sometimes you feel), yeah, things are bad but I am just tired of this crap, tired of divorce and probably also if you get remarried or have a significant other in your life, there is always, "Hey don't worry about that–you are with me now and . . ." So, if you are in another relationship, that has issues, too. (Your new love interest might say) "Why are you taking time off to go do that, but you don't take time off to do this with me?" You end up in the same trap as you were before, you don't want to go there. So that whole thing is difficult; (it is difficult) to find another significant other who is also compassionate around that topic. –Elliot

According to these members, then, most men want to go on with their lives after a painful family separation. The existence of new life priorities simply adds increased momentum to the often powerful drive to move forward emotionally without looking back.

Lack of Exposure

Other members and leaders argued that the lack of participation on behalf of many men was simply due to a paucity of information on the availability of local groups. In other words, a sizeable percentage of men simply do not know that fathers' rights groups are active and fighting on behalf of the issues that impact them directly.

> I think it's a non-exposure (issue), not knowing (that) the groups exist. Even today, (our group has) made a lot of strides in the last year. (But) basically, (I) at 42 didn't know (the group) existed. And I'm very political. I work with U.S. Congressmen, and state

legislators, and I didn't know it existed. People are just finding out about it. –Jules

Another respondent echoed similar sentiments about the need to distribute information about the group more effectively.

> (Most men) don't know there is help out there. I didn't know about it until just a few years ago. I guess I'd like to see (publicity about the group) more. I don't know how we can promote it more, but there are a lot of guys out there that don't know (about) it. . . . You talk to more guys (and) they have the same kind of problems (that) I do. –Tomas

Inherent in many of these perspectives was a twofold sense of responsibility. Men had to do more to learn about resources in their geographical areas, as their quotes demonstrate. However, many respondents also argued that fathers' rights groups needed to do a better job of getting their message out as well.

Men Are Not "Natural Organizers"

One of the most interesting explanations as to why more men are not joining fathers' rights groups had to do with members' perspectives on the differing propensity of men versus women to organize. For these respondents, men are not "natural-born" organizers in the same way that women are. This puts them at a relative disadvantage when it comes to advocacy work in the political arena. Part of what inhibits men from political action is also gender-based socialization when it comes to showing emotions. According to several respondents, joining a group signals weakness, something most men want to avoid.

> Men have a stigma of being male, being dominant, and our society teaches us to be tough and to tough it out. This is something (that) you have to go through. . . . When I played football and got hurt, you showed your toughness by not admitting to the pain. You got through it as best you can, but I think men, especially nowadays, need to talk about it. –Lukas

Beyond the notion that actively seeking out a group indicates male weakness, other respondents indicated that certain men do not become involved in fathers' rights groups because they believe that help should come to them rather than the other way around. To current members, this common attitude again works to the detriment of men in comparison to women as organizers.

> If you look at most men, so many men are so stubborn. . . . Like my dad when my mother passed away a couple of years ago. Hospice sent stuff to my dad saying (that) there were support groups to go to. Of course, my dad is saying, I am not going to those support groups, blah, blah, blah. I just think some men have that attitude that they want the help, but they don't want to have to go get it. They think it should come to them, kind of. . . . Some men are that way that they just don't want it. They want to put that big tough side on. They walk around saying, I can handle it, I don't need anybody's help. That's why (fewer) men join these groups. I think that is why the women's movement was so great because women can bond like that, but I think men have trouble doing that. –Harry

Still other respondents argued that men do not join these groups because there is a deep shame associated with bringing issues related to the loss of one's children to the public's attention.

> I think I said it at the beginning . . . people say men don't join groups . . . I'm sorry, (but) I go to football games on weekends and there are a lot of men. Men will go join billiard clubs, they join bowling leagues. . . . It's about if you join these (fathers' rights) groups, you are held up to social stigma that is really difficult. You stand up and identify yourself as someone who has lost your children and in this society, God knows what runs through the people's minds as for the reasons why. –Burt

Continuing this theme, other fathers pointed to men's inability to see the larger picture of fathers' rights as a cause, and instead focused solely on their own cases. This "inward-looking" tendency of many fathers, then, as compared with the "outward-looking" tendency of most women, has prevented these groups from enlarging their scope of membership.

Lack of Resources

Finally, for other respondents, the critical issue impeding more men from joining fathers' rights groups is a lack of resources. In order to participate actively in a group, fathers have to make certain financial sacrifices. Not only are there transportation costs, but there are also opportunity costs associated with attending these meetings.

> I think (that there are) two reasons (as to why more people do not join fathers' groups): (1) The same reason I am not super active–I don't have the time, I have to work a lot of times during the meetings. (2) It costs money to be able to have that free time and do things with these people–it costs you money. . . . I attended a little rally protest march at the State House here last winter and we had people coming from (all over the state). . . . That cost them money to drive from (all over the state) to spend the day down here, feed themselves, the kids, and then drive back. That is a cost. –Sean

Fathers' rights groups, for the most part, are cash-poor. They tend to rely on volunteers to conduct the majority of their business, and members are expected to incur most of the direct and indirect costs of participating. For many, even a minor contribution to the cause in the form of meeting attendance may simply be prohibitive.

Despite all of the above-mentioned barriers to growth, most respondents remained cautiously optimistic that they could be eventually overcome. Indeed, numerous members described these barriers as simply temporary roadblocks to their success and offered concrete ways to meet these challenges. More specifically, these respondents maintained that in order to jump-start the membership rolls, the chief objectives for these groups should be to provide quality information about the judicial system, offer emotional support for members, and make incremental, father-friendly changes in public policy so that ultimate success–true equality with mothers–becomes a more tangible and attainable goal. Success in these areas, in their view, would breed further success in terms of membership growth.

CONCLUSIONS

In recent years, policymakers have paid increased attention to certain aspects of the fatherlessness debate–that is, those issues that tend to impact low-income fathers. After President Clinton called father-absence "the single biggest social policy problem" in our society in 1995, President George W. Bush committed his Administration to restoring the prestige of fathers in American families. For example, the Bush Administration recently encouraged the states to introduce increased flexibility within their Temporary Assistance to Needy Families (TANF) programs in order to promote father-friendly families. By 2002, states like Mississippi, North Dakota, and Oklahoma responded by disregarding the income of a new spouse in calculating welfare benefits during a post-wedding period of between three and six months. Bush also supported new economic empowerment and faith-based initiatives of up to $64 million for fiscal year 2002 and up to $315 million in five future years, lending political weight to organizations that attempt to attack these specific root causes of fatherlessness.

But these initiatives do nothing for the more socioeconomically and demographically advantaged yet nonetheless disaffected fathers who tend to join fathers' rights groups, the organizations that were studied here. These fathers have different concerns. First, they lack information about child support and child custody policies. And when they seek out this information, many feel that both sets of policies are unfair to men. Second, they experience this perceived injustice in emotional isolation, finding it challenging to connect with others who will understand their plight. Third, they clearly want to affect public policy in the area of family law, but are only beginning to identify the organizational hurdles that they must first clear in advocating for change. In sum, the common theme that unites all three of these concerns is the sense of being voiceless during a period of major upheaval in their lives. Their organizational affiliation is one way to speak out to others regarding the complex and turbulent issues that they are experiencing on a daily basis, and they hope that others will soon overcome any negative attitudes that they have regarding participation.

What types of policies, if any, should be designed in response to these concerns? As a starting point, new efforts should be made to not only provide information to these fathers regarding their rights and responsibilities with respect to child support and custody, but also to fully demonstrate how these laws were formulated with each person's well-being in mind. For example, all parents might be required to complete a workshop or view a special video on the legal process concerning child support and custody prior to their entry into the court system. Furthermore, existing and/or new father-oriented programs should also promote the idea that seeking out others in a time of need does not demonstrate weakness, as many men presume, and that organizational participation can be a healthy outlet for sharing and expression. Finally, policymakers should be open to hearing about the ways in which these groups–if they continue to mobilize–might alter the current direction of family policy. Only through the first step of listening will public officials then be able to assess the relative strengths and weaknesses of these groups' claims.

NOTES

1. Living Arrangements of Children Under 18 Years Old, 1960-Present, U.S. Census Bureau, Table CH-1. Accessed from *http://www.census.gov/population/socdemo/hh-fam/tabCH-1.pdf* on 11/8/04.

2. These 26 groups constitute the total of each respondent's primary affiliation. Some were members of multiple groups at one point in time–belonging to other groups in my study or, in most cases, groups that I did not have permission to study. Counting these second and third affiliations would bring the groups studied total to 34.

3. Sometimes I inserted words for grammatical clarity or to protect the identity/personal characteristic of a person/organization; these word insertions are always noted by parentheses. Punctuation marks were often added to clarify the meaning of the quote.

4. One individual chose not to report his age.

5. Note that respondents frequently offered more than one answer to this question, and this overlap is reflected in the percentages reported here.

REFERENCES

Arendell, T. (1995). *Fathers and divorce*. Thousand Oaks, CA: Sage.

Baker-Fletcher, G.K. (1998). Keeping the promises of the Million Man March. In G.K. Baker-Fletcher (Ed.), *Black religion after the Million Man March* (pp. 102-111). Maryknoll, NY: Orbis Books.

Baskerville, S. (2002). The politics of fatherhood, *PS: Political Science and Politics, 35*, 695-699.

Bertoia, C. & J. Drakich. (1993). The fathers' rights movement: Contradictions in rhetoric and practice, *Journal of Family Issues, 14*, 592-615.

Blankenhorn, D. (1995). *Fatherless America: Confronting our most urgent social problem*. New York: Basic Books.

Coltrane, S. (2001). Marketing the marriage "solution": Misplaced simplicity in the politics of fatherhood, *Sociological Perspectives, 44*, 387-418.

Coltrane, S. & N. Hickman. (1992). The rhetoric of rights and needs: Moral discourse in the reform of child custody and child support laws, *Social Problems, 39*, 400-420.

Comanor, W.S. & Phillips, L. (2002). The impact of income and family structure on delinquency, *Journal of Applied Economics, 5*, 209-232.

Crowley, J.E. (2003). *The politics of child support in America*. New York: Cambridge.

Doolittle, F., V. Knox, C. Miller, & S. Rowser (1998). *Building opportunities, enforcing obligations: Implementation and interim impacts of Parents' Fair Share*. New York: Manpower Demonstration Research Corporation.

Doolittle, F. & S. Lynn. (1998). *Working with low-income cases: Lessons for the child support enforcement system from Parents' Fair Share*. New York: Manpower Demonstration Research Corporation.

Dowd, N. (2000). *Redefining fatherhood*. New York: New York University Press.

Fineman, M.A. (1991). *The illusion of equality*. Chicago: University of Chicago Press.

Gabbidon, S. (2000). African American male college students after the Million Man March: An exploratory study, *Journal of African American Men, 5*, 15-26.

Gavanas, A. (2004). *Fatherhood politics in the United States: Masculinity, sexuality, race and marriage.* Urbana: University of Illinois Press.

Johnson, S. (2000). Who Supports the Promise Keepers? *Sociology of Religion, 61,* 93-104.

Kiernan, K. (1992). The impact of family disruptions in childhood on transitions made in young adult life, *Population Studies, 46,* 213-234.

Krein, S.F. & A. H. Beller. (1988). Educational attainment of children from single-parent families: Differences by exposure, gender, and race, *Demography, 25,* 221-234.

Lauritsen, J. L. (2003). How families and communities influence youth victimization, *Juvenile Justice Bulletin.* Washington, DC: Office of Juvenile Justice and Delinquency Prevention.

McLanahan, S. (1985). Family structure and the reproduction of poverty, *American Journal of Sociology, 90,* 873-901.

McLanahan, S. (1998). Growing up without a father. In C. Daniels (Ed.), *Lost fathers: The politics of fatherlessness in America* (pp. 85-108). New York: St. Martin's Press.

Messner, M. A. (1997). *Politics of masculinities: Men in movements.* Thousand Oaks, CA: Sage.

Mincy, R. & H. Pouncy. (1997). Paternalism, child support enforcement, and fragile families. In L. Mead (Ed.), *The new paternalism: Supervisory approaches to poverty* (pp. 130-160). Washington, DC: The Brookings Institution.

Mincy, R. & H. Pouncy. (1999). There must be 50 ways to start a family. In W. Horn, D. Blankenhorn, & M. B. Pearlstein (Eds.), *The fatherhood movement: A call to action* (pp. 83-104). New York: Lexington Books.

Painter, G. & Levine, D. (2004). Daddies, devotion, and dollars, *American Journal of Economics and Sociology, 63,* 813-850.

Popenoe, D. (1996). *Life without father: Compelling new evidence that fatherhood and marriage are indispensable for the good of children and society.* New York: Free Press.

Quicke, A. & K. Robinson. (2000). Keeping the promise of the Moral Majority? A historical/critical comparison of the Promise Keepers and the Christian Coalition, 1989-98. In D. Claussen (Ed.), *The Promise Keepers: Essays on masculinity and Christianity* (pp. 7-19). Jefferson, NC: McFarland & Company.

Simons, R. L. (1996). *Understanding differences between divorced and intact families: Stress, interaction and child outcomes.* Thousand Oaks, CA: Sage.

Sorenson, E. & C. Zibman. (2001). Getting to know poor fathers who do not pay child support, *Social Service Review, 75,* 420-434.

Strauss, A. & J. Corbin. (1990). *Basics of grounded theory: Grounded theory procedures and techniques.* Newbury Park, CA: Sage.

Waller, M. (2002). *My baby's father: Unmarried parents and paternal responsibility.* Ithaca, NY: Cornell.

Williams, G.I. & R. H. Williams. (1995). "All we want is equality": Rhetorical framing in the fathers' rights movement. In J. Best (Ed.), *Images of issues: Typifying contemporary social problems* (pp. 191-212). New York: Aldine De Gruyter.

Wilson, W.J. (1996). *When work disappears: The world of the new urban poor.* New York: Knopf.

Gender Equality and Fertility in Sweden: A Study on the Impact of the Father's Uptake of Parental Leave on Continued Childbearing

Ann-Zofie Duvander

Gunnar Andersson

SUMMARY. In Sweden, the birth or adoption of a child is accompanied by the right to more than one year of paid parental leave that can be shared between parents. This article examines the relationship between the father's and the mother's respective use of such leave and the continued childbearing of a couple. Our investigation is based on longitudinal information on registered parental leave use and childbearing of all intact unions in Sweden during 1988-99. We analyze our data by means of event-history analysis. We expected an extended paternal involvement in leave-taking to be positively associated with continued childbearing,

Ann-Zofie Duvander is affiliated with Statistics Sweden/SCB, Demographic Analysis and Gender Equality, Box 24300, SE-104 51 Stockholm. Gunnar Andersson is affiliated with the Max Planck Institute for Demographic Research, Rostock, Germany.

The authors are grateful to Statistics Sweden for providing them with the demographic raw data, to Jonathan MacGill for assistance in organizing the data, and to the Max Planck Institute for Demographic Research for providing its facilities to Ann-Zofie Duvander while she and Andersson worked together on this project at the aforementioned institute.

[Haworth co-indexing entry note]: "Gender Equality and Fertility in Sweden: A Study on the Impact of the Father's Uptake of Parental Leave on Continued Childbearing." Duvander, Ann-Zofie, and Gunnar Andersson. Co-published simultaneously in *Marriage & Family Review* (The Haworth Press, Inc.) Vol. 39, No. 1/2, 2006, pp. 121-142; and: *Families and Social Policy: National and International Perspectives* (ed: Linda Haas, and Steven K. Wisensale) The Haworth Press, Inc., 2006, pp. 121-142. Single or multiple copies of this article are available for a fee from The Haworth Document Delivery Service [1-800-HAWORTH, 9:00 a.m. - 5:00 p.m. (EST). E-mail address: docdelivery@haworthpress.com].

since it makes family building more compatible with the mother's labor force participation. In addition, such commitment to childrearing from the father's side is likely to signal his greater interest for continued family building. Around 85% of fathers take some leave but in most cases for a brief time. We find a positive effect of a father's taking moderately long leave on a couple's second- and third-birth propensity, but no such effect of a father's taking very long parental leave. *[Article copies available for a fee from The Haworth Document Delivery Service: 1-800-HAWORTH. E-mail address: <docdelivery@haworthpress.com> Website: <http://www.HaworthPress.com> © 2006 by The Haworth Press, Inc. All rights reserved.]*

KEYWORDS. Family policy, fertility, gender equality, parental leave, parenthood, Sweden

The main goal of Swedish family policy has been to support the reconciliation of active labor force participation and family life of women and men (Statens Offentliga Utredningar, 1972). Public policies have been seen as an instrument in promoting gender equality both at the household level and in the labor market. A scheme of paid parental leave, which can be shared between parents, is a crucial component of these policies.

The Swedish parental leave system affects gendered behavior in two ways. First, it enhances the reconciliation of work and family life for women as its income-replacement character provides incentives for them to become established in the labor market before considering childbearing. It also allows women to keep a foothold in the labor market while taking care of new-born children so that they can continue with labor market work after the leave. Secondly, the parental leave system encourages fathers to take parental leave, mainly through the months that are reserved for father's use. In this respect, Sweden is the first country in the EU which really can be considered as developing a system with the potential of altering gendered behavior in breadwinning and child care (Haas, 2003; Haas & Hwang, 1999).

While the first impact of the parental leave system has been quite successful, the second goal is still to be fulfilled. In comparison to men in other countries, Swedish men take parental leave relatively frequently (Kamerman, 2000), but they have certainly not entered the realm of household activities to the extent as women have entered the labor market. Fathers still use only a fraction of the total leave periods covered by the parental leave insurance system (Sundström & Duvander, 2002). In response to the slow increase in fathers' uptake of parental leave, Swedish authorities have tried to promote a faster change in behavior. Increased paternal involvement in childrearing has been emphasized not only as a means to promote gender equality at the couple level but also to strengthen the emotional bonds between fathers and their children (Rostgaard, 2002). In our study, we ask whether a more active paternal involvement in terms of parental leave also can be related to a couple's subsequent childbearing behavior. Such involvement may enhance the compatibility between childrearing and labor force participation of the mother and thereby make it easier for her to have another child. It signals the father's commitment to childrearing and possibly also to continued family building. In short, we wonder whether a higher degree of gender equality at the individual level, as measured by a more gender equal division of the parental leave, can be connected with higher fertility.

Swedish family policy has no explicit pronatalist goal, but often contains an assumption that gender equality indeed has a positive effect on fertility. The policy is otherwise formulated as a welfare issue, with the purpose of enabling couples to have the number of children they actually want to have (Andersson, 2005; Ministry of Health and Social Affairs, 2001). A positive impact of gender equality on fertility is nowadays often assumed in family-demographic research (e.g., Bernhard, 1993; Joshi, 1998; McDonald, 2000a,b). In this respect, fathers' uptake of parental leave reflects one important aspect of gender equality at the couple level.

Our study thus deals with the issue of whether public policies can have an impact on childbearing behavior. Previous studies of possible relationships between family policy and fertility in Scandinavia have frequently focused on how childbearing trends have been related to the implementation of some changes in that policy. Family policy is then treated as an aggregate-level factor. (For examples, see Andersson, 2004a; Hoem, 1990, 1993; Oláh, 2003; Rönsen, 2004; Sundström & Stafford, 1992.) More rarely has the effect of the variation in individual use of a policy been studied (two important exceptions are given by Oláh, 2001, 2003). In our study, we use individual-level data on use of parental leave benefits and subsequent childbearing of Swedish couples with one or two common children in order to estimate the possible effect of the uptake of parental leave on continued childbearing. With this approach, we can distinguish between individuals who have used the policy option we want to study and individuals who have not. This better allows us to detect any effects of the particular policy on individual childbearing behavior.

We begin with an overview of the Swedish parental leave system and of fertility developments in Sweden. This is followed by a discussion of the possible connection between gender equality and childbearing. We then describe our data before turning to the results and our concluding discussion.

THE SWEDISH PARENTAL LEAVE PROGRAM

The Swedish parental leave program was introduced in 1974. It then gave the right to six months of paid leave from work after the birth of a child. Sweden was the first country in the world to introduce a gender neutral parental leave scheme (for an international overview of parental leave policies and their consequences, see Ferrarini, 2003; Kamerman, 2000; Moss & Deven, 1999). Employed mothers and fathers were granted an income replacement of 90% of their previous earnings up to a relatively high ceiling. Parents who have had no earnings prior to the use of the leave receive only a low flat rate. During the 1990s, this rate was equivalent to 6 Euro or US $8 per day. All parents permanently residing in Sweden are entitled to parental leave. Such leave can be used in various ways: full-time, half-time, or quarter-time by either of the parents until the child turns eight. Benefits are paid out of the general tax system with no direct cost to employers. The parental leave policy also includes benefits for care of sick children to be used when parents have resumed labor market activity. In 1980, ten additional so called "daddy days" to be used exclusively by the father in connection with childbirth were introduced.

The entitlement period was stepwise prolonged during the 1970s and 1980s. In 1989 it was extended to 15 months of which three months were paid at a low flat rate. Originally parents could split the leave between them as they preferred. In 1995, one month of the leave became reserved for each parent, which popularly has been labeled as the introduction of a "daddy month." The intention was to increase fathers' use of parental leave. In 2002 a second month reserved for each parent was introduced as the leave was prolonged to 16 months. In 1995, 1996 and 1997 the income-replacement level was stepwise reduced to 75%, as public finances were strained, but was raised again to the present level of 80% in 1998. However, since the ceiling of the income replacement has not followed increases in incomes, today a larger minority of parents are replaced at a lower level than the stipulated 80%. This applies especially to fathers who more often than mothers have earnings above the ceiling. In the early 1990s, around a tenth of fathers earned more than that level, which at present amounts to around 32,000 Euro or US $38,000, on an annual basis (counted as earnings before tax but after social-security contributions).

In sum, the Swedish parental leave system is very generous in terms of income replacement, length, and flexibility (it can, for example, be prolonged by accepting a lower replacement level during a longer time), but fathers still use only a fraction of total leave. Table 1 demonstrates that fathers' share of all benefit days has increased from only a half percent in 1974 when the policy was introduced to 12% of leave days 25 years later. After 1995, when the daddy month was introduced, the fraction of male leave users increased, but fathers on leave then took fewer days on average. This may be due to an influx of less motivated fathers, who used a few benefit days that would otherwise have been forfeited (Sundström & Duvander, 2002). The situation can still be described in terms of fathers choosing whether to take leave, and if so, when and for how long, while mothers mainly consider the length of their leave (Bekkengen, 2002).

Economic characteristics are important determinants of Swedish fathers' use of parental leave. Both mother's and father's earnings have a positive impact on father's uptake; father's earnings have the strongest impact (Nyman & Pettersson, 2002; Sundström & Duvander, 2002). However, father's uptake does not seem to increase with earnings above the ceiling of the income replacement, which could be interpreted as sensitivity to the cost of parental leave (Sundström & Duvander, 2002). Furthermore, fathers with more education, employed in the public sector, and with partners with more education take more leave than other fathers (Bygren & Duvander, 2005; Haas, 1992; Näsman, 1992; Nyman & Pettersson, 2002; Sundström & Duvander, 2002).

The huge impact of the level of earned income before childbirth on the benefit level during parental leave is a strong incentive to establish oneself in the labor market before considering becoming a parent. Indeed, earned income is positively related to Swedish women's entry into motherhood (Andersson, 2000; Duvander & Olsson, 2001; Hoem, 2000). The same holds when entry into fatherhood is studied (Duvander & Olsson, 2001). In Sweden, labor force participation of women at childbearing ages is high and almost parallel to that of men (Bygren, Gähler & Nermo, 2004).

TABLE 1. Fathers' Share of Parental Leave Use in Sweden, 1974-2004

	Fraction of Benefit Days Used by Fathers (Percent)	Fraction of Men of Parental Leave Users (Percent)	Average Number of Days Used by Fathers Who Took Leave in a Year
1974	0.5	2.8	21
1975	0.9	4.0	30
1976	1.4	5.2	36
1977	2.2	7.0	42
1978	4.3	N.A.	N.A.
1979	4.8	N.A.	N.A.
1980	5.2	N.A.	N.A.
1981	5.0	N.A.	N.A.
1982	5.1	N.A.	N.A.
1983	5.2	N.A.	N.A.
1984	5.1	N.A.	N.A.
1985	5.5	N.A.	N.A.
1986	6.2	23.0	26
1987	7.5	24.5	29
1988	6.5	23.1	31
1989	6.9	24.6	32
1990	7.1	26.1	33
1991	8.1	26.5	39
1992	9.1	26.9	43
1993	10.1	27.4	45
1994	11.4	28.3	44
1995	9.6	27.9	34
1996	10.6	31.1	30
1997	9.9	30.9	28
1998	10.4	32.4	27
1999	11.9	36.2	29
2000	12.7	37.7	28
2001	14.1	39.9	29
2002	15.9	41.6	30
2003	17.6	42.7	32
2004	18.7	43.2	32

Source: Calculations based on data from the National Social Insurance Agency

FERTILITY DEVELOPMENTS IN SWEDEN

During recent decades, Swedish fertility has evolved in a roller-coaster fashion (Hoem & Hoem, 1996), being positively related to the business cycle (Andersson, 2000). After an increase in fertility during the economic boom by the end of the 1980s and early 1990s, Sweden experienced a sharp decline in fertility during the 1990s. In 1990, the total fertility (TFR) of Sweden was 2.1 children per woman and this was among the highest rates in Europe. It subsequently fell to an unprecedented low of 1.5 children per woman in 1997-99. Fertility has started to increase again (Andersson, 2004b). In 2004, the TFR of Sweden was close to 1.8, which is similar to that of the other Nordic countries.

The mid-1990s was a period of economic hardship and the labor force participation of both women and men dropped. Many young women and men stayed in school longer when unemployment increased. The weaker attachment of young adults to the labor market was one of the reasons why fertility decreased during that period (Andersson, 2000; Hoem, 2000). The fertility decline was mainly due to young women postponing becoming mothers and two-child parents deciding not to have a third child. First births of women above 30 and second births were less affected. It has been suggested that the overall economic climate of the 1990s had a further role to play in the fertility decline than that given merely by the negative changes in individual labor market attachment of young Swedes. Hoem (2000) found that the unemployment level in the local municipality mattered for women's first-birth patterns also when the individual's own labor market status was considered. Cut-backs in family policies, like the aforementioned reductions in income-replacement levels during parental leave, may also have affected fertility adversely. A reversal of such policy changes as the economy improved again by the turn of the century is likely to be positively related to the most recent increases in fertility.

FATHER'S USE OF PARENTAL LEAVE
AND CONTINUED CHILDBEARING

A positive correlation between gender equality in the home and fertility is often suggested (e.g., Bernhard, 1993; Joshi, 1998; McDonald, 2000a,b) and sometimes even found in empirical studies based on individual-level data (for supportive evidence see, e.g., Buber, 2002; Mencarini & Tanturri, 2004). In our case, the sharing of parental leave between parents can be considered as one measure of such equality. A finding in a study by Oláh (2003) indeed suggests that there was a positive impact of the father's uptake of parental leave on second births in Swedish couples during the 1970s to 1980s.

The major argument put forward for why gender equality would increase fertility is that a more equal division of labor in the household would ease women's work burden at home and thus enhance the degree of compatibility between childrearing and their labor force participation. Such compatibility makes it easier to realize childbearing plans. Parental leave taken by the father can, for example, facilitate a faster return to work of the mother. More crucial might be that a shared parental leave indicates a shared responsibility for childcare during the child's first year(s), and that it signals the father's commitment to share the care of children. The sharing of childcare in the child's early life is important, as patterns and divisions of such care are unlikely to change when the child grows older (Hwang & Lamb, 1997). A higher degree of gender equality might also affect fertility positively, in a more indirect way, if it affects women's well-being (Blair, 1993; Glass & Fujimuto, 1994) and marital stability (Oláh, 2001) positively. Women in gender equal relationships may be more prone to continue childbearing in their present relationship.

It is equally important to consider the role of the father's desire for more children as both parents' childbearing plans are decisive for continued childbearing (Thomson, 1997; Thomson & Hoem, 1998). In this respect, a more gender equal division of parental leave is likely to be positively related to the father's desire for more children. Kaufman (2000) finds that in U.S. men with egalitarian attitudes are more likely to intend to have a child than other men. Bulanda (2004) demonstrates how U.S. fathers with more egalitarian attitudes are also more likely than traditional fathers to be involved with their children, and Hyde, Essex, and Horton (1993) show that such men take relatively longer parental leave than other men.[1]

In other words, a selection of men with preferences for children are likely to use a larger share of the parental leave and be more likely to continue childbearing. A father's uptake of parental leave signals an interest in children and childrearing, which is likely to be positively related to his childbearing intentions. The actual experience of parental leave can both be negatively and positively related to the desire for more children. Men who share the leave may gain further interest in children so that their desire for more children is strengthened. On the other hand, the work burden of childrearing noticed while on leave may impede these men's desire for further children. The same holds with respect to the mother's experience of parental leave and her childbearing desires. When studying the relationship between the division of parental leave and the continued childbearing of a couple, we also need to consider that a father's unusually large uptake of parental leave may mirror the mother's reduced interest in childrearing and future children, and vice versa. A very large uptake of parental leave, especially of the father, might also be due to a situation where the other parent is not entitled to a decent level of wage replacement.

In a discussion of the impact of gender equality on childbearing, we want to underline that only an equal–or close to equal–sharing of the parental leave indicates true gender equality. As long as the father's share of the parental leave is as small as it normally is today, it cannot really be seen as a reflection of gender equality in the family, nor in the labor market. Bekkengen (2002) argues that fathers may well use parental leave without challenging the gender-based structure in the couple relationship and often do so when it fits their own situation and needs. Björnberg (1998) finds that men involved in childcare explain that they do so because it is rewarding for their self-fulfillment, rather than because they are concerned about achieving gender equality. In our study, we see fathers' uptake of parental leave as important in the way it signals (a) a commitment to share the duties of childrearing with the mother, and (b) an interest in children and the father-child relation as such.

Finally, our study provides complementary insight into how mothers' patterns of parental leave use are related to couples' continued childbearing. Practically all women in Sweden take extensive parental leave and the impact of their leave use on childbearing is likely to have other consequences and implications, in addition to men's use of leave. For example, an unusually short uptake of parental leave on behalf of the mother might either indicate a quick return to the labor market due to her strong career orientation or reflect a situation where she is not entitled to a high level parental leave benefit, given her prior weak attachment to the labor market.

DATA AND METHODS

Our data are derived from Swedish population registers and cover the period 1988-99. They comprise demographic information on all co-residing couples with one or two common children who ever lived in

Sweden during that period. The demographic data have been merged with information on registered earned income of these parents stemming from Swedish tax registers. Information on educational attainment has been added from other administrative registers. The data cover all couples where both partners are Swedish-born and where the couple's first common child also is the first child of the mother. Observations are censored when parents separate. The data on earned income are given on a yearly basis and include income replacement during periods of sickness and parental leave. (Parental leave benefits are specified separately as well.) As the information is yearly, we are not able to sort out spells of parental leave and labor market work within a given year. We use the information on paid parental leave benefits during the period following childbirth as a determinant of the propensity to have another child during subsequent years.

As the information on income is given on a yearly basis and we want to follow parents' uptake of parental leave immediately after childbirth, we have restricted our data set to couples with a child born in January. Our data comprise 34,000 one-child couples and 27,000 two-child couples in 1988-99. We study the amount of parental leave benefit paid to fathers and mothers of such children during the first two years following childbirth and relate these amounts to the total earnings of the same parents during the same period. This gives the fraction of earnings that comes from the income replacement of the parental leave system. This amount, the fraction of earnings that comes from taking parental leave, is used as a proxy for the fraction of time parents were on leave during that period. Unfortunately, in our data, we have no information on the actual number of days that parents were on leave. We use a reference period of two years after childbirth since most parents are able to take the main part of their parental leave within that time. Fathers who participate more actively in the parental leave program often take most of their leave towards the end of the couple's parental leave period, which is likely to occur more than one year after childbirth. Our design means that couples who have another birth within this two-year period necessarily had to be excluded from our study. Almost one-fourth (24%) of second births and 17% of third births occurred during this time period, two years immediately after the birth of the first or second child. Swedish parental leave policy gives incentives to parents to have children at relatively short birth intervals. This reduced our sample size from 34,000 one-child couples to 28,500 such couples and from 27,000 two-child couples to 26,000 couples of that kind.

In our analyses of the impact of parents' uptake of parental leave on continued childbearing, we relate subsequent registered births to the corresponding exposure times of "risk" of having another child. This amounts to an event-history analysis of childbearing behavior where we estimate the impact of different levels of parental leave use on the propensity to have another child, when controlling for the simultaneous effect of other demographic and socio-economic variables known to be related to both leave use and childbearing. The estimated risks reflect both the timing and the quantum of the event we study. This technique is a standard tool in analyses of time-dependent data like ours. (For an introduction to event-history analysis, see Allison, 1984.)

We estimate models for second and third births separately, since we know that fertility patterns differ by parity. Almost all one-child parents proceed to have a second birth, which means that models for that parity progression mainly cover the timing of such births (see Oláh, 2003, for further analyses of second births in Sweden). Around half of two-child couples also proceed to have a third child which means that the latter models measure the timing of such births as well as distinguish between those who eventually have such a child and those who do not (see Berinde, 1999; Corman, 2001 on third births in Sweden).

Our demographic control variables include *age of woman* in three-year age groups from 19-21 to 40-42 years, *age difference between parents*, and *time since previous birth*, that is, age of the youngest child. We also control for *calendar year period* with two-year groups from 1988-89 to 1998-99. The estimates of these control variables are not presented in this article but are available in Duvander and Andersson (2004). As both continued childbearing and parents' use of parental leave are influenced by human capital and economic resources, we present models with and without controlling for the earned income of the couple and for parents' educational attainment. The *couple income*, recalculated at the price level of 1995, is categorized into low level of annual earnings (0-250,000 Swedish kronor),[2] medium earnings, (250-400,000 Swedish kronor), high earnings (400-550,000 Swedish kronor), and top earnings (more than 550,000 Swedish kronor). We include the *educational level* of both father and mother, for which information is updated every year and categorized into primary, secondary, and higher education.

Our primary independent variables are father's and mother's uptake of parental leave benefits. As patterns in parental leave use differ between men and women, we have categorized the variables for fathers and mothers differently. *Father's use of parental leave* is categorized into (a) no leave benefit, (b) leave benefit amounting to up to 3% of the earned income during the two years following childbirth, (c) leave benefit equivalent to 3-10% of his income, (d) leave benefit equivalent to 11-25% of his earned income, and (e) benefit equivalent to more than a quarter of that income. A situation where the father has received less than 3% of his earned income from the parental leave insurance means that he probably only has used the so called "daddy days." These days are taken in immediate connection to the birth and do not imply a situation where the father is at home with the child on his own. More extensive uptake of parental leave is more likely to refer to situations where the father stays at home as the primary caregiver of the child.

Mother's use of parental leave is categorized into (a) leave benefit equivalent to less than 25% of her earned income during the two years following childbirth, (b) leave benefit equivalent to 25-50% of that income, (c) leave benefit equivalent to 51-75% of her earned income, and (d) more than 75% of the earned income being an income replacement from the parental leave system. The latter category is likely to reflect a situation where a mother only shortly (or not at all) returned to work during the two-year period immediately following childbirth.

Table 2 describes our study population of one- and two-child parents by providing the distributions of exposure time to the risk of a second and a third birth, respectively, over the various categories of father's and mother's uptake of parental leave, couple income, and educational attainment. Patterns are very similar for the two birth orders. Slightly more than a tenth of fathers used no leave at all. The largest categories are those of fathers who received less than 3 or 3-10% of their income from the parental leave insurance. Only 3-4% of fathers fall into the category where more than a quarter of their income came from such benefits. The category of mothers where less than a quarter of the earned income came from the parental leave insurance is equally small. Only 4-5% of mothers fall into that category. The categories where up to half and up to three quarters of the income came from parental leave benefits are the most common for mothers. The exposures corresponding to the highest dependence on the parental leave insurance, where more than three quarters of earnings were of that character, comprise only 14-15% of Swedish mothers' after-birth periods.

TABLE 2. Characteristics of Study Populations of One- and Two-Child Parents in Sweden: Exposures of Risk to a Second and a Third Birth. Fractions of Couple Months for Each Variable (Percentages)

Variable	One-Child Parents	Two-Child Parents
Father's Uptake of Parental Leave During the First/Second Child's First Two Years		
No Leave Benefit	13.8	11.7
Less than 3% of Earned Income	38.6	39.6
3-10% of Earnings	31.0	33.2
11-25% of Earnings	12.7	12.6
More than 25% of Earnings	3.9	2.9
Mother's Uptake of Parental Leave During the First/Second Child's First Two Years		
Less than 25% of Earned Income	5.0	3.9
25-50% of Earnings	40.1	40.3
51-75% of Earnings	40.7	40.8
More than 75% of Earnings	14.1	15.0
Couple Earnings		
Low	24.2	20.3
Medium	55.4	63.7
High	16.4	13.2
Top	4.1	2.8
Woman's Educational Level		
Primary	12.6	11.2
Secondary	59.9	58.5
Higher	27.5	30.3
Man's Educational Level		
Primary	19.4	18.8
Secondary	55.5	52.8
Higher	25.1	28.3

RESULTS

The results of our models are presented in Tables 3a and 3b. The estimates are expressed in terms of relative risks for the various categories of our variables. A risk value greater than one indicates that the propensity to have another child is higher than for parents of the reference category of the same variable; a risk value lower than one indicates a reduced risk of having another child when the effects of the other covariates of the model are held constant.

The models on second births (Table 3a) reveal a positive impact of father's uptake of parental leave on that parity progression. Couples where the father takes parental leave have considerably higher second-birth intensities than couples where the father takes no leave at all, and second-birth risks increase with an increasing level of paternal parental leave use. However, for the small category of one-child couples where the father took very extensive leave, there is reduced second-birth intensity. The basic relationship between father's parental leave use and second birth is relatively unaffected by the control for socio-economic variables.

The relationship between mother's parental leave use and second births is also not so strongly affected by the controls for couple income and educational characteristics. Second-birth risks are highest for the most common categories of couples where the woman has received between one and three quarters of her earnings from the parental leave system. Very low and very high levels of maternal uptake of leave are related to a reduced risk of second birth. It is thus the normative pattern of behavior that is related to the highest second-birth risk. The extreme users, be they men or women, have the lowest risks of having a second child.

Table 3b indicates that couples where the father took a relatively large amount of parental leave had the highest third-birth fertility. Such couples have about 10% higher third-birth fertility than other couples (Model 1b). However, in this case the relationship is strongly affected by the control for parents' educational characteristics and couple income. Educational groups with high third-birth risks, i.e., mothers and fathers with high educational levels,[3] are over-represented in the group where fathers take extended leave. With the control for educational characteristics, the positive effect of paternal leave use on third-birth risks vanishes (Model 3b). The control for couple income has the opposite effect, and when both types of socio-economic variables are included in the model, we find a weak but still clearly positive impact of father's uptake of parental leave, except for the small category where he received more than a quarter of his income from the parental leave system (Model 4b).

For third births, the impact of the mother's use of parental leave is quite the opposite of what we found for second births. There is a J-shaped pattern in the relationship between mother's leave use after the

TABLE 3a. Relative Risk of a Second Birth of Swedish Couples with One Common Child, by Parents' Parental Leave Use and Socio-Economic Characteristics, Standardized for Mother's Age, Age Difference Between Parents, Time Since First Birth, and Calendar Year

Variable	Model 1a	Model 2a	Model 3a	Model 4a
Father's Uptake of Parental Leave During First Child's First Two Years				
No Leave Benefit	1	1	1	1
Less than 3% of Earned Income	1.16	1.13	1.16	1.13
3-10% of Earnings	1.23	1.19	1.21	1.18
11-25% of Earnings	1.26	1.23	1.21	1.17
More than 25% of Earnings	0.93	0.97	0.90	0.94
Mother's Uptake of Parental Leave During First Child's First Two Years				
Less than 25% of Earned Income	0.91	0.89	0.84	0.84
25-50% of Earnings	1	1	1	1
51-75% of Earnings	1.04	1.05	1.05	1.06
More than 75% of Earnings	0.93	0.96	0.93	0.96
Couple Earnings				
Low		0.84		0.83
Medium		1		1
High		1.08		0.98
Top		1.26		1.05
Woman's Educational Level				
Primary			0.75	0.75
Secondary			1	1
Higher			1.23	1.23
Man's Educational Level				
Primary			0.89	0.89
Secondary			1	1
Higher			1.20	1.18

Note: Reference level of each variable given without decimals

TABLE 3b. Relative Risk of a Third Birth of Swedish Couples with Two Common Children, by Parents' Parental Leave Use and Socio-Economic Characteristics, Standardized for Mother's Age, Age Difference Between Parents, Time Since Second Birth, and Calendar Year

Variable	Model 1b	Model 2b	Model 3b	Model 4b
Father's Uptake of Parental Leave During Second Child's First Two Years				
No Leave Benefit	1	1	1	1
Less than 3% of Earned Income	1.01	1.06	0.99	1.04
3-10% of Earnings	1.04	1.10	1.00	1.07
11-25% of Earnings	1.13	1.18	1.02	1.07
More than 25% of Earnings	1.11	1.10	1.00	0.99
Mother's Uptake of Parental Leave During Second Child's First Two Years				
Less than 25% of Earned Income	1.11	1.08	1.06	1.03
25-50% of Earnings	1	1	1	1
51-75% of Earnings	1.11	1.10	1.10	1.09
More than 75% of Earnings	1.39	1.33	1.42	1.34
Couple Earnings				
Low		1.24		1.26
Medium		1		1
High		1.10		0.94
Top		1.42		1.10
Woman's Educational Level				
Primary			0.86	0.85
Secondary			1	1
Higher			1.54	1.55
Man's Educational Level				
Primary			0.94	0.92
Secondary			1	1
Higher			1.22	1.22

Note: Reference level of each variable given without decimals

second birth and third-birth fertility. Couples where the mother got more than three quarters of her income from leave benefits have by far the highest third-birth intensities; they are around a third higher than for other couples with two children. In many cases, such an extensive up-take is likely to reflect a situation where the mother never returned to the labor market as the couple was waiting for the arrival of a third child.

DISCUSSION

The purpose of this study was to examine how paternal participation in the parental leave after the birth of a child is related to the subsequent fertility of Swedish couples. This amounts to the study of the impact of individual use of an important family policy component on individual fertility. More specifically, we consider a father's involvement in pa-rental leave as one crucial aspect of the degree of gender equality in the parental couple. We expect a higher degree of such equality to be posi-tively correlated with couple fertility. Indeed, we find that father's up-take of parental leave is positively related to continued childbearing. Couples where the father took some leave have higher second- and third-birth propensities than couples where the father took no leave at all, and couples where the father took a leave corresponding to more than the one to two weeks of so called "daddy days" have higher fertility than couples where the father only took very brief leave. The positive relationship disappears, however, in the small group of couples where the father took really extensive leave, comprising 25% or more of his income for the period.

When interpreting these results, we have to be aware that present lev-els of paternal parental leave use in Sweden cannot really be taken as a reflection of true gender equality. Fathers still take only a fraction of all parental leave, and we regard the patterns we find as more indicative of positive effects of the father's commitment to share the responsibilities and joys of childrearing than of any true gender equity in the couple. In terms of policy effects, however, our results give some support for the possibility that active paternal involvement in a parental leave scheme like that in Sweden can be positively related to individual fertility.

Nevertheless, we need to be aware that the patterns we find cannot be taken as firm support for the existence of causal effects of parental leave use on couple fertility. Selection effects are likely to be at play where fa-thers who are more inclined to have further children also are more likely to take parental leave and have a higher propensity to have another child. Other underlying factors may affect both parental leave use and continued childbearing. The possibility of such an impact of unobserved characteristics also holds for the negative effect we found of father's very extensive parental leave use on couple childbearing. Couples where the father received an unusually large fraction of his income from the parental leave system commonly are low-income earners. The low income of these couples might mask some further characteristics that are negative for continued childbearing, such as non-qualification of the mother for a high level of parental leave benefit or the drop-out of the father from labor market activity.[4]

In our study, we could also demonstrate that one-child couples where the mother took an average amount of parental leave had the highest second-birth fertility. This is likely to indicate a connection between normative use of parental leave and the norm to have a second child. For two-child couples, we found a polarization in the relationship between mother's use of parental leave and third-birth propensities, with mothers with the most extensive leaves and those with the shortest leaves being the most likely to have a third child. This supports the notion of different pathways to a third child in Sweden, with higher third-birth fertility of mothers with strong as well as reduced attachment to the labor market (Berinde, 1999; Corman, 2001). The situation with an extended parental leave of the mother is likely to reflect a temporary withdrawal from labor market activity in anticipation of a third child. This pattern in behavior shows that third-birth fertility need not always be related to more egalitarian family dynamics.

CONCLUSION

We found some evidence that increased paternal involvement in childrearing indeed is positively related to continued childbearing, but we are careful in not claiming that our findings necessarily reflect the causal impact of gender-equal behavior on couple fertility. To address issues of possible endogeneity, that is when some common factors affect both the processes of parental leave use and childbearing, we would need to apply more sophisticated models where we also try to control for various selection effects. In addition, to study the effect of true gender equality on couple fertility would require that it is much more common that fathers take extensive periods of parental leave than what it is today. A development towards a more symmetrical division of parental leave will also put some pressure on Swedish mothers to give up a larger fraction of this generous benefit. Swedish fathers' share of parental leave use is increasing steadily and it is plausible that further increases will be connected to a more gender equal and child friendly Swedish society. These developments will call for continued research on the impact of leave taking on fertility.

NOTES

1. In the U.S., periods of parental leave are very brief and often unpaid. For an update of recent developments, see Han and Waldfogel (2003).

2. The value of one Swedish krona is approximately 11 Euro cents and 13 U.S. cents.

3. In studies on educational gradients in second- and third-birth risks it is common to find positive effects of educational attainment like we find here. People have spent much energy explaining, or explaining away the positive pattern for women, which contradicts common theory about education and fertility. Among procedures applied are sophisticated uses of the covariate "age at first birth" (see in particular B. Hoem, 1996) and arguments involving differential childbearing selectivity at different educational attainments (see, e.g., Hoem, Prskawetz, & Neyer, 2001; Kravdal, 2001; Kreyenfeld, 2002).

4. In general, childbearing of Swedish parents is more sensitive to weak labor market attachment of the mother than to weak attachment of the father. Weak paternal labor market performance can even be positively related to couple fertility (Andersson, Duvander, & Hank, 2005; Duvander & Andersson, 2003).

REFERENCES

Allison, P. (1984). *Event history analysis. Regression for longitudinal event data.* Sage University Paper 46. Series: Quantitative Applications in the Social Sciences. Newbury Park, CA: Sage Publications.

Andersson, G. (2000). The impact of labor-force participation on childbearing behavior: Pro-cyclical fertility in Sweden during the 1980s and the 1990s. *European Journal of Population, 16,* 293-333.

Andersson, G. (2004a). Childbearing developments in Denmark, Norway, and Sweden from the 1970s to the 1990s: A comparison. *Demographic Research Special Collection, 3,* 155-176. Available http://www.demographic-research.org.

Andersson, G. (2004b). Demographic trends in Sweden: An update of childbearing and nuptiality up to 2002. *Demographic Research, 11,* 95-110. Available http://www. demographic-research.org/Volumes/Vol11/4.

Andersson, G. (2005). A study on policies and practices in selected countries that encourage childbirth: the case of Sweden. Contribution to the "Consultancy Study on Population Related Matters–A Study on Policies and Practices in Selected Countries that Encourage Childbirth" for the Government of Hong Kong Special Administrative Region. MPIDR Working Paper 2005-05. Rostock, Germany: Max Planck Institute for Demographic Research.

Andersson, G., Duvander, A.-Z., & Hank, K. (2005). Erwerbsstatus und Familienentwicklung in Schweden aus paarbezogener Perspektive [Labor market status and continued childbearing of couples in Sweden]. In A. Tölke, & K. Hank (Ed.), *Männer–Das ‚vernachlässigte’ Geschlecht in der Familienforschung [Men–The neglected sex in family research]* [Sonderheft 4 der *Zeitschrift für Familienforschung*] (pp. 220-234). Wiesbaden, Germany: VS Verlag für Sozialwissenschaften.

Bekkengen, L. (2002). *Man får välja–om föräldraskap och föräldraledighet i arbetsliv och familjeliv [One has to choose–on parenthood and parental leave in work and family life]*. Malmö, Sweden: Liber.

Berinde, D. (1999). Pathways to a third child in Sweden. *European Journal of Population, 15*, 349-378.

Bernhardt, E. (1993). Fertility and employment. *European Sociological Review, 9*, 25-42.

Björnberg, U. (1998). Family orientation among men: A process of change in Sweden. In E. Drew, E. Emerek, E., & E. Mahon. (Ed.), *Women, work and the family in Europe* (pp. 200-207). London, U.K.: Routledge.

Blair, S. L. (1993). Employment, family, and perceptions of marital quality among husbands and wives. *Journal of Family Issues, 14*, 189-212.

Buber, I. (2002). The influence of the distribution of household and childrearing tasks between men and women on childbearing intentions in Austria. MPIDR Working Paper 2002-004. Rostock, Germany: Max Planck Institute for Demographic Research.

Bulanda, R. E. (2004). Paternal involvement with children: The influence of gender ideologies. *Journal of Marriage and Family, 66*, 40-45.

Bygren, M., & Duvander, A.-Z. (2005). Couples’ workplace situation and their division of the parental leave. Working Paper in Social Insurance 2005:2. Stockholm, Sweden: Swedish Social Insurance Agency.

Bygren, M., Gähler, M., & Nermo, M. (2004). Familj och arbete–Vardagsliv i förändring [Family and work–Everyday life in transition]. In M. Bygren, M. Gähler, & and M. Nermo, (Ed.), *Familj och arbete–Vardagsliv i förändring* (pp. 11-55). Stockholm, Sweden: SNS Förlag.

Corman, D. (2001). *Success at work and in family life: Studies in selected western fertility and family dynamics*. Demography Unit Dissertation Series 4. Stockholm, Sweden: Stockholm University.

Duvander, A.-Z., & Olsson, S. (2001). När har vi råd att skaffa barn? [When can we afford to have a child?] *RFV analyserar*, Rapport 2001:8. Stockholm, Sweden: National Social Insurance Board.

Duvander, A-Z., & Andersson, G. (2003). När har vi råd att skaffa fler barn? En studie om hur inkomst påverkar fortsatt barnafödande [When can we afford to have more children? A study on how income affects continued childbearing]. *RFV analyserar*, Rapport 2003:8. Stockholm, Sweden: National Social Insurance Board.

Duvander, A-Z., & Andersson, G. (2004). Leder delad föräldraledighet till fler barn? En studie om hur pappors och mammors föräldrapenninguttag påverkar benägenheten att skaffa ytterligare barn [Does shared parental leave lead to more children? A study on how fathers’ and mothers’ uptake of parental leave affects the propensity to have another child]. *RFV analyserar,* Rapport 2004:15. Stockholm, Sweden: National Social Insurance Board.

Ferrarini, T. (2003). *Parental leave institutions in eighteen post-war welfare states.* Swedish Institute for Social Research, Dissertation Series. Stockholm, Sweden: Stockholm University.

Glass, J., & Fujimoto, T. (1994). Housework, paid work, and depression among husbands and wives. *Journal of Health and Social Behavior, 35,* 179-191.

Haas, L. (1992). *Equal parenthood and social policy: A study of parental leave in Sweden.* Albany, NY: State University of New York Press.

Haas, L. (2003). Parental leave and gender equality: Lessons from the European Union. *Review of Policy Research, 20,* 89-114.

Haas, L., & Hwang, P. (1999). Parental leave in Sweden. In P. Moss, & Deven, F. (Ed.), *Parental leave: progress or pitfall?* (pp. 45-68). The Hague/Brussels, The Netherlands/Belgium: NIDI/CBGS Publications, Vol. 35.

Han, W.-J., & Waldfogel, J. (2003). Parental leave: The impact of recent legislation on parents leave taking. *Demography, 40,* 191-200.

Hoem, B. (1996). The social meaning of the age at second birth for third-birth fertility: A methodological note on the need to sometimes respecify an intermediate variable. *Yearbook of Population Research in Finland, 33,* 333-339.

Hoem, B. (2000). Entry into motherhood in Sweden: The influence of economic factors on the rise and fall in fertility, 1986-1997. *Demographic Research, 2.* Available http://www.demographic-research.org/Volumes/Vol2/4.

Hoem, B., & Hoem, J. M. (1996). Sweden's family policies and roller-coaster fertility. *Jinko Mondai Kenkyu [Journal of Population Problems], 52,* 1-22.

Hoem, J. M. (1990). Social policy and recent fertility change in Sweden. *Population and Development Review, 16,* 735-748.

Hoem, J. M. (1993). Public policy as the fuel of fertility: Effects of a policy reform on the pace of childbearing in Sweden in the 1980s. *Acta Sociologica, 36,* 19-31.

Hoem, J. M., Prskawetz, A., & Neyer, G. (2001). Autonomy or conservative adjustment? The effect of public policies and educational attainment on third births in Austria, 1975-96. *Population Studies, 55,* 249-261.

Hwang, C-P., & Lamb, M. E. (1997). Father involvement in Sweden: A longitudinal study of its stability and correlates. *International Journal of Behavioral Development, 21,* 621-632.

Hyde, J. S., Essex, M., & Horton, F. (1993). Fathers and parental leave: Attitudes and experiences. *Journal of Family Issues, 14,* 616-641.

Joshi, H. (1998). The opportunity costs of childbearing: More than mothers' business. *Journal of Population Economics, 11,* 161-183.

Kamerman, S. (2000). Parental leave policies: An essential ingredient in early childhood education and care policies. *Social Policy Report, 14,* 3-15.

Kaufman, G. (2000). Do gender role attitudes matter? Family formation and dissolution among traditional and egalitarian men and women. *Journal of Family Issues, 21,* 128-144.

Kravdal, Ø. (2001). The high fertility of college educated women in Norway: An artifact of the separate modelling of each parity transition. *Demographic Research, 5,* 187-216. Available http://www.demographic-research.org/Volumes/Vol5/6.

Kreyenfeld, M. (2002). Time-squeeze, partner effect or self-selection? An investigation into the positive effect of women's education on second birth risks in West Germany. *Demographic Research, 7,* 15-47. Available http://www.demographic-research.org/Volumes/vol7/2.

McDonald, P. (2000a). Gender equity, social institutions and the future of fertility. *Journal of Population Research, 17,* 1-16.

McDonald, P. (2000b). Gender equity in theories of fertility transition. *Population and Development Review, 26,* 427-439.

Mencarini, L., & Tanturri, M. L. (2004). Time use, family role-set and childbearing among Italian working women. *Genus LX* (1): 111-137.

Ministry of Health and Social Affairs. (2001). *Barnafödande i fokus: Från befolkningspolitik till ett barnvänligt samhälle [Childbearing in focus: From population policy to a child friendly society].* Ministry Publications Series Ds 2001, 57. Stockholm, Sweden: Fritzes.

Moss, P., & Deven, F. (1999). *Parental leave: Progress or pitfall?* The Hague/ Brussels, The Netherlands/Belgium: NIDI/CBGS Publications, Vol. 35.

Näsman, E. (1992). Parental leave in Sweden–a workplace issue? Stockholm Research Reports in Demography 73. Stockholm, Sweden: Stockholm University.

Nyman, H., & Pettersson, J. (2002). Spelade pappamånaden någon roll? [Did the daddy month have any impact?] *RFV analyserar,* Rapport 2002:14. Stockholm, Sweden: National Social Insurance Board.

Oláh, L. Sz. (2001). Gender and family stability: Dissolution of the first parental union in Sweden and Hungary. *Demographic Research, 4,* 27-96. Available http://www. demographic-research.org/Volumes/Vol4/2/.

Oláh, L. Sz. (2003). Gendering fertility: Second births in Sweden and Hungary. *Population Research and Policy Review, 22,* 171-200.

Rønsen, M. (2004). Fertility and family policy in Norway–A reflection on trends and possible connections. *Demographic Research, 10,* 266-286. Available http://www. demographic-research.org/Volumes/Vo10/10/.

Rostgaard, T. (2002). Setting time aside for the father: Father's leave in Scandinavia. *Community, Work & Family, 5,* 343-364.

Statens Offentliga Utredningar. (1972). *Familjestöd [Family support].* Rapport 1972:34. Stockholm, Sweden: Regeringskansliet.

Sundström, M., & Duvander, A.-Z. (2002). Gender division of childcare and the sharing of parental leave among new parents in Sweden. *European Sociological Review, 18,* 433-447.

Sundström, M., & Stafford, F. (1992). Female labour force participation, fertility and public policy in Sweden. *European Journal of Population, 8,* 199-215.

Thomson, E. (1997). Couple childbearing desires, intentions, and births. *Demography, 34,* 343-354.

Thomson, E., & Hoem, J. M. (1998). Couple childbearing plans and births in Sweden. *Demography, 35,* 315-322.

Social Policy for Family Caregivers of Elderly: A Canadian, Japanese, and Australian Comparison

Carol D. H. Harvey
Satomi Yoshino

SUMMARY. Elders in Canada, Japan and Australia are an increasing proportion of the population. This research focused on (1) the expected familial roles for care provision of frail elderly and (2) the relationship of expected familial roles to social policy toward elder care. Using a case study method, analysis of government documents such as annual reports, white papers, and Web sites was undertaken. Results show that elders in Australia and Canada desire independence from offspring, whereas filial responsibility for elders in Japan is a cultural ideal. In all three countries, societal expectations fit the current federal governmen-

Carol D. H. Harvey is affiliated with the Department of Family Social Sciences, University of Manitoba, Winnipeg, Manitoba, Canada R3T 2N2 (E-mail: charvey@ cc.umanitoba.ca). Satomi Yoshino is affiliated with the Department of Human Ecology, University of Alberta, Edmonton, Canada AB T6G2N1.

Earlier versions of this research were presented at the XXIII Congress of the International Federation for Home Economics, Kyoto, Japan, August 2004, and the Social Development and Family Changes Seminar, sponsored by the Committee on Family Research, International Sociological Association and the research group FLACSO, Mexico City, March 2005.

[Haworth co-indexing entry note]: "Social Policy for Family Caregivers of Elderly: A Canadian, Japanese, and Australian Comparison." Harvey, Carol D. H., and Satomi Yoshino. Co-published simultaneously in *Marriage & Family Review* (The Haworth Press, Inc.) Vol. 39, No. 1/2, 2006, pp. 143-158; and: *Families and Social Policy: National and International Perspectives* (ed: Linda Haas, and Steven K. Wisensale) The Haworth Press, Inc., 2006, pp. 143-158. Single or multiple copies of this article are available for a fee from The Haworth Document Delivery Service [1-800-HAWORTH, 9:00 a.m. - 5:00 p.m. (EST). E-mail address: docdelivery@haworthpress.com].

tal policies of shifting the burden of care to families, but families in need find limited societal assistance. *[Article copies available for a fee from The Haworth Document Delivery Service: 1-800-HAWORTH. E-mail address: <docdelivery@haworthpress.com> Website: <http://www.HaworthPress. com> © 2006 by The Haworth Press, Inc. All rights reserved.]*

KEYWORDS. Australia, Canada, elderly, family caregivers, social policy

Elders in Canada, Japan and Australia, like in other industrialized countries, are increasing in number and in population proportion, and yet relatively little has been done to examine national social policies that can help families assist their frail members. Cross-cultural comparisons can bring insight into policy analysis, and this case study of carer policy in three countries is designed to show points of similarity and contrast. Comparative analysis can show what future policy directions are needed. By knowing what policies are being implemented, practitioners can help families with their important roles as carers of frail elderly and can become advocates for alternative services and funding.

These three countries were chosen for a number of reasons. They are alike as they are all experiencing rapid population aging, about which people are concerned (Cabinet Office, 2003; Keating, Fast, Frederick, Cranswick & Perrier, 1999; Weston, Qu & Soriano, 2003); they are all industrialized, have highly educated citizens, and are highly urbanized. They are dissimilar in that Canada and Australia have small populations which are geographically dispersed, whereas Japan is densely populated. Canada and Australia have ethnically diverse populations, with a large proportion of immigrants, whereas Japan is culturally and racially more homogeneous. The countries are also different in the values held by elderly people and their offspring as to the roles and responsibilities of families toward care of frail elders. The three countries, therefore, provide points of comparison and contrast, both in attitudes toward family care of elders and in social policy to meet the challenges of population aging.

ELDERLY POPULATIONS IN CANADA, JAPAN AND AUSTRALIA

In Canada, Japan and Australia the number and proportion of the population age 60 and older is increasing rapidly. In 1921 in Canada, only 5% of the population was over 65 years of age; corresponding figures for 1971 and 2001 were 8% and 13% (Statistics Canada, 2001). The United Nations shows that 17% of Canadians were over age 60 in 2002; by 2050, that figure is projected to be 30% (United Nations, 2002). The fastest growing segment of the elderly group is aged 85 and over; centurions are also increasing in number.

In Japan one in every six Japanese was over 65 years of age in 2000; by the year 2050 one in every three Japanese is expected to be elderly (Ministry of Health, Labour & Welfare, 2002). The United Nations reports elders in Japan age 60 and above were 24% of the population in 2005, and projected to be 42% in 2050 (United Nations, 2002).

Australia has a falling birth rate and an increased life expectancy (Weston et al., 2003). The median age of Australians increased in the 10-year period from 1988 to 1998 by 3 years, from 31.6 to 34.6, and the median is anticipated to be 44.1 in 2051 (McCormack, 2000). Of Australia's 19 million inhabitants, 12% are age 65 or older, and that proportion is expected to double by 2051 (McCormack, 2000). For elders age 60 and over, who constituted 17% of Australia's population in 2005, projections are that the figure will rise to 28% in 2050 (United Nations, 2002). Like Canadian elderly, the Australian elders are diverse, with a third born abroad, and half of the foreign-born coming from non-English speaking countries (McCormack, 2000; Weston et al., 2003). Although the numbers of elderly in Australia is increasing, the proportion of the elderly population that is classified as poor is decreasing. McCormack (2000) estimates 3.6% of Australian women and 2.4% of men over 65 are poor; the reason for the decrease, he says, is "the increase in non-cash benefits of the social wage" (p. 624).

Many researchers and politicians alike in all three countries view these population trends with alarm. Some are worried about the increasing costs to sustain an elderly population, when the dependency ratio is climbing and the number of workers to support the old is shrinking (Weston et al., 2003). As Canada and Australia have increased transfer payments to elderly recipients, the relative wealth of the elderly has increased, and thus Ozanne (1996) notes some Australians think that elders can afford their own care, particularly when other groups like children are at economic risk. At the same time, women, the traditional carers, have increasingly less time available with work and family responsibilities. Finally, the electoral mood in both Canada and Australia stresses independence and self-reliance (Ozanne, 1996). In Japan, where traditional values have emphasized that elder care should be provided within families, particularly by daughters-in-law, family changes, such as decreasing multigenerational residency patterns, have made that goal more difficult to reach (Hirayama & Mizaki, 1996; Maeda & Nakatani, 1992).

The definition of who is an informal "carer" is not clear in all studies across all countries. A general operational definition is "a person who provides personal services, transportation, or advice to another for 10 hours per week or more" (Personal communication, Australian Institute for Family Studies research staff, March, 2004). The carer, according to this definition, can be a friend, neighbor or family member, and the care recipient can be of any age. In this research we use the term "family carer" to mean someone providing service, generally without remuneration, to another person related by kinship, and the "care recipient" to mean a relative over the age of 65. Such family carers are most commonly spouses or offspring, particularly daughters or daughters-in-law. Social policies offered by the national governments in all three countries were scanned, with an eye to ascertaining which policies assist families in their roles caring for frail elderly members.

Current carer policy in all countries arises from the social context, and it is important to first examine how Canadians, Japanese and Australians have cared for elders in the past 50 years or so. Second, current policies will be presented and analyzed. Finally, comparison and contrast among Canada, Japan and Australia will be made.

METHODOLOGY

A case study method was used here. It is a way of examining "a contemporary phenomenon within its real-life context" (Yin, 1989, p. 23) and is appropriate when the investigator has little or no control over questions being asked. By intensely exploring a single example, in this case supports for caregivers of frail elderly family members, and comparing three country examples within the case we were able to understand policy details (Rothe, 2000).

National social policy in Canada, Japan and Australia was examined by reviewing research reports and policy documents. Reports and legislation at the national level were deemed most important, since they cover all families in the respective countries. Since Canada and Australia have a number of local or state/provincial differences, delving into local differences is beyond the scope of a single article and therefore local policies are omitted. We used annual reports of governments and lobby groups, postings on governmental Web sites, and legislation. To present the findings we used a classification system by Chambers

(1993), focusing on goals and objectives, forms of benefits or services delivered, entitlement rules, and financing method.

HISTORY OF ELDER CARE

Canada

Prior to the 1920s Canadians felt people should prepare themselves for old age, and, if frail, families should be responsible for elder care (Novak, 1997). As urbanization and industrialization occurred, family ties weakened, and family responsibility toward elders waned (Novak, 1997). However, most of Canada's elder care is still done by families, in conjunction with programs and facilities paid with public monies. To assist elders and others a universal health care system was established in the 1960s, designed to assist acute cases. Residential care facilities were also built to help chronically ill elders. Old Age Assistance and Guaranteed Income Supplement policies also were developed to support financial independence of the elderly (Novak, 1997).

Recent demographic trends in society and governments' deficits of health care funding increased attention paid to community-based services. Home care of the elderly developed as a way to keep people in their homes, which they desire, and as a way to reduce long-term care costs (Organization for Economic Co-operation and Development, 1996). These home care services vary from one province to another in terms of services provided and funding sources. Canada's spending on home care has been increasing, particularly on subacute care, while provinces have been trying to cut hospital and long-term care costs. Informal caregivers, largely family members, provide the most care of frail elderly (Harlton, Keating & Fast, 1998).

Japan

After World War II the General Headquarters of the Supreme Commander of the Allied Forces (GHQ) directed and supervised Japanese social policies for several years (Adachi, 2000). Social security changes instituted by the GHQ included promotion of social welfare and security, as well as public health (Ministry of Health & Welfare, 1996). Services for elderly Japanese were developed, including health, education and recreation, modeled after public services of Western Europe and

North America (Maeda, 2000). Japan established national pension plans and health care system in 1961 (Maeda, 2000).

However, prior to the 1960s, responsibility for elder care was entirely on families, and there was no public support system for families providing elder care in Japan. In 1963, the Law of Welfare of the Elderly (LWE) was enacted, which became the foundation for supporting elder people in Japan. From the 1960s the government created several programs to support family caregiving at home, but in-home nursing services took a long time to develop (Maeda & Shimizu, 1991).

By the 1980s a large number of frail elders in Japan were cared for in hospitals, since sons and daughters-in-law were increasingly living apart from elders and could not always care for them. In the 1980s and 1990s Japan began a shift from hospital institutional care of frail elders back to care at home, in order to support people in familiar circumstances and to reduce the government's health care expenditures (Ministry of Health & Welfare, 1996). The government of the time wanted to control costs, and shifting more care back to families could do exactly that. Policy makers realized the necessity of improving home care services in order to support family caregiving at home and gain the support of the Japanese population for the shift away from costly hospitalization. The national government introduced the Gold Plan in 1989, and the establishment of the Long-term Care Insurance (LTCI) was set as the main objective (Ministry of Health, Labour & Welfare, 2002).

Australia

From the Colonial period to World War I Australians viewed elderly people as poor (Ozanne, 1996). Outside families, most assistance to frail elderly came from religious or charity groups, with limited roles of federal and local governments (Ozanne, 1996). By the 1920s Australia established basic public health services and pensions. Some housing programs, which were means tested, were also established.

After World War II aged persons were seen as "a social problem worthy of state public policy focus" (Ozanne, 1996, p. 191). Most of the money spent was for nursing care in residential facilities. There were also a number of state and charity programs for elderly people, and these were done in what Ozanne calls "a fairly patchwork ad hoc manner" (p. 191).

By the 1980s Australia had established both Federal and State Ministries for the Aged, and public perception of the health of aged members of society increased (Ozanne, 1996). In 1983 Australian governmental aged policy shifted from residential to community care (Howe, 2001), bringing regulation of residential facilities and introduction of assessment teams to evaluate potential residents. New home care services were established (Ozanne, 1996), and people were encouraged to stay in their own homes as long as possible.

In 1985 Australia established the Home and Community Care (HACC) Programme which was designed to support people at home, shift public expenditures from institutional to community care, and assist carers with "respite care, information, advice and support" (Jenson & Jacobzone, 2000). Funded with a split between federal (60%) and state governments (40%) the HACC program is still supported (Jenson & Jacobzone, 2000).

CURRENT AGED CARE POLICIES

An overview of the policies studied in this research is shown in Table 1. A country-by-country comparison is made, together with a description of the policies and their intended recipients.

Philosophy

Public policies on elder care in Japan have been significantly influenced by the cultural belief that elder care should be provided by family members (Kiefer, 1987; Maeda & Shimizu, 1991). As a result of this belief, the development of both nursing homes and home care services for elderly people was significantly delayed. Traditionally, the Japanese view of the aged is one of respect and admiration (Cinelli, McConatha & McConatha, 1991). This cultural view came from "the indigenous culture of Asian society, particularly respect for age and filial piety derived from Confucian ethics, which originated in China" (Kamo, 1988, pp. 300, 301). Additionally, the Japanese dislike asking for outside help on family issues because traditionally it is considered to be shameful to expose family problems to strangers (Hirayama & Miyazaki, 1996). Even today, a strong belief remains that families should provide care for their elderly members. Unlike both Canada and Australia, where independence and autonomy are considered to be very important, it is considered to be normal for elderly Japanese to be dependent on their offspring once they become frail (Hirayama & Miyazaki, 1996; Kamo, 1988).

In contrast to Japan, Canadians value independence and individualism in old age. This freedom is protected by law and reinforced by so-

TABLE 1. Overview of Social Policy and Current Programs, by Country

	Canada	Japan	Australia
Philosophy	Shift from institutional to community based care. Individual automomy and independence valued.	Family support of frail elders is a cultural ideal, and policy is designed to supplement it.	Policy designed to "enhance the well being of older people" via independence, health, care and support (McCormack, 2000).
Caregiver leave	Caregiver Leave: Compassionate Care Benefits through Employment Insurance and job protection through Canadian Labour Code for work absence for caregiving (began in January, 2004).	Long-term care and home care are covered by a federal program, Long Term Care Insurance (LTCI). –Caregiver Leave: Started in 1999, 40% of usual salary through EI. Available to a limited number of people (Ministry of Health, Labour, and Welfare, 2004).	1985: Home and Community Care established (Jenson & Jacobzone, 2000). 60% federal and 40% state funding. Still in effect. –"Pyramid" structure of formal care (Howe, 2001).
Caregiver support	Caregiver Support: indirect and direct financial compensation available to qualified recipients (Keefe & Fancey, 1998).	Caregiver Support: Indirect and direct financial compensation available to qualified recipients.	Carers Package (Keefe, 2004).

cial policies (Wengner, 1991). Although family members in Canada rely on one another, many of the decisions of elders are influenced by the values of independence and individualism (Wenger, 1991). Similar to Canada, Plath (2002) cites research showing that "independence is strongly held by older Australians" (p. 40).

Policies in Canada

Family care is emphasized in government reports, as well as in studies of Canadian elderly. Most care of frail elderly is by family members, although friends have some limited involvement; hence, the term "informal care" is used to indicate people outside the formal care providers who help frail elders (Keating, 2001; Romanow, 2002). Canadian caregivers are primarily between the ages of 30 and 59; 18% of women and 27% of men aged 60 and over are carers (Keating et al., 1999).

A shift in emphasis in the health system from institutional to community-based care has had implications for informal carers. Not only is de-institutionalization occurring, but also early discharge and short hospital stays have increased the demand for home care, which in turn has shifted the responsibility toward informal caregivers, who provide 85 to 90% of home care (Romanow, 2002). Family caregivers save the health system over $5 billion (Canadian) per year; they also provide services equivalent to 276,000 full-time employees (Family Caregivers Association of Nova Scotia, 2002).

By January 2004 the federal government instituted Compassionate Care Benefits to provide support to a "family member who is seriously ill with a significant risk of death" (Liberal Task Force on Seniors, 2004, p. 14). In order to be eligible carers have to have (1) more than a 40% decrease in weekly earnings due to caregiving responsibilities and (2) at least 600 hours of Employment Insurance (EI) insured hours in the last year. Beneficiaries can get up to 55% of their usual earnings through EI to a maximum of six weeks. This legislation will not cover carers of care recipients who have long-term disabilities and are not in imminent danger of death. Due to stringent eligibility requirements recipients are fewer than anticipated (Picard, 2005). Rather than the 270,000 recipients Human Resources Canada expected in the year following the enactment of the legislation, fewer than 5,000 Canadians received benefits in 2004. The 2005 budget for the program is the same dollar amount as the 2004 expenditures, suggesting stringent eligibility requirements will stay in place (Picard, 2005).

The federal government also provides tax benefits for caregivers (Finance Canada, 2004). Like all tax benefits the carer has to earn sufficient income to make the benefit apply. Family members who give at-home care can reduce federal tax up to $605 (Finance Canada, 2004). In the area of long-term and home care, provincial and territorial variation occurs. There is no national standard for either long-term care or home care (Health Canada, 1999). Services generally include personal care, nursing, and home making services, but payments to service providers vary and may include a mix of public and private sector workers (Health Canada, 1999). As mentioned earlier, so many local policies exist in this area that they are outside the scope of this article; instead, we are concentrating on national policies.

Policies in Japan

Because families' abilities to provide care for their frail elderly members have been declining, the major concern of the government in recent years has been how to maintain the tradition of family care. The government launched Long Term Care Insurance (LTCI) in 2000 to support family caregivers to stay in the elder care system, and the LTCI continued to be expanded in order to provide support toward family caregivers who are facing ever increasing demands from their frail elderly family members (Cabinet Office, 2003).

Long term and home care services are the responsibility of the national Japanese government (OECD, 1996). LTCI in Japan has three objectives, including restructuring previous care systems into an integrated health, medical and welfare system, launching a system understandable for users, and facilitating financial responsibility for elder care among members of society (Ministry of Health, Labour & Welfare, 2002). After screening judgments are made, eligible Japanese are provided services by municipalities and benefits are based on level of need (Ministry of Health, Labour & Welfare, 2002). Co-payment by recipients is necessary, including a 10% user fee, although the fees can be waived in the case of poverty. Given the traditional Japanese feeling that families should care for frail elders, the LTCI was a step forward; however, whether families receive enough care is questionable due to the requirement for government assessment tests.

The LTCI theoretically made a great contribution to expand governmental support to family caregivers. The LTCI not only gave families alternatives to provide care for their frail family members by supplying formal services, but it also made financial services available to them in the form of insurance. However, because the amount of service covered by the insurance is decided by governmental assessment, whether or not families are satisfied with services they receive is inconclusive (Arai & Kumamoto, 2004; Sodei, 2004).

Caregiver leave is also available in Japan, starting in 1999 (Ministry of Health, Labour & Welfare, 2004). Caregivers who are working may have three months leave (six months for public workers), in which return to their jobs is guaranteed after the leave is completed. Employment Insurance provides 40% of the usual salary of the worker while on leave (Ministry of Health, Labour & Welfare, 2004). Since this leave is available to a limited number of people and one's income while on leave is lowered, it does not provide widespread public assistance to family caregivers.

Additionally, caregiver support is available in Japan. Tax credits provide indirect financial benefits to those who qualify, and various amounts of payments, which are determined by the condition of care receiver, to family caregivers are available (Ministry of Health, Labour & Welfare, 2000).

Policies in Australia

The Australian federal government's strategy for "enhancing the well-being of older people" (McCormack, 2000, p. 629) has a four-fold theme, emphasizing independence, health, care, and support. This policy is in keeping with the conservative government in power, which stresses individualism, a decreased role for the state, and an increased role for private enterprise. The independence part of the policy suggests that "older people should make greater efforts to be financially responsible for themselves in old age" (McCormack, 2000, p. 629), despite the fact that the OECD estimates Australia spends proportionately less on elder care than other industrialized countries analyzed (Jenson & Jacobzone, 2000).

The value of independence, cited by Plath (2002), means different things to different people: It may in fact signal the public's worry about older people draining the public purse. Castles (2000) argues this concern is a "moral panic" (p. 301), which is unfounded. Castles states Australia already spends less per capita on older people than other OECD nations, and any increases in transfer payments are expensive because they are funded by public borrowing rather than tax increases. Borrowing at high interest rates means the financing costs of transfer payment increases are burdensome for the public, not the increases themselves.

One could visualize Australia's policy toward care of elders as a pyramid, Howe (2001) argues. At the bottom of the pyramid are large numbers of independent elderly, living in the community and receiving services mainly from family and friends and with little additional support from the Home and Community Care Program (HACC). In the middle are more programs of support, with fewer recipients, who require more care of family members as well. At the top are the relatively few people in high cost residential care (Howe, 2001).

With the current emphasis on cost reduction and the push for independence and individual responsibility for aging, Ozanne (2000) argues that younger, more disabled and more dependent recipients are being neglected in favor of the larger numbers of the relatively well and financial stable elderly population.

The Australian Bureau of Statistics (ABS) defines carers as persons who provide regular and sustained informal assistance to a family member or friend without remuneration (Creelman, 2002). Primary carers are defined as those who provide more inclusive services and are likely to continue to do so for another six months. Based on those definitions the ABS suggested in 1998 carers numbered 2.3 million. About 2% of these provided primary care, the largest group of whom were providing for a spouse or partner. Women make up 70% of primary carers, and over one in five are age 65 or older (Creelman, 2002).

COMPARISON AND CONTRAST AMONG CANADIAN, JAPANESE AND AUSTRALIAN POLICIES

The proportion of elderly is rising in all three countries. Canada, Japan and Australia have public health and publicly funded pension systems; only in Japan has the pension system recently been revised to reflect changes in both the economy and the number of elderly people who receive pensions now and in the immediate future. Public health involves co-pay in Australia and Japan, while public health issues dominate Canadian politicians and policy makers, including various proposals to reduce waiting time and keep the system publicly financed.

All three countries have recently introduced legislation for financial compensation to carers of frail family members. The earliest entry into this area was Australia in the mid 1980s; Japan provides limited financial support only for low-income caregivers; Canada has introduced financial support only if the care recipient is within six months of death. In all three countries carer coverage is limited by small payments to carers and by strict eligibility requirements. If carers of frail elderly are old themselves, financial compensation tied to earnings are not applicable.

It appears that the shift from institutional to community care of frail elders has meant that family members are responsible, despite the fact that some families are ill-equipped to provide care. If a spouse is doing the care, he or she may also be elderly and frail. In all three countries advocates for families need to watch the level of funding available, the wait times, and the eligibility criteria; only legislation that covers more carers, with short wait times and sufficient funds will make a difference to families. In Australia, the situation has been to enact the legislation for carers and then make eligibility so restrictive and funding so low that its effect is not significant.

In the area of home care we see that the Japanese public definitely wants more government involvement. The proposed national legislation in Canada for home care is needed; again, it is important to ensure that its provisions are broad enough to be of real assistance to familial caregivers, particularly elderly (and possibly frail) spouses. As the Brotherhood of St. Laurence (2003) cautions in Australia, making eligibility requirements restrictive and forcing people to admit dependency may chase potential clients from the programs designed to help them.

LIMITATIONS AND IMPLICATIONS

This case study was limited to information provided in official documents and research reports. We do not have data available to evaluate adequacy of coverage nor public perceptions of policies. The LTCI in Japan is under review in 2005, but the data on that review are not available at this writing.

Official documents and research reports, used here, are in the public domain. We have an audit trail that other scholars may use, in the form of this article and its bibliography, as well as an earlier one (Harvey & Yoshino, 2004), and research extensions to other countries is needed. Future research that assesses public opinion is needed also. It is important for future research to ascertain the quality of services that are available and investigate the gaps in services from the viewpoint of family caregivers, as has been done in the United States by Silverstein and Parrott (2001).

Finally, we think that practitioners may want to use our research, as they often act as opinion leaders in their communities. Informational forums could be held in which people advocate for help from all levels of government for family carers. Informed citizens can pressure politicians to act to supplement and aid the work of families in caring for frail elders.

REFERENCES

Adachi, K. (2000). The development of social welfare services in Japan. In S. O. Long (Ed.), *Caring for the elderly in Japan and the US* (pp. 191-205). London, UK: Routledge.

Arai, Y. & Kumamoto, K. (2004). Caregiver burden not 'worse' after new public long term care (LTC) insurance scheme took over in Japan. *International Journal of Geriatric Psychiatry, 19*, 1205-1206.

Brotherhood of St. Laurence (2003). In their own homes: Challenges of caring for low-income older Australians. *Brotherhood Comment*, November, 1-2.

Cabinet Office (2003). *Koureihakusyo.* [Public opinion poll on elder care.] Retrieved March 25, 2004, from http://www8.cao.go.jp/survey/h15/h15-kourei/images/zu06.gif

Castles, F. G. (2000). Population ageing and the public purse: Australia in comparative perspective. *Australian Journal of Social Issues, 35*, 301-315.

Chambers, D. E. (1993). *Social policy and social programs* (2nd ed.). Toronto, Canada: Maxwell Macmillan Canada.

Cinelli, B., McConatha, D. & McConatha, J. (1991). Japan's coming crisis: Problems for the Honorable Elders. *Journal of Applied Gerontology, 10*, 224-235.

Creelman, A. (2002). Carer policy in aged care: A structural interests perspective. In H. Gardner & S. Barraclough (Eds.), *Health and Social Policy in Australia,* 2nd ed. (pp. 275-293). Melbourne, Australia: Oxford University Press.

Family Caregivers Association of Nova Scotia (2001). *Recognition and support for family caregivers as an integral part of health care.* Retrieved February 4, 2004, from http://www.hc-sc.gc.ca/english/pdf/romanow/pdfs/Family%20Caregivers%20 Association%20of%20Nova%Scotia.pdf

Finance Canada (2002). Taxes. Retrieved March 3, 2004 from http://www.fin.gc. ca.fag/gag4c.html

Harlton, S. V., Keating, N. & Fast, J. (1998). Defining eldercare for policy and practices: Perspectives matter. *Family Relations, 47*, 281-289.

Harvey, C. D. H. & Yoshino, S. (2004). *Who helps families with caregiving of frail elders? Comparison of Canadian and Australian policy.* Presented at the annual conference of the Canadian Association for Research in Home Economics, Winnipeg, Manitoba, Canada, June 2.

Health Canada (1999). *Report on the national roundtable on home and community care.* Ottawa, Canada: Ministry of Public Works and Government Services Canada.

Hirayama, H. & Miyazaki, A. (1996). Implementing public policies and service in rural Japan: Issues and problems. *Journal of Aging and Social Policy, 8*, 133-146.

Howe, A. L. (2001). Recent developments in aged care policy in Australia. In Chi, I., Mehta, K. K. & Howe, A. L. (Eds.), *Long-term care in the 21st century: Perspectives from around the Asia-Pacific rim* (pp. 101-116). Binghamton, NY: The Haworth Press, Inc.

Jenson, J. & Jacobzone, S. (2000). *Care allowances for the frail elderly and their impact on women care-givers.* Paris, France: Organization for Economic Co-operation and Development, Labour Market and Social Policy Occasional Papers No. 41.

Kamo, Y. (1988). A note on elderly living arrangements in Japan and the United States. *Research on Aging, 10*, 297-305.

Keating, N. (2001). *Informal care networks of Canadian seniors with long-term health problems.* Retrieved February 4, 2004, from http://www.hc-sc.gc.ca/iacb-dgiac/ arad-draa/english/mdd/finalreport/ekeating.pdf

Keating, N., Fast, J., Frederick, J., Cranswick, K. & Perrier, C. (1999). *Eldercare in Canada: Context, content and consequences.* Ottawa, Canada: Minister of Industry.

Keefe, J. M. (2004). Policy profile for compensating family caregivers. Retrieved October 20, 2005, from http://www.msvu.ca/mdcaging/PDFs/Policy_Profile_ Australia_October_2004.pdf

Keefe, J. M. & Fancey, M. A. (1998). *Financial compensation versus community supports: An analysis of the effects on caregiving and care receivers.* Ottawa, Canada: Health Canada.

Kiefer, C. W. (1987). Care of the aged in Japan. In E. Norbeck & M. Lock (Eds.), *Health, illness and medical care in Japan* (pp. 89-109). Honolulu, HA: University of Hawaii.

Liberal Task Force Report for Seniors (2004). Retrieved on March 30, 2004, from www.liberal.parl.gc.ca/seniors

Maeda, D. (2000). The socioeconomic context of Japanese policy for aging. In S. O. Long (Ed.), *Caring for the elderly in Japan and the US* (pp. 28-51). London, UK: Routledge.

Maeda, D. & Nakatani, Y. (1992). Family care of the elderly in Japan. In J. Kosberg (Ed.), *Family care of the elderly* (pp. 196-209). Newbury Park, CA: Sage.

Maeda, D. & Shimizu, Y. (1991). Family support for elderly people in Japan. In H. L. Kending, A. Hashimoto & L. C. Coppard (Eds.), *Family support for the elderly* (pp. 235-249). Oxford, UK: Oxford University Press.

McCormack, J. (2000). Looking back and moving forward? Ageing in Australia 2000. *Ageing and Society, 20,* 623-631.

Ministry of Health and Welfare (1996). *Social security policies in Japan.* Retrieved July 25, 2002, from http://www.mhlw.go.jp/english/ssp_in_j/index.html

Ministry of Health, Labour & Welfare (2000). *Zenkoku Kousei Kankei Shiryo.* [National data on social welfare.] Retrieved April 4, 2004, from http://ww1.mhlw go.jp/topics/h12-kyoku_2/roujin-h/tp0119-1.html

Ministry of Health, Labour & Welfare (2002). *Long-term insurance in Japan.* Retrieved July 25, 2002, from http://www.mhlw.go.jp/English/topics/elderly/care/ 1.html

Ministry of Health, Labour & Welfare (2004). *Shyokugyou seikatu to kazaoku seikatu tono ryouritu no tameni.* [Balancing work and family life.] Retrieved April 2, 2004, from http://www.mhlw.go.jp/general/seido/koyou/ryouritu/index.html

Novak, M. W. (1997). *Aging and society: A Canadian perspective* (3rd ed.). Scarborough, ON: ITP Nelson.

Organization for Economic Co-operation and Development (1994). *The reform of health care systems: A review of seventeen OECD countries.* Health policy studies, no. 5. Paris: France: OECD.

Organization for Economic Co-operation and Development (1996). *Caring for frail elderly people: Policies in evolution* (OECD social policy studies; no. 19). Paris, France: Author.

Ozanne, E. (1996). Constructing and reconstructing old age: The evaluation of aged policy in Australia. In A. McMahon, J. Thomson, & C. Williams (Eds.), *Understanding the Australian welfare state: Key documents and themes* (pp. 185-198). Croydon, VI: Macmillan Education Australia.

Picard, A. (2005). Caregiver program lacks heart. *Globe and Mail,* September 29, p. A19.

Plath, D. (2002). Independence in old age: Shifting meanings in Australian social policy. *Just Policy, 26*, 40-47.

Romanow, R. J. (2002). *Commission on the future of health care in Canada: Final report.* Ottawa, Canada: Health Canada.

Rothe, J. P. (2000). *Understanding qualitative research.* Edmonton, AB: The University of Alberta Press.

Silverstein, M. & Parrott, T. M. (2001). Attitudes toward government policies that assist informal caregivers: The link between personal troubles and public issues. *Research on Aging, 23*, 349-374.

Sodei, T. (2004). Kaigohokenseidoka no kaigosa-bisuhyouka ni kansuru henk. [Changes in the evaluation of care services under the long-term care insurance]. *Kosei no shihyou [Journal of Health and Welfare Statistics]*, 51, 1-6.

Statistics Canada (2001). *Report on the demographic situation in Canada.* Ottawa, Canada: Statistics Canada. United Nations Population Information Network (2002). Population Division Wall Chart 2002. Retrieved October 24, 2005 from http://www.un.org/esa/socdev/ageing/resources.htm

Wenger, G. C. (1991). The major English-speaking countries. In H. L. Kending, A. Hashimoto, & L. C. Coppard (Eds.), *Family support for the elderly* (pp.117-137). Oxford, UK: Oxford University Press.

Weston, R., Qu, L. & Soriano, G. (2003). Australia's ageing yet diverse population. *Family Matters, 66* (Spring), 6-13. Melbourne, Australia: Australian Institute for Family Relations.

Yin, R. (1989). *Case study research: Design and methods.* Newbury Park, CA: Sage.

The Child and Dependent Care Tax Credit: A Policy Analysis

Nicole D. Forry

Elaine A. Anderson

SUMMARY. The Child and Dependent Care Tax Credit (CDCTC) is a federal program designed to facilitate the employment of persons with dependents. This article uses incremental theory as a framework for outlining the legislative process through which the CDCTC was developed and alterations the tax credit has endured from 1954 to the present. The effect of the CDCTC on families with diverse incomes is explored, revealing inequitable benefits favoring higher income families. Despite nominal targeting of this credit to low-income families, such families were found to rarely claim the credit. A discussion of barriers to and limitations of the credit for low-income families is provided and recommendations to improve the CDCTC are offered. *[Article copies available for a fee from The Haworth Document Delivery Service: 1-800-HAWORTH. E-mail address: <docdelivery@haworthpress.com> Website: <http://www.HaworthPress.com> © 2006 by The Haworth Press, Inc. All rights reserved.]*

Nicole D. Forry is a doctoral candidate in the Department of Family Studies, University of Maryland, 1204 Marie Mount Hall, College Park, MD 20742 (E-mail: forry@wam.umd.edu). Elaine A. Anderson is Professor in the Department of Family Studies, University of Maryland, 1203 Marie Mount Hall, College Park, MD 20742 (E-mail: eanders@umd.edu).

[Haworth co-indexing entry note]: "The Child and Dependent Care Tax Credit: A Policy Analysis." Forry, Nicole D., and Elaine A. Anderson. Co-published simultaneously in *Marriage & Family Review* (The Haworth Press, Inc.) Vol. 39, No. 1/2, 2006, pp. 159-176; and: *Families and Social Policy: National and International Perspectives* (ed: Linda Haas, and Steven K. Wisensale) The Haworth Press, Inc., 2006, pp. 159-176. Single or multiple copies of this article are available for a fee from The Haworth Document Delivery Service [1-800-HAWORTH, 9:00 a.m. - 5:00 p.m. (EST). E-mail address: docdelivery@haworthpress.com].

KEYWORDS. Child and Dependent Care Tax Credit, child care, dependent care, legislative process, policy

The dilemma of finding affordable, quality child care has been an issue of increasing concern since women entered the workforce during World War II. Prior to the 1940s there was little emphasis placed on public child care. Although there was some interest in enhancing children's development through nursery schools and providing child care services to low-income mothers who had difficulty caring for their own children, there was little question that child care was, for the most part, the responsibility of the mother (Cohen, 1996).

World War II altered American discourse regarding child care. As the available labor force in the United States dwindled due to the draft, the country's traditional view of women's place being in the home shifted and women were recruited to work outside the home, mostly in war-related industries. As both an incentive to work and in an effort to fill the gap left by women who were no longer home to care for their children, the United States provided temporary child care aid to mothers working in the defense industry through the Lanham Act of 1940 (Cohen, 1996). Much to the surprise of the nation's leaders, this trend of women entering the workforce did not immediately cease following the end of the war, nor did the demand for child care subside (Cohen, 1996). For a more complete review of the history of child care in the United States we refer the reader to the works of Berry (1993), Michel (1999) and Michel and Mahon (2002).

Due to the steady rise of women in the labor force, combined with the growth of single parenthood, child care remains an issue of national significance today. According to the U.S. Bureau of Labor Statistics (2004), among families with children under the age of six both parents worked in 53% of two-parent families, 64% of single mothers worked and 85% of single fathers worked. To address parental needs, various types of child care have emerged over the years. Examples include child care centers; family day care providers, or persons who provide care out of their homes; preschool programs such as Head Start and public or private nursery schools; kith or kin care; and self-care. There is also much variability in quality among child care providers of all types (Fuller, Kagan, Loeb, & Chang, 2004; Kontos, Howes, Shinn, & Galinsky, 1995). Most studies conclude that center-based care and preschool programs generally offer the best quality care as measured by provider qualifications, intensity of structured activities, and positive child outcomes (e.g., enhanced cognitive growth, strong social skills, and fewer behavior problems) (Fuller et al., 2004; Loeb, Fuller, Kagan, & Carrol, 2004; Spieker, Nelson, Petras, Jolley, & Barnard, 2003).

Concern in the child care field continues, however, over the ability to access high quality care, due partly to families' financial constraints and the high cost of the service (Brandon, 1999; Brayfield & Hofferth, 1995; Burchinal & Nelson, 2000; Chin & Phillips, 2004). For families with children under five, weekly child care costs averaged $94/week in 1999 (U.S. Census Bureau, 2005). This cost has increased since 1999 and does not accurately reflect the higher cost of care for infants or families living in urban areas. However, more recent figures have not been released by the U.S. Census Bureau, a universally accepted source for data.

With respect to costs, a high percentage of family income is spent on child care, especially for low-income families and for those where parents have low educational achievement (Anderson & Levine, 1999; Brayfield & Hofferth, 1995; Hofferth, 1999; U.S. Department of Health and Human Services [USDHHS], 1999). For families with employed mothers and children under five, the U.S. Census Bureau (2005) reports that those at less than 100% of the poverty threshold paid 33.95% of their monthly income on child care. In contrast, higher income families, despite spending more than the national average on child care, allocate a much smaller percentage of their income for the service (6.6%) (U.S. Census Bureau, 2005). Given the high percentage of income paid for child care by impoverished and low-income families, it is not surprising that low-income families are more likely to use less expensive informal kith and kin care than more expensive high quality center-based care (Chin & Phillips, 2004; Henly & Lyons, 2000; Hofferth, 1999; Zinsser, 2001). This phenomenon has generated debate and political action in recent years due to research findings that demonstrate low-income children benefit more from high-quality care than higher-income children (Votruba-Drzal, Coley, & Chase-Lansdale, 2004).

Numerous social programs have been developed to enhance the affordability and quality of child care, particularly for low-income families in the U.S. Some of these programs provide direct services to families. These include the Child Care Development Fund, Head Start, Early Head Start, and state-implemented pre-kindergarten programs. Other programs offer families temporary relief from the expense of child care by allowing parents to stay home with their children. Federal and state Family and Medical Leave Act policies as well as state At-Home Infant Care programs fall into this category. Finally, there are two tax programs designed to absorb some of the expense associated with raising children: the Child Tax Credit (CTC) and the Child and Dependent Care Tax Credit (CDCTC). In addition to these child specific programs, there are means tested programs designed to increase low-income families' net incomes, thereby indirectly affecting the proportion of income spent on child care expenses. These programs include Temporary Aid to Needy Families (TANF) and the Earned Income Tax Credit (EITC) (Ellwood, 2000). For a brief description of each of these programs, see Table 1.

The purpose of this article is to examine in more detail the Child and Dependent Care Tax Credit. This program was chosen because it is the least researched child care specific program in existence. Information on this program is important in order to provide policy makers and administrators with a better understanding of the continuity and gaps in child care services. Presented here is a brief description of the CDCTC as well as a framework for understanding the evolution of the program. The legislative history of the CDCTC, its impact on families with diverse incomes, as well as an analysis of barriers to its utilization and limitations are also presented. Recommendations for improving the CDCTC within the context of the incremental theoretical framework are presented at the conclusion of the article.

DESCRIPTION OF CURRENT CHILD
AND DEPENDENT CARE TAX CREDIT

The CDCTC is a non-refundable tax credit that covers a portion of one's employment-related child and dependent care expenses. Expenses are allowable for the care of children under thirteen and dependents of any age that are physically or mentally incapable of caring for themselves. The amount a family can claim with the CDCTC is delimited in four ways. First, the total amount of allowable expenses a family can claim is limited. Currently, the expense limit is $3,000 for families with one child in care and $6,000 for families with two or more children in care. Second, the amount a family claims cannot exceed the earned income of the lower earning taxpayer/spouse. Third, because the tax credit is not refundable, a family cannot benefit from the tax credit in excess of the amount they owe in federal income taxes. Finally, the credit is graduated on a sliding scale ranging from 20% for higher-income taxpayers to 35% for low-income taxpayers. (See Table 2 for details.)

TABLE 1. U.S. Social Programs Affecting Child Care

Program	Purpose	Service Offered
Child Care Development Fund (CCDF)	(a) Provide low-income families with child care and (b) enhance the quality of child care	Child care vouchers/certificates, 4% of CCDF funds are set aside for quality improvement
Head Start/Early Head Start	Enhance the development and school readiness of children in low-income families through education and support services	Preschool education, parent involvement, family support and access to a variety of health services for pregnant mothers and children
Pre-Kindergarten Programs	Enhance children's school readiness	Part-time/full-time instruction in a classroom setting for 3-4 year olds
Family and Medical Leave	Protect employees temporarily unable to work due to the need to care for a child, spouse or parent, or to recover from a serious illness	Twelve weeks unpaid leave with continued coverage in employer-sponsored group health insurance
At-Home Infant Care	Support parental choice to stay home with infants	Parents receive a subsidy in exchange for caring for their infants at home
Child Tax Credit	Ease families' financial burden of raising children	A partially refundable federal tax credit of $1,000[a]
Child and Dependent Care Tax Credit	Support families' ability to work by alleviating child care expenses	Tax credit between 20% and 35% of one's work-related child care expenses
Temporary Aid to Needy Families	Promote self-sufficiency among needy families	Provides financial aid and work support services
Earned Income Tax Credit	Facilitate employment among low-income workers	Provides a tax credit up to $4,300 depending on family type and income

Notes. [a]Benefit phases out starting at $75,000 for single parents and $110,000 for married couples.
Sources. The Finance Project. (n.d.). *The Child Tax Credit.* Available at: http://www.financeprojectinfo.org/mww/childtaxcredit.asp; State Policy Documentation Project. (2001). *Summary of policy issues: Categorical eligibility for TANF cash assistance.* Available at: http://www.spdp.org/tanf/categorical/categsumm.htm; U.S. Department of Health and Human Services [U.S. DHHS]. (2002). *Income guidelines for participation in Head Start programs.* Available at: http://www.acf.hhs.gov/programs/hsb/about/incomeguidelines/; U.S. DHHS. (2004). *Child Care Development Fund.* Available at: http://www.acf.hhs.gov/programs/ccb/geninfo/ccdfdesc.htm; U.S. DHHS. (2005). *At-Home Infant Care initiatives sponsored by the states.* Available at: http://www.nccic.org/poptopics/stateathome.html; U.S. DHHS. (2005). *Head Start Bureau programs and services.* Available at: http://www.acf.hhs.gov/programs/hsb/programs/index.htm; U.S. Department of Labor. (2005). Compliance Assistance Family and Medical Leave Act (FMLA). Available at: http://www.dol.gov/esa/whd/fmla/; U.S. Internal Revenue Service [U.S. IRS]. (2003). *Child and dependent care expenses* (Cat. No. 15004M). Washington, DC: Author; U.S. IRS. (2005). *Publication 596, Earned Income Tax Credit.* (Cat. No. 15173A). Available at: http://www.irs.gov/pub/irs-pdf/p596.pdf.

TABLE 2. Child and Dependent Care Tax Credit Maximum Claims by Income and Number of Children

If adjusted earned income is:		Then the percentage of expenses allowed to be claimed is:	Maximum that can be claimed for one dependent	Maximum that can be claimed for two or more dependents
Over	But not over			
$0	$15,000	35%	$1,050	$2,100
15,000	17,000	34%	1,020	2,040
17,000	19,000	33%	990	1,980
19,000	21,000	32%	960	1,920
21,000	23,000	31%	930	1,860
23,000	25,000	30%	900	1,800
25,000	27,000	29%	870	1,740
27,000	29,000	28%	840	1,680
29,000	31,000	27%	810	1,620
31,000	33,000	26%	780	1,560
33,000	35,000	25%	750	1,500
35,000	37,000	24%	720	1,440
37,000	39,000	23%	690	1,380
39,000	41,000	22%	660	1,320
41,000	43,000	21%	630	1,260
43,000	No limit	20%	600	1,200

Note. From U.S. IRS (2003).*Child and Dependent Care Expenses*, p. 12. (Cat. No. 15004M). Washington, DC: Author

The CDCTC is designed to have differential impacts on families depending on the family's income level, with the maximum benefit targeted to the lowest income group of families (annual income of $15,000 or less) and declining proportionally for families with higher incomes. Despite the CDCTC being designed to maximize benefits for the lowest income families, in reality, the opposite is often true. As this credit is non-refundable, the only families who can fully realize the benefit of the credit are those with tax liability equal to or greater than the value of the credit. Thus, only moderate- and high-income families can obtain the full CDCTC for which they are eligible.

CONCEPTUAL FRAMEWORK

The CDCTC has undergone great change in mission, scope, benefit level and structure since its implementation in 1954. In order to understand the logic behind these changes, it is useful to apply incremental theory, based on the tenets of rational choice theory. Rational choice theory suggests actions in the political process often are chosen in increments to maximize benefits and minimize costs (White & Klein, 2002). Further, incremental theory highlights the importance of continuity on policy decisions (Zimmerman, 2001). For example, according to incremental theory, policies and programs are more often built upon than disbanded. This approach is partly due to policymakers' desire to appease constituents, who would likely balk at losing a program to which they may feel entitled. Also, policymakers rely on existing policies and programs to serve as a framework for understanding the social problems they address. Thus, it may be difficult for policymakers to think outside of the box and create a new program when their understanding of a social problem and response to it is shaped by existing policy. Finally, because stakeholders advocate for programs providing evidence about effectiveness, existing programs profit from a sense of legitimacy that is difficult to establish with new programs. Consequently, according to incremental theory, policy decisions are likely to be based on incremental changes to existing policies that will benefit the most influential constituents (Zimmerman, 2001). The evolution of the CDCTC is an example of the application of incremental theory.

LEGISLATIVE HISTORY OF THE CHILD AND THE CHILD AND DEPENDENT CARE TAX CREDITS: 1954-2004

Child care was historically viewed as a maternal responsibility. Despite a man's ability to deduct many employment-related expenses from his taxable income, both in 1939 and again in 1949, the United States tax court ruled that a mother could not deduct from her income for tax purposes the expense of child care (Cohen, 1996). By the early 1950s there was increasing pressure on legislators to provide a tax deduction for the child care expenses of working women ("Children and Taxes," 1953). In 1954, such a deduction was created.

The child and dependent care tax deduction, proposed as part of the 1954 Revision of the Tax Code, was introduced with the purpose of supporting single parents, primarily mothers, with child care expenses (Albright, 1953; Brown, 1953). This bill was designed to address the problem of unemployment among single parents through the alleviation of work-related child care expenses. The House version of the bill (H.R. 8300) did just that, supporting widows, widowers, divorced persons, and wives whose husbands were incapable of work. The bill provided a $600 tax deduction for the child care expenses associated with children under 10 ("Revision," 1954). However, as the bill moved through the legislature, the purpose and focus of the child and dependent care tax deduction changed significantly.

A politically savvy women's group, the Gold Star Wives Club, advocated before the Senate for the application of the tax deduction to all working women ("Revision," 1954). The Senate incorporated this amendment into its passed version of the bill with the stipulation that working wives receiving the tax deduction file taxes jointly with their husbands and have a joint annual income no greater than $4,500 ("Revision," 1954). The final version of the tax bill, named the Revision of Internal Revenue Laws of 1954 (P.L. 591) was passed and signed into law by President Eisenhower on August 16, 1954 ("Revision," 1954). Applying the tax deduction for all working women regardless of income was an incremental step away from the original purpose of the bill, facilitating the employment of low-income single parents. This action set the stage for future policy developments.

The next significant change of the child and dependent care tax deduction occurred through the Tax Reform Act of 1976. Prior to this reform, families were unable to claim child and dependent care tax benefits unless they itemized deductions. Families who had no deductions except for the child and dependent care benefit were better off by claiming the standardized deduction. Consequently the Child and Dependent Care Tax Deduction (CDCTD) was largely underutilized.

In order to make the CDCTD more accessible, the Tax Reform Act of 1976 altered the benefit structure of the program from a tax deduction to a tax credit. Also under this reform, the child and dependent care tax deduction was altered in scope to include all working parents, regardless of income. Thus, all working parents became eligible for a 20% tax credit of employment-related child care expenses. The allowable expenses for calculating the CDCTC of 1976 could not exceed $2,000 for one child or $4,000 for two or more children and the amount of credit received could not exceed $400 for each of the taxpayers' first two dependents (Dunbar, 1999). Altering the scope of the CDCTC to include all families regardless of income, the Tax Reform Act of 1976 represented the second major incremental step away from a child and dependent care tax provision designed to support low-income single parents' employment.

A third revision of the CDCTC came in the early 1980s when Congress implemented a sliding scale on the tax credit. According to this policy, families earning $10,000 or less were able to claim a 30% credit for eligible child care expenses, with a maximum credit of $720 for one child and $1,449 for two or more children (Dunbar, 1999). The tax credit was then reduced by 1% for every $2,000 if one's income exceeded $10,000. For families with an income over $28,000, the credit maximized at 20% of one's eligible child and dependent care expenses with a maximum credit of $480 for one child and $960 for two children (Dunbar, 1999). The sliding scale revision, designed to make the tax credit more progressive, was an incremental step back towards addressing the original social problem of supporting low-income families' employment through a reduction in work-related child care expenses.

In 2001 the most recent revision to the CDCTC was implemented. As part of the Economic Growth and Tax Relief Reconciliation Act of 2001 (EGTRRA), the CDCTC was expanded in two ways. First, EGTRRA increased the maximum allowable expenses for child/dependent care to $3,000 for one child and $6,000 for two or more children in order to account for inflation (Maag, 2003). Second, the credit rates for the CDCTC were expanded by EGTRRA. Prior to this legislation, the credit rate families were eligible to receive maximized at 30% for families earning $10,000 or less and gradually declined 1% for every $2,000 over that income with the minimum credit rate of 20% available to families earning over $28,000 (Dunbar, 1999). EGTRRA increased the credit rate for low-income families to 35% for families earning $15,000 or less and decreasing 1% for every $2,000 with a minimum credit rate of 20% for families with incomes of $43,000 or over (Maag, 2003).

The justifications for these changes were twofold. First, the changes implemented by EGTRRA adjust for some inflation in incomes over the last 20 years, when the CDCTC was last updated (National Women's Law Center [NWLC], 2003). Second, the legislation increased the percentage of tax credit available to many families by slowing the decline per income of the tax rate (Maag, 2003). This credit alteration was particularly beneficial for working poor families with incomes between $18,000 and $33,000 (NWLC, 2003), a group that is often on the cusp of income ineligibility for other social programs.

To summarize, the legislative history of the CDCTC in the U.S. can be understood best in the framework of incremental theory. From the introduction of the child and dependent care tax deduction in the 1954 Revision of the Tax Code, to the CDCTC of today; the mission, scope, benefit level and structure of the tax program shifted gradually but significantly. The current CDCTC has evolved as a reflection of past policies (Lindblom, 1959) and resulted in several incremental changes (Frohock, 1979). Throughout all of the changes the CDCTC has endured, the program has remained intact. In the next sections, the current impact of the CDCTC on families with diverse incomes will be examined as will the barriers to and limitations of this credit for low-income families.

EFFECT OF THE CHILD AND DEPENDENT CARE TAX CREDIT ON FAMILIES WITH DIVERSE INCOMES

Eligible low-income families have historically underutilized child and dependent care tax benefits (Blau, 2001). Despite the low utilization rate of this benefit among low-income families, the CDCTC claimed the majority of federal dollars targeted toward public child care from the late 1970s through the late 1980s (Rich, 1988). As of 2003, a smaller proportion of the federal budget was allocated to the CDCTC, though it remained the third largest child care program, following the Child Care Development Fund and Head Start (Gish, 2003).

Consistent with historical utilization patterns, the CDCTC is currently used predominantly by middle- and upper-income families. Data from the IRS on tax credits filed in 2002 reveal that the majority of persons claiming the CDCTC (57.1%) and the majority of the country's revenue paid out by the credit (54%) goes to families with combined incomes of $50,000 or more, families to whom the tax credit is not nominally targeted (U.S. Internal Revenue Service [USIRS], 2004a). (See Figure 1 for breakdown by income categories.) Families with incomes under $15,000, the group to whom this program is nominally targeted, filed only 1.4% of CDCTCs and received only 0.4% of the dollars paid out by this program in 2002 (USIRS, 2004a).

Although it is impossible to determine the exact number of credits and percentage of CDCTC dollars going to families in the bottom and top 10% income brackets (defined in 2002 as $5,392 and $92,663, respectively) due to limitations in available data, estimates using the categories of $5,000 or less and $100,000 or more are possible (USIRS, 2004b). Using these categories, of the dollars paid out by the CDCTC in

FIGURE 1. Dollar Amounts Paid Out by Child and Dependent Care Tax Credit, 2002

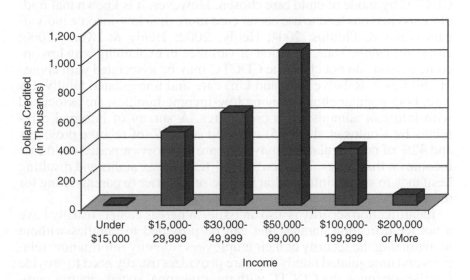

Source. U.S. Internal Revenue Service [IRS]. (2004). *Table 2. 2002, Individual Income Tax, All Returns; Tax Liability, Tax Credits, and Tax Payments, by size of adjusted gross income.* Retrieved February 23, 2005, from http://www.irs.gov/pub/irs-soi/02in02ar.xls

2002, less than 1% went to taxpayers in the bottom decile income bracket and more than 17% went to taxpayers in the top decile bracket.

In conclusion, the CDCTC has differential utilization rates for families of varied incomes. Moderate to high-income families are most likely to claim the tax benefit. Low-income families, for whom this program was originally developed, seldom claim the credit. In the following sections, within the context of incremental theory, barriers faced by low-income earners applying for the CDCTC, limitations of the credit, and recommendations to overcome these challenges are discussed.

BARRIERS TO CLAIMING THE CHILD AND DEPENDENT CARE TAX CREDITS

In addition to the relative lack of benefit received from the CDCTC for low-income families, other factors including low-income families' child care choices and relative lack of familiarity with the tax system serve as barriers to claiming the credit. Unfortunately, there are no reliable data to date that would allow one to analyze the utilization of the CDCTC by mode of child care chosen. However, it is known that middle-class persons tend to use center care more than low-income individuals (Chin & Phillips, 2004; Henly, 2002; Henly & Lyons, 2000; Hofferth, 1999). Thus, a portion of variance in explaining why low-income persons do not claim the CDCTC may be associated with choice of child care. Relative (kith and kin) care and unregulated family day care, both popular choices among low-income families, are associated with informal administrative procedures. A survey of informal caregivers by Kontos et al. (1995) revealed only 5% of relative providers and 42% of non-regulated family day care providers reported child care income on their taxes. Thus, providers' fears of tax audits and resulting hesitancy to supply information may be one barrier to parents filing for the CDCTC.

Identification security is also an issue. Whereas centers usually have a tax identification number that can be provided to families without jeopardizing the security of their employees' identity information, relatives and unregulated family day care providers usually need to provide families claiming the CDCTC with their personal social security number. According to Kontos et al. (1995), only 12% of relatives and 46% of unregulated family day care providers reported giving their social security number to parents. Additionally, 70% of relatives and 35% of unregulated family day care providers reported not wanting to give parents their social security number (Kontos et al.,1995).

In addition to comparisons of administrative practices between centers, family day care providers, and paid informal providers, it is important to note additional considerations related to the child care choices of low-income persons that may affect their propensity to claim the CDCTC. First, low-income families use unpaid relative care more often than middle- and upper-income families (Zinsser, 2001). Families using non-paid child care arrangements are not eligible to receive the CDCTC. Second, families using paid informal caregivers and possibly some family day care centers may not keep a record of their child care expenditures and therefore may not have the proof of purchase necessary to claim the CDCTC.

Finally, low-income families may not be as savvy at navigating the tax system as higher income families. Middle- and upper-income individuals are often socialized by their peers regarding the value of tax breaks and how to claim tax benefits. There is evidence to suggest that many low-income individuals do not even know they are eligible for tax benefits such as the CDCTC (personal communication, Children's Defense Fund, February 23, 2005). As described earlier, there are a plethora of reasons why the CDCTC may be underutilized by low-income families. These reasons include parents' inability to obtain needed information from providers, use of unpaid providers, and lack of awareness regarding the CDCTC.

LIMITATION OF THE CHILD AND DEPENDENT CARE TAX CREDIT

In addition to the barriers listed above, the CDCTC also has some important limitations. First and foremost, the CDCTC is not refundable. Thus, many low-income families do not fully benefit from the tax credit because they lack sufficient tax liability. Second, the allowable child care expenses on which the CDCTC is based do not completely cover the cost of child care that families face each year (Cohen, 1996; Donahue & Campbell, 2002). In 2003, the average cost of child care for one child was $303 per month or $3,636 per year (Giannarelli, Adelman, & Schmidt, 2003). The CDCTC limits allowable expenses to $3,000 for one child and $6,000 for two or more children. This gap between allowable expenses and average child care expenses is partly due to the lack of a provision that would keep the CDCTC indexed for inflation and partly due to political conservatism (NWLC, 2003). Third, the CDCTC does not help families who are struggling to afford child care at the time when they must pay for it (Cohen, 1996). Given the structure of the tax credit, families need to pay for their child care upfront. Low-income families often live paycheck to paycheck. Therefore, the notion of getting a tax credit sometime in the future benefits families little when expenses are due.

RECOMMENDATIONS FOR IMPROVING THE CHILD AND DEPENDENT CARE TAX CREDIT

With several adjustments to the program, the CDCTC could be a more valuable benefit for low-income working families. In order for these adjustments to be more politically feasible, however, an incremental strategy must be employed. Following are five steps that could be undertaken to improve the CDCTC.

The most important adjustment would be to make the CDCTC refundable (NWLC, 2000). Making this credit refundable would allow poor and low-income families to fully benefit from the tax program. As previously stated, currently families with incomes over $100,000 gain more financial benefits from the CDCTC than families earning under $15,000. If the credit were made refundable, low-income families would receive a tax refund for the difference between the amount they owed in taxes and the worth of their CDCTC. Adjusting the credit to be refundable would be of particular importance for families that do not qualify for other child care programs, or despite being eligible, do not receive them due to program waiting lists (Giannarelli et al., 2003). If the credit were made refundable, the utility of the CDCTC for low-income families could also be improved by providing families with an opportunity to project their annual child care costs and receive their CDCTC throughout the year, rather than in a lump sum tax return. This provision could be modeled after the Earned Income Tax Credit's advance payment delivery system (Romich, 2000).

The second set of adjustments to improve the CDCTC would be to (a) raise the allowable expenses for child care and (b) eliminate the two-child limit (NWLC, 2000). Although states vary in average child care expenses, the national average child care expenditure surpasses the $3,000/$6,000 child care expense limits of the CDCTC by $636 per year for one child. Additionally, because $6,000 is the allowable expense for two or more children, this allowance is *at least* $1,272 short of the average cost of care for an eligible family with more than one child. Increasing the maximum allowable child care expense commensurate with the average child care expense for the state reporting the highest expenses would accomplish two things. First, it would allow most families to claim all of their child care expenses, regardless of where they lived. Second, this change would enable families to choose higher quality child care.

In addition to adjusting the allowable child care expenses to coincide with child care prices, restructuring the CDCTC to include incremental adjustments regardless of the number of children in a family, would improve the value and fairness of this credit. Currently, the CDCTC has one benefit level for families with one child in care and a second for families with two or more children in care. Families with more than two children in care are thus unable to benefit from child care expense claims for their additional children.

Another adjustment to improve the CDCTC would be to index all aspects of the program to inflation (NWLC, 2003). As is currently legislated, the CDCTC is not indexed to inflation, thus over time the allowable child care expenses lose value and the number of families eligible for the greatest percentage of credit decreases (i.e., as families' earnings increase commensurate with inflation fewer become eligible to receive the 35% credit) (Maag, 2003; NWLC, 2003).

Lastly, the accessibility of this tax credit to low-income working families could be enhanced through education and outreach efforts targeted to low-income/poor families and family/informal child care providers. Perhaps if low-income families and the providers who serve them were more aware of the CDCTC and eligibility requirements were made more visible, some of the barriers to accessing the program would be eliminated.

CONCLUSIONS

The CDCTC, a tax credit originally aimed at facilitating low-income single parents' employment, has undergone numerous changes since its inception. Throughout the credit's tenure, the families most heavily targeted for assistance have underutilized the benefit. In this article, incremental theory was applied as a framework for understanding the legislative history of the CDCTC. Utilization patterns, barriers and limitations of the credit were then presented and recommendations to improve the credit were offered. As suggested by incremental theory, the policy recommendations have emerged from the data and the impact of the existing policy. However, additional research on the CDCTC needs to be conducted. Research questions regarding the CDCTC that remain unanswered include: (a) how utilization patterns of this tax credit differ by families' level of poverty (e.g., 100% FPL (federal poverty level) and below, 100-200% FPL, 200% FPL and above), (b) what benefits families at various levels of poverty receive from the program, and (c) at what poverty levels service gaps exist between the CDCTC and CCDF subsidies.

REFERENCES

Albright, R. C. (1953, June 17). House tax revision hearings started. *The Washington Post*, p. 2.

Anderson, P. M., & Levine, P. B. (1999). *Child care and mothers' employment decisions. Working Paper 7058, National Bureau of Economic Research*. Retrieved September 12, 2004, from http://papers.nber.org/papers/w7058.v5.pdf

Berry, M. F. (1993). *The politics of parenthood.* New York: Penguin.

Blau, D. M. (2001). *The child care problem: An economic analysis.* New York: Russell Sage.

Brandon, P. D. (1999). Income-pooling arrangements, economic constraints, and married mothers' child care choices. *Journal of Family Issues, 20,* 350-370.

Brayfield, A., & Hofferth, S. (1995). Balancing the family budget: Differences in child care expenditures by race/ethnicity, economic status, and family structure. *Social Science Quarterly, 76,* 158-177.

Brown, L. (1953, March 25). Defends tax relief bill for mothers who work. *The Washington Post,* p. 23.

Burchinal, M. R., & Nelson, L. (2000). Family selection and child care experiences: Implications for studies of child outcomes. *Early Childhood Research Quarterly, 15,* 385-411.

Children and taxes. (1953, June 7). *The Washington Post,* p. B4.

Chin, T., & Phillips, M. (2004). Social reproduction and child-rearing practices: Social class, children's agency, and the summer activity gap. *Sociology of Education, 77,* 185-210.

Cohen, A. J. (1996). A brief history of federal financing for child care in the United States. *The Future of Children, 6,* 26-40.

Donahue, E. H., & Campbell, N. D. (2002). *Making care less taxing: Improving state child and dependent care tax provisions.* Washington, DC: National Women's Law Center.

Dunbar, A. E. (1999). Child care expenses: The child care credit. In R. D. Ebel, J. J. Cordes, & J. G. Gravelle (Eds.), *The encyclopedia of taxation and tax policy* (pp. 66-68). Washington, DC: The Urban Institute.

Ellwood, D. T. (2000). The impact of the earned income tax credit and social policy reforms on work, marriage, and living arrangements. *National Tax Journal, 53,* 1063-1106.

Frohock, F. (1979). *Public policy: Scope and logic.* Englewood Cliffs, NJ: Prentice Hall.

Fuller, B., Kagan, S. L., Loeb, S., & Chang, Y. (2004). Child care quality: Centers and home settings that serve poor families. *Early Childhood Research Quarterly, 19,* 505-527.

Giannarelli, L., Adelman, S., & Schmidt, S. (2003). *Getting help with child care expenses. Occasional Paper Number 62.* Washington, DC: The Urban Institute.

Gish, M. (2003). *Child Care Issues in the 108th Congress.* Washington, DC: Congressional Research Service.

Henly, J. R. (2002). Informal support networks and the maintenance of low-wage jobs. In F. Munger (Ed.), *Laboring below the line: The new ethnography of poverty, low-wage work, and survival in the global economy* (pp. 179-203). New York: Russell Sage.

Henly, J. R., & Lyons, S. (2000). The negotiation of child care and employment demands among low-income parents. *Journal of Social Issues, 56,* 683-706.

Hofferth, S. (1999). Child care, maternal employment, and public policy. *The Annals of the American Academy of Political and Social Science, 563,* 20-38.

Kontos, S., Howes, C., Shinn, M., & Galinsky, E. (1995). *Quality in family child care and relative care.* New York: Teachers College Press.

Lindblom, C. (1959). The science of "muddling through." *Public Administration Review, 19,* 79-88.

Loeb, S., Fuller, B., Kagan, S. L., & Carrol, B. (2004). Child care in poor communities: Early learning effects of type, quality, and stability. *Child Development, 75,* 47-65.

Maag, E. (2003). *Recent expansions to Child and Dependent Care Tax Credit.* Retrieved September 13, 2004, from http://www.urban.org/urlprint.cfm?ID=8660

Michel, S. (1999). *Children's interests/mothers' rights: The shaping of America's child care policy.* New Haven, CT: Yale University Press.

Michel, S., & Mahon, R. (2002). *Child care at the crossroads: Gender and the welfare state restructuring.* New York: Routledge.

National Women's Law Center [NWLC]. (2000). *Tax relief for employed families: Improving the dependent care tax credit.* Retrieved September 22, 2004, from http://www.nwlc.org/pdf/TaxReliefDCTCJuly2000.pdf

National Women's Law Center [NWLC]. (2003). *Indexing the DCTC is necessary to prevent further erosion of the credit's value to low-income families.* Retrieved September 23, 2004, from http://www.nwlc.org/pdf/IndexingDCTCFactSheet2003.pdf

Revision of internal revenue laws. (1954). In *Congressional Almanac* (Vol. 10, pp. 476-489). Washington, DC: Congressional Quarterly News Features.

Rich, S. (1988, August 5). Federal Child Care Funds Have Ballooned. *The Washington Post,* p. A25.

Romich, J. L. (2000). How families view and use the EITC: Advance payments versus lump sum delivery. *National Tax Journal, 53,* 1245-1266.

Spieker, S. J., Nelson, D. C., Petras, A., Jolley, S. N., & Barnard, K. E. (2003). Joint influence of child care and infant attachment security for cognitive and language outcomes of low-income toddlers. *Infant Behavior & Development, 26,* 326-345.

U.S. Bureau of Labor Statistics. (2004). *Table 4. Families with own children: Employment status of parents by age of youngest child and family type, 2002-03 annual averages.* Retrieved February 23, 2005, from http://www.bls.gov/news.release/famee.t04.htm

U.S. Census Bureau. (2005). *PPL Table 5: Weekly child care payments by employed mothers with children under 5.* Retrieved June 5, 2005, from http://www.census.gov/population/socdemo/child/ppl-168/tab06.xls

U. S. Department of Health and Human Services [USDHHS]. (1999). *Access to child care for low-income working families.* Retrieved October 14, 2004, from http://www.acf.hhs.gov/programs/ccb/research/ccreport/ccreport.htm

U.S. Internal Revenue Service [USIRS]. (2003). *Child and dependent care expenses* (Cat. No. 15004M). Washington, DC: Author.

U.S. Internal Revenue Service [USIRS]. (2004a). *Table 2.–2002, Individual Income Tax, all returns: Tax liability, tax credits, and tax payments, by size of adjusted gross income.* Retrieved February 25, 2005, from http://www.irs.gov/pub/irs-soi/02in02ar.xls

U.S. Internal Revenue Service [USIRS]. (2004b). *Tax states at a glance: Individual returns.* Retrieved October 27, 2004, from http://www.irs.gov/taxstats/article/0,,id = 102886,00.html

Votruba-Drzal, E., Coley, R. L., & Chase-Lansdale, P. L. (2004). Child care and low-income children's development: Direct and moderated effects. *Child Development, 75*, 296-312.

White, J. M., & Klein, D. M. (2002). *Family theories* (2nd ed.). Thousand Oaks, CA: Sage.

Zimmerman, S. L. (2001). *Family policy: Constructed solutions to family problems.* Thousand Oaks, CA: Sage.

Zinsser, C. (2001). Child care within the family. *The Future of Children, 11*, 123-127.

California's Paid Leave Law:
A Model for Other States?

Steven K. Wisensale

SUMMARY. On July 1, 2004 California implemented the first and only paid family leave bill in the nation's history. This article explores the formulation and passage of the law and reviews its utilization patterns and impact one year later. Included is a brief historical overview of the Family and Medical Leave Act of 1993; the role of the states in the development of leave policy before and after the passage of the FMLA; the unique political and economic circumstances surrounding the adoption of California's law in 2002; and a discussion of whether or not the nation's only paid family leave law is a model for other states to follow. *[Article copies available for a fee from The Haworth Document Delivery Service: 1-800-HAWORTH. E-mail address: <docdelivery@haworthpress.com> Website: <http://www.HaworthPress.com> © 2006 by The Haworth Press, Inc. All rights reserved.]*

KEYWORDS. California's paid leave law, Family and Medical Leave Act, family leave, paid leave, work and family

Steven K. Wisensale, PhD, is affiliated with the University of Connecticut.

Address correspondence to: Steven K. Wisensale, Professor of Public Policy, School of Family Studies, U-2058, 348 Mansfield Road, University of Connecticut, Storrs, CT 06269-2058 (E-mail: steven.wisensale@uconn.edu).

[Haworth co-indexing entry note]: "California's Paid Leave Law: A Model for Other States?" Wisensale, Steven K. Co-published simultaneously in *Marriage & Family Review* (The Haworth Press, Inc.) Vol. 39, No. 1/2, 2006, pp. 177-195; and: *Families and Social Policy: National and International Perspectives* (ed: Linda Haas, and Steven K. Wisensale) The Haworth Press, Inc., 2006, pp. 177-195. Single or multiple copies of this article are available for a fee from The Haworth Document Delivery Service [1-800-HAWORTH, 9:00 a.m. - 5:00 p.m. (EST). E-mail address: docdelivery@haworthpress.com].

Within the last quarter century, the challenge of balancing work and family has become a major topic of debate among policymakers who, simultaneously, wrestle with the questions of state versus federal power, and private versus public responsibility when it comes to designing and implementing social policy. In short, should the family or the state assume responsibility for balancing work and family? And, if it is the latter, should it be the state or the federal government that shoulders the burden?

The purpose of this paper is fourfold: First, to provide a brief historical overview of the Family and Medical Leave Act; second, to identify the role of the states in the development of leave policy both before and after the passage of the FMLA in 1993; third, to focus on California's version of family-leave policy by discussing how its 2002 paid family leave law was formulated and passed; and fourth, to respond to the following question: Is California's paid family leave law (CPFL) a model for other states? Each of these will be discussed in detail.

HISTORICAL OVERVIEW OF THE FAMILY AND MEDICAL LEAVE ACT

On August 5, 2003 supporters of the Family and Medical Leave Act (FMLA) celebrated the tenth anniversary of the law's implementation. Signed by President Clinton on February 5, 1993, the FMLA grants workers in companies of 50 or more employees up to twelve weeks of unpaid leave for the birth or adoption of a child and for the care of a sick child, spouse, or parent with a serious health condition. It also guarantees job security in that an employee is entitled to return to the same or comparable job and requires the employer to maintain health benefits as if the employee never took leave. To be eligible under the law, a worker must be employed for at least one year or 1,250 hours. However, a company may deny leave to a salaried employee who falls within the highest 10 percent of the company's payroll if the worker's leave would create "substantial and grievous injury" to the business operations.

The passage of the FMLA may have appeased those critics who reminded policymakers that the United States was one of a few industrialized nations without such a policy (Hyde, Essex, Clark et al., 1996). However, the law is quite limited in scope, does not apply to all family types, nor does it cover all caregiving scenarios. Because it is unpaid, most single parents and lower income couples cannot afford to take time off from work even if given the opportunity (Gornick & Meyers, 2003; Heymann, 2005).

Also, although the law is touted as an example of intergenerational policy making, it does not cover grandchildren who care for grandparents, nor does it cover in-law care. That is, a wife may care for her elderly mother or father but she cannot provide such care to her mother-in-law or father-in-law and be covered under the law. And further, the FMLA is totally insensitive to same-sex partners. Despite the fact that more than a thousand communities, corporations, nonprofit organizations, and universities have adopted domestic partnership policies that grant equal status to same-sex couples with respect to benefit coverage, the FMLA does not apply to this type of nontraditional family (Elving, 1995).

The law also has three characteristics that place it in sharp contrast to typical models in other industrialized nations. One, it is unpaid. A large majority of industrialized countries provide some form of wage replacement for those who take leave from work. Two, the American model has a family focus. That is, unlike its European counterparts that are designed for new parents, the U.S. law is intergenerational in structure, thus allowing time off from work for the birth or care of a child as well as an elderly parent. And three, unlike most other industrialized countries, the United States links eligibility for leave to company size (50 or more employees). Consequently, the FMLA only applies to about 6 percent of the corporations and covers only about 60 percent of the labor force (Department of Labor, 2000).

But despite these obvious shortcomings, it is not surprising that many Democrats hailed Clinton's election victory and the signing of the FMLA as an end to 12 years of Republican rule and the conservatives' version of new federalism (now known as devolution) under presidents Reagan and Bush. The FMLA was soon championed as the first major sign of a resurrection of federal power, and the national government, it was believed, would be destined to play a more aggressive role in creating and enforcing national standards, such as those incorporated in the FMLA (Bernstein, 2001; Elving, 1995).

THE ROLE OF THE STATES BEFORE AND AFTER THE FMLA

It is important to emphasize here that by the time Bill Clinton had affixed his signature to the 1993 law, about 34 states had already adopted some form of leave policy, with some producing comparable or stronger legislation than the Clinton version (Wisensale, 2001). Twenty-three states covered both private and state employees; 11 states applied their policies to state employees only. Nineteen of the states gave time off only for childbirth and pregnancy, whereas 15 states had adopted broader types of legislation, permitting leave for more general family reasons. There was also much variation among the states in duration of leave and the size of companies to which the law applied (Wisensale, 2001).

Within the first eight years of its adoption, the FMLA was evaluated twice by the Department of Labor: in 1996 and 2000. On April 30, 1996, the Commission on Leave issued its first report: *A Workable Balance: Report to Congress on Family and Medical Leave Policies.* The 314-page document concluded that the FMLA had a positive impact on employees overall and was not the burden on businesses that some had predicted. Ninety percent of companies covered by the law reported no negative impact. "For most employers, compliance is easy, the costs are non-existent or small and the effects are minimal," states the report. "Most periods of leave are short, most employees return to work, and reduced turnover seems to be a tangible effect" (Commission on Leave, 1996, p. xxii).

More specifically, between 1993 and 1995, nearly 15 million people used the FMLA for either personal reasons or to care for a family member. By 2004 more than 40 million employees had used it (National Partnership for Women and Families, 2004). However, it was also reported that 3.4% of eligible employees who needed leave did not take it. And, of those, about 66% indicated that the reason they did not use the FMLA was because they could not afford it (Commission on Leave, 1996). This finding was later confirmed by the second major evaluation of the FMLA conducted by the Department of Labor: *Balancing the Needs of Families and Employers: Family and Medical Leave Surveys.* This study concluded that the major reason workers needed leave and did not take it was due to cost. Simply put, they could not afford to take time off (Department of Labor, 2000). Such findings prompted both Congress and the Clinton administration to propose expanding the FMLA in two respects: accessibility and affordability.

Between 1993 and 1999, almost 20 initiatives to expand the Family and Medical Leave Act were put forth by members of Congress. Some wanted the law to apply to smaller companies, and others wanted to include additional hours to address basic family needs, such as taking children to dental appointments or for attending parent-teacher meetings (Wisensale, 2003). Others proposed that the coverage be expanded to include domestic partners, parents-in-law, and grandparents. Several proposals were extremely narrow in focus and specific in structure, such as allowing employees to take leave for literacy training, to make living organ donations, and to prevent employers from requiring employees to take FMLA disputes to arbitration instead of court. However, all legislative proposals failed (Gladstone, 1999; Jordan, 1999). The reasons for their failure were not unfamiliar to political observers. Most proposals emerged from a Democratic administration confronting a Republican-controlled congress during a president's lame-duck term. They were considered either too costly or very disruptive for businesses to implement properly (Waldfogel, 1999). In the meantime, a new White House strategy was slowly emerging.

Confronted with a Republican Congress in the second half of his first term, the lame duck and beleaguered president, who survived an impeachment trial in the Senate, realized that few of his legislative proposals would succeed. To overcome this obstacle, President Clinton followed a path not unfamiliar to his predecessors. He deliberately bypassed Congress by issuing orders to his federal agencies. Frustrated over Congress's inability to expand the FMLA, Clinton chose to change the venue of the debate in the spring of 1999 from Capitol Hill to the Department of Labor (Wisensale, 2003).

In his commencement address at Grambling State University in Louisiana on May 23, 1999, the president announced two new initiatives aimed at the FMLA. First, he directed the Department of Labor to explore the ways states may use surplus Unemployment Insurance (UI) funds to subsidize parents who use the FMLA to care for a newborn or newly adopted child (thus "Baby UI"). The second initiative recommended that federal employees be permitted to use up to 12 weeks of accrued sick leave to care for a seriously ill child, parent, or spouse. Prior to 1999, federal workers could only use up to 13 days of accrued sick leave per year to care for seriously ill family members. "I believe it is imperative that your country give you the tools to succeed not only in the workplace but also at home. If you or any American has to choose between being a good parent and successful in your careers, you have paid a terrible price, and so has your country," he told the Grambling graduates (President's Commencement Address, 1999).

The following day Clinton issued an Executive Memorandum entitled "New Tools to Help Parents Balance Work and Family." In the memo, the president ordered the secretary of labor, Alexis Herman, to propose regulations that would allow states to use UI funds to support parents on leave after the birth or adoption of a child. He also called upon the secretary to develop model legislation that states could adopt in following these new regulations (Presidential Memorandum, 1999).

Under the president's proposal, states were permitted to tap the surpluses of their UI trust funds to cover 12 weeks of parental leave. In short, any employee leaving work under the FMLA for the birth or adoption of a child would be classified as temporarily laid off, and therefore declared eligible for unemployment compensation. The idea runs parallel to the use of Temporary Disability Insurance (TDI) which provides a wage replacement for new mothers in five states (California, Hawaii, New Jersey, New York, and Rhode Island). Companies in TDI states are required to offer paid leave to new mothers, just as it would be offered to other employees who are ill or temporarily disabled (Meyers, 1995).

However, there is much variation, both in the funding mechanisms used and the amount of benefits provided under these five TDI models (California refers to it as SDI or State Disability Insurance). For example, in three states (Hawaii, New Jersey, and New York), employee and employer contributions, though not necessarily equal, support the TDI trust funds. In two states (California and Rhode Island), the employers make no contributions. With respect to the amount of benefits available to workers who take leave, there is also much variation among the five models. The wage replacement levels start at about 50% of an employee's salary in New York and climb to about 66% in Hawaii. All states maintain a maximum weekly cap calculated on the basis of average wages, but no state's maximum benefit per worker per week exceeds $800 (Wisensale, 2001).

Spurred on by Clinton's initiative, 13 states, between May 23, 1999 and July 2000, introduced legislation that included a provision for some type of paid family leave. These included California, Connecticut, Georgia, Illinois, Indiana, Maine, Massachusetts, Maryland, Minnesota, New Hampshire, New Jersey, Vermont, and Washington. No state succeeded in passing paid leave legislation, and only three states (Connecticut, Massachusetts, and New Jersey) proposed coverage that extended beyond "baby care" (Baby UI) and included coverage for elder care. Connecticut's proposal, for example, was designed to use only UI funds to cover the birth or adoption of a child, whereas other leaves, such as time off for elder care, would be funded through a new Medical Leave Insurance Fund (MLIF). Both Massachusetts and New Jersey produced similar hybrid proposals that would allow UI to cover childbirth and adoption, but care of other family members would be funded through separate mechanisms. Massachusetts referred to its elder care component as a "family employment trust fund," whereas New Jersey named its version "Family temporary disability" or FTD leave (National Partnership for Women and Families, 2002).

One year later, in 2001, the number of states proposing paid leave doubled from 13 to 26 and by early 2002 it had risen to 28 states. Although there was much activity in the states, not one succeeded in passing paid leave legislation until California in September of 2002. Perhaps a primary reason for such a massive failure across the board can be attributed to legislators' lack of confidence in a fairly novel funding mechanism, the use of unemployment insurance. Only a few states had completed studies that included projected costs under various models, be it UI or TDI. Concerns were also raised about the long-term viability of the UI model, in particular, if there was a steady economic decline for an extended period of time–even though Canada had employed the UI model on a national scale for nearly a decade despite occasional economic downturns (Trzcinski, 1994). The economic decline began about 2000 and, consequently, the push for paid leave under the UI model weakened considerably. Instead, many states began to focus on converting accrued sick and vacation leave to a watered down version of paid family leave. California, however, chose a different path.

CALIFORNIA'S PAID FAMILY LEAVE LAW

On September 23, 2002 Governor Gray Davis (D) signed the nation's first paid family leave law; SB 1661 was sponsored and engineered through the General Assembly by Senator Sheila Kuehl (D) of Santa Monica. Beginning July 1, 2004, 13 million of 16 million California workers became eligible for six weeks of paid family leave per year to care for a new child (birth, adoption, or foster care) or a seriously ill family member (parent, child, spouse, or domestic partner). The specific components of this landmark legislation are:

- Beginning in 2004, workers who qualify receive up to 55% of their wages for up to six weeks, with a cap of $728 per week. The cap will be adjusted each year according to the state's average weekly wage.
- The average worker pays less than $3 per month, or an estimated $27 per year, for this new benefit. Employers are not required to contribute.

- All workers applying for paid leave must wait for at least one week.
- Employers can require employees to use a maximum of two weeks of vacation time before receiving paid leave and one week includes the waiting period.
- The paid leave benefit is funded under California's State Disability Insurance Program (SDI)–a program that is funded 100% by employee contributions.
- Job security is not guaranteed under the new law. However, depending on individual cases, employee job retention may be secured through other pre-existing statutes.

According to the Labor Project for Working Families (2003) at the University of California-Berkeley, three major factors made California particularly fertile territory for a paid family leave program.

First, there was already in existence a benefits infrastructure that could shoulder the burden of a new paid leave policy. That is, California, along with four other states (Hawaii, New Jersey, New York, and Rhode Island) already employed the concept of temporary disability insurance as a vehicle for providing paid leave during pregnancy. California's initiative was to simply add *family* care to that model. Also, in 1999 and as a precursor to SB 1661, a new California law required employers to permit employees to use up to half of their annual accrued sick leave to care for ill family members.

Second, over a ten-year period a strong advocacy base formed that focused on work and family issues. Leading the charge was the Work and Family Coalition, an assortment of labor unions pulled together by the Labor Project for Working Families. Unions negotiated for child care and argued for paid leave in their labor contracts. Also included was the California Labor Federation, which is the state version of the AFL-CIO. The CFRA had played a crucial role in previous legislative battles over pregnancy rights and sick leave benefits (Carsten, 2004; Labor Project for Working Families, 2003).

And third, the political climate was ripe for an initiative on paid leave. The Democrats had controlled the Assembly, the Senate, and the Governor's office since 1998. Historically, California Democrats maintained strong ties with labor organizations and the types of advocacy groups referred to earlier. Also, in retrospect, most analysts contend that because the paid leave bill was introduced during an election year, with the governor running for a second term, voters confronted with their own personal work and family conflicts would resonate toward politicians who supported paid leave.

A fourth factor may be included here as well. Although the California economy was not necessarily the healthiest in the nation, its status was far from the huge $38 billion deficit it faced less than a year after the law's enactment. Nor was Governor Davis in a particularly vulnerable position politically. He certainly was not the target of a recall election scheduled for October 2003, a year after the enactment of the law. In short, had SB 1611 been introduced a year later than it was, one can speculate that the odds of its passing would be fairly slim. Both the political and economic climate of California changed drastically within a very short period of time, which ultimately culminated in Arnold Schwarzenegger being elected governor.

In late 1999 Governor Davis signed a bill that not only raised California's SDI benefit but it also directed the Employment Development Department (EDD) "to study the potential costs of providing paid family leave through SDI" (Labor Project for Working Families, 2003). Following the publication of the EDD report which indicated that paid family leave could be offered at a relatively modest cost, a two-year campaign by advocacy groups for paid leave began. In February 2002, Senator Kuehl introduced SB 1661, also known as "Disability Compensation: Family Temporary Disability Insurance."

The bill's journey through the legislative process was not unlike that of the FMLA's experience in the 1980s or numerous state initiatives over the last two decades. By the time it was sent to Governor Davis's desk for his signature, more than 20 different compromises had been struck and strong arguments on both sides of the issue had been heard. In the Assembly, supporters testifying before the Insurance and Appropriations committees included representatives from the American Association of University Women, California Catholic Conference, California Child Care Resource and Referral Network, California Labor Federation, California National Organization for Women, Congress of California Seniors, and the State Parent and Teachers Association. Generally speaking, their arguments revolved around three major points. First, families are over-burdened with caregiving responsibilities across generations and they need support. Second, they cannot afford to take leave without some form of wage replacement. And third, because the private sector is slow to respond to work and family conflicts, it is the government's responsibility to take action (California Assembly Insurance Committee Hearing, 2002).

The primary opponents testifying during Assembly hearings were the California Chamber of Commerce, California Manufacturing Technical Association, and the National Federation of Independent Businesses. Their major arguments were that the legislation would be too costly, that it would hurt small businesses in particular, and that it would ultimately cost California jobs, as businesses would cut personnel costs under an expanded SDI by simply hiring fewer workers (California Assembly Appropriations Committee Hearing, 2002).

Following a lively debate on the Assembly floor on August 27, 2002, SB 1661 passed by a margin of 45 to 27. But more importantly, three major changes were made in the bill that would shape the debate in the Senate. First, the original proposal that called for a 50-50 sharing of the cost between employer and employee was dropped. The employees would shoulder the entire cost burden. Second, it was agreed that the employee must use two weeks of vacation leave prior to applying for paid leave. And third, unlike the FMLA, job security for leave takers would not be guaranteed because existing laws would cover workers anyway (California Assembly Floor Debate, 2002).

With respect to the Senate, the bill was subject to hearings before the Labor and Industrial Relations Committee and the Appropriations Committee. Speaking in support of the proposal were representatives from the American Association of University Women, California Children and Families Commission, California Labor Federation, California Permanent Commission on the Status of Women, National Partnership for Women and Families and several witnesses who provided personal hardship stories as family caregivers. Opponents of SB 1661 who testified in the Senate hearings included representatives from the California Chamber of Commerce and the California Manufacturers and Technology Association (California Senate Appropriations Committee Hearing, 2002; California Senate Labor and Industrial Relations Committee Hearing, 2002).

Although the arguments put forth in the Senate debate were similar to those expressed in the Assembly, the opponents' arguments were somewhat diffused by the three major compromises that were struck in the house. That is, it would be funded solely by employee contributions, that employees would have to first use two weeks of vacation leave, and that there would be no job guarantee. Still, even during the Senate floor debate, Republican opponents, led by Senator Haynes, argued that the bill would place an undue tax burden on the employee and raised concerns about the likelihood of fraud being committed by unscrupulous workers. "It's a bad idea, the wrong way to go, and it's not necessary," argued Haynes as the Senate floor debate drew to a close (California Senate Floor Debate, 2002). Somewhat surprising was the lack of economic impact studies put forth by opponents of the bill. Proponents of SB 1661 argued strongly through the use of several studies, including one from the University of Chicago, that the financial impact on businesses would be relatively light. Nonetheless, on August 30, 2002, the bill passed the Senate by a margin of 21 to 9 and was sent on to Governor Davis's desk for his signature. After nearly a month of contemplation, a block of time that worried both supporters and opponents, the Governor signed the bill into law on September 23, 2002. The California paid leave law compared to the FMLA is presented in Table 1.

California's Leave Law One Year Later

Passing a law is one thing, measuring its effectiveness is quite another matter. In July, 2005 California's Employment Development Department (EDD) issued a special report, *The Paid Family Leave Insurance Program Year in Review July 1, 2004-June 30, 2005*. The new program paid nearly 138,000 workers about $300 million in its inaugural year. Benefits averaged $409 a week, with leaves averaging about five weeks. A summary of claims and costs is presented in Table 2.

TABLE 1. California's Paid Leave Law and the FMLA

California Paid Leave Law	Federal FMLA
Applies to seriously ill spouse, child, parents, and domestic partner	Applies to seriously ill spouse, child, parents, and the employee's own illness
6 weeks paid leave	12 weeks unpaid leave
6 weeks of no job protection	Job protected
Employer may require a worker use up to 2 weeks vacation	Employer may require use of all accrued vacation and paid personal time
Applies to all employers no matter how many workers are employed	Only applies to employers of 50 or more employees
No minimum period of service required to be eligible for leave	Requires 12 months of work to be eligible for leave
No exemption for key workers	Allows exemption for key workers (top 10% in salary)
Employee and the state determine eligibility	Employer determines eligibility

As deduced from the figures presented in Table 2, more than 88 percent of claims were for bonding with a new child. Of those, 83 percent were from mothers, 17 percent from fathers. About 12 percent took leave to care for a seriously ill family member, with 70 percent by women and 30 percent by men. However, the numbers of people applying for the benefit fell short of initial expectations. California estimated that 300,000 people would receive benefits within the first year, but only about half that number applied and even fewer received benefits (Quinn, 2005). Reasons for the lower numbers may range from many people being unaware of the program to workers viewing the average wage replacement of $409 as too small. However, pregnant women in particular may be more likely to apply for paid leave because they are already enrolled in the state disability system (SDI) that provides a wage replacement.

Opponents of the legislation, such as the California Chamber of Commerce and others, who initially argued that paid leave would harm business and make the state less appealing to investors, have not officially commented on the EDD report, other than to state that it is too

TABLE 2. Paid Family Leave Claims and Benefits
(July 1, 2004 through June 30, 2005)

Total Claims Received:	176,085
Total Benefits Paid:	$299,287,454
Average Weekly Benefit Amount:	$409.24
Average Weeks Per Claim:	4.84
Total Bonding Claims:	155,483
Type	*Percentage*
Females	83%
Males	17%
Biological	98.5%
Adoption/Foster	1.5%
Total Care Claims:	20,602
Type	*Percentage*
Females Providing Care	70%
Males Providing Care	30%
Caring for Spouse	36.3%
Caring for Child	22.1%
Caring for Parent	21.6%
Caring for Domestic Partner	1.3%
Caring for All Others	18.7%

Source: California State Employment Development Department (2005)

early to pass judgment. Efforts by Nevada and other states to encourage California's businesses to move to a "more friendly environment" where mandatory paid leave laws do not exist have not been successful (Quinn, 2005). However, it is likely that perhaps the law's utilization patterns and its impact on corporations will become more visible with each passing year. The California Development Department will report on the program annually.

IS CALIFORNIA'S PAID FAMILY LEAVE LAW A MODEL FOR OTHER STATES?

Following the passage of SB 1661 and its eventual signing by Governor Gray Davis, there was much euphoria among an assortment of advocacy groups that had fought hard for paid leave for more than a decade. Not surprisingly, the question as to whether or not California's success could be duplicated in other states quickly moved to the top of legislative agendas. However, as will be argued here, it is highly unlikely the California model can and will be replicated in more than a mere handful of states. The reasons supporting this conclusion are spelled out in some detail below.

First, only four other states have infrastructures and funding mechanisms similar to California's that could support paid family leave. That is, only five states in all (California, Hawaii, New Jersey, New York, and Rhode Island) have state mandated Temporary Disability Insurance (TDI). Therefore, if any of the other 45 states desire to adopt the California paid leave model, they will first have to create a TDI type of funding mechanism. It should be emphasized that the first state to adopt such a model for paid maternity leave (not family leave) was Rhode Island in 1942. Hawaii was the last state to adopt its TDI law in 1969 and no other state has done so for more than 35 years. It is somewhat of a curiosity that only five states adopted this model, none of them abandoned it, and yet no other state has adopted it. One of the oddities in the history of public policy, this unique phenomenon has yet to be explained adequately.

Second, whatever window of opportunity was open during 2002 for the enactment of paid leave, closed quickly. Since the passage of SB 1661, both the political and economic climate in California has changed drastically. In a recall election, Gray Davis was replaced by Arnold Schwarzenegger, who responded to a massive deficit by calling for major budget cuts. So too has the economic climate changed in other states and so too has the window of opportunity closed for them as well. Rising unemployment, combined with decreasing revenues, has created a retrenchment mentality on the part of policy makers in almost every state. Consequently, expanding leave policy to include a wage replacement is highly unlikely. And, therefore, with states having to dip into their Unemployment Insurance trust funds on a daily basis, the UI model for funding paid leave appears to be no longer feasible. Instead, many states are reduced to tinkering with employees' accrued sick leave and vacation time to serve as a proxy for paid leave.

And third, even if other states do pursue a strategy for adopting paid leave, it appears that most have veered away from the "family" (intergenerational) component that is at the very heart of the federal FMLA and have, instead, narrowed paid leave to "baby care." To its credit, particularly in light of the demographic forecasts that predict a growing aging population that will demand more family care, California maintained the intergenerational component in SB 1661. But of the 27 states that put forth paid leave initiatives over the last three years, only six (including California) inserted care of an elderly parent in their proposed bills. In a previous work I concluded that this phenomenon is representative of "two steps forward and one step back." That is, the first step forward was passage of the FMLA in 1993. The second step forward was Clinton's recommendation in 1999 that states adopt paid leave. And the one step backward, was the dropping of parent care ("family care") and limiting leave to care of newborns (Wisensale, 2003). In short, with such a widespread development among almost half the states, it is highly unlikely that a successful paid leave policy would resemble California's model anyway. It simply would not be "family care." Nor have other states included coverage for same-sex domestic partners in their proposals as has California. In fact, the FMLA does not include such coverage either.

Moving Forward or Sliding Backwards?

With few states succeeding in adopting paid leave laws, a more recent strategy has been to focus on paid sick leave. In a study conducted by the National Partnership for Women and Families in 2004, it was learned that 47 percent of private sector workers and 59 million total workers in the U.S. have no paid sick leave at all, although government workers do have paid sick leave (National Partnership for Women and Families, 2004). Without sick days, employees often come to work ill, decreasing productivity and infecting co-workers. The situation is even worse for workers with children. Nearly 86 million Americans do not have paid sick days that they can use to care for a sick child. Consequently, parents are often forced to send the ill child off to school, leave the child home alone, ask an older sibling to miss school to stay home and care for the child, or take time off from work with the possibility of losing their pay or their job.

To address this deficiency, more than half the states introduced legislation between 2002 and 2004 that would guarantee paid sick leave to employees. However, to date, only six states require employers to allow their workers to use their own sick leave to care for ill family members. Meanwhile, at the federal level, an initiative has been put forth to establish mandatory paid sick leave. Introduced by Senator Ted Kennedy (D-MA) and Representative Rosa DeLauro (D-CT) in April, 2005, the Healthy Families Act would guarantee seven paid sick days per year for full-time employees, and a pro-rata amount for part-time employees. It would cover public and private sector employers with at least 15 employees.

Some may argue that such developments represent progress. However, an equally strong argument can be made that sick leave is little more than incremental policymaking that, if adopted, will prevent the development of a more comprehensive paid leave policy that is comparable to many of the European models. After all, why should someone be required to use their own sick days to care for a family member? Should there not be a separate policy in place to support caregivers who need to take time off from work to care for their loved ones? In short, are we moving forward or backward with respect to paid leave policy in America? And what price will we pay as a society if we choose not to act at all?

Toward the Future: The Cost of Inaction

It is clear that the debate over paid leave will continue well into the future. Although it is argued here that few, if any, states will adopt a paid leave model similar to California's, this does not mean that other models will not emerge. And surely, the debates that follow will focus on cost estimates. But until the methodology employed is acceptable to both sides, the controversy surrounding the fiscal impact of paid leave will continue. An area often overlooked by researchers, however, particularly economists, is the cost of inaction. That is, can the absence of a particular policy be measured in terms of "cost" or economic "loss"? At least two studies completed so far concerning family care address this very question.

In their study, *Unnecessary Losses: Costs to America for the Lack of Family and Medical Leave*, Spalter-Roth and Hartmann (1990) concluded that employees, employers, and government all lose if family leave is either unavailable or unpaid. For example, women lacking maternity leave who returned to the job market after childbirth were unemployed longer and earned lower wages, amounting to a total of nearly $607 million in lost earnings in one year, compared to women who could take leave and return to their jobs. Employers also benefit from family leave through lower worker absenteeism, reduced turnover rates, enhanced productivity, higher morale, and greater company loyalty. Spalter-Rother and Hartmann also argue that government costs are reduced as well if a family-leave policy, preferably a paid one, is in place. Women who give birth, but cannot take leave (paid or unpaid), will require more income assistance in the form of government transfer payments. This is particularly true for lower-income workers. "At the lower end of the labor market social welfare policies to some extent operate as paid maternity leave," writes Kristin Weaver (1996, p. 20).

Another study that examined the costs of family care was the "1999 MetLife Juggling Act Study," produced for the MetLife Mature Market Institute in conjunction with the National Alliance for Caregiving and the National Center for Women and Aging at Brandeis University. According to the findings, family care costs individuals as much as $659,000 over their lifetimes in lost wages, lost Social Security benefits, and pension contributions because they take leave, quit their jobs entirely, or pass up opportunities for training, promotions, and choice assignments. When the $659,000 figure is broken down further, the caregivers studied lost $566,500 in wages, $67,000 in retirement contributions, and $25,500 in Social Security benefits. Twenty-nine percent reported that they declined promotions. Twenty-nine percent turned down transfer or relocation opportunities, and 22% claimed they missed out on opportunities to develop new job skills (MetLife, 1999).

Two years earlier, MetLife (1997) completed a study on the financial impact of family care on business. In the "MetLife Study of Employer Costs for Working Caregivers," it was reported that lost productivity due to family care costs U.S. businesses between $11 billion and $29 billion annually, not to mention lower morale among employees and declining retention rates. Lost also are lower turnover costs and higher productivity.

But is there another question to be asked? How much money has family caregiving saved American taxpayers? A 2004 MetLife study on caregiving nationwide reported that the value of family caregiving to society is estimated at $257 billion annually. The survey concluded that 44.4 million caregivers provide unpaid care to another adult. Almost six in ten (59%) of these caregivers either work or have worked while providing care, and about 62% have had to make some adjustments to their work life, from reporting late to work to giving up work entirely. Furthermore, with respect to elder care in particular, it is not just women who are the caregivers. Almost four in ten (39%) caregivers are men and 60% of them are working full time (MetLife, 2004).

Unfortunately, without appropriate supports, such as paid leave, many family caregivers will be unable to sustain their commitment, choosing instead to shift the costs of care onto society as a whole. This is further complicated by the fact that the real challenge of family care may still be in front of us. In 2010, the 78 million baby boomers in the United States will begin to turn sixty-five. Multiple chronic illnesses will become commonplace among this population and their caregiving demands will increase as they age. Clearly, this development will have a severe impact on families, corporations, and government. It is unlikely that either 12 weeks of paid parental leave (this is baby care, not elder care) or seven paid sick days will address this challenge.

In an era of conservative politics that tolerates little or no intervention by the federal government, states will be expected to put forth paid leave initiatives on their own but cost citizens and corporations little or nothing in taxes. While California represents a model of success, few states will or should replicate its actions because they will differ in political culture, economic stability, and policy history with respect to work and family issues. Consequently, each will have to develop its own unique funding mechanism that provides an adequate wage replacement for those employees who need to address family concerns.

REFERENCES

Bernstein, A. (2001). *The moderation dilemma: Legislative coalitions and the politics of family and medical leave.* Pittsburgh, PA: University of Pittsburgh Press.
California Assembly Appropriations Committee Hearing (2002). June 26, 2002. Sacramento, CA: California Assembly Television (video).
California Assembly Floor Debate (2002). Assembly Floor Debate on SB 1661, August 27, 2002. Sacramento, CA: California Assembly Television (video).

California Assembly Insurance Committee Hearing (2002). August 22, 2002. Sacramento, CA: California Assembly Television (video).
California Senate Appropriations Committee Hearing (2002). May 23, 2002. Sacramento, CA: California Senate Television (video).
California Senate Floor Debate (2002). Senate Floor Debate on SB 1661, August 30, 2002. Sacramento, CA: California Senate Television (video).
California Senate Labor and Industrial Relations Committee Hearing (2002). May 14, 2002. Sacramento, CA: California Senate Television (video).
California State Employment Development Department (2005). *Paid family leave insurance program year in review–July 1, 2004-June 30, 2005.* Sacramento: California State Employment Development Department.
Carsten, M. (2004). *Update on the California paid family leave studies.* Claremont, CA: Berger Institute for Work, Family and Children.
Commission on Leave (1996). *A workable balance: Report to Congress on family and medical leave policies.* Washington, DC: U.S.
Department of Labor. Department of Labor (2000). *Balancing the needs of families and employers: Family and medical leave surveys.* Washington, DC: Department of Labor.
Elving, R. (1995). *Conflict and compromise: How Congress makes the law.* New York, NY Simon and Schuster.
Gladstone, L. (1999). *Maternity and parental leave policies: A comparative analysis.* Washington, DC: Congressional Research Service Report, no. 85-148.
Gornick, J. & Meyers M. (2003). *Families that work: Policies for reconciling parenthood and employment.* New York, NY: Russell Foundation.
Heymann, J. (2005). Inequalities at work and at home: Social class and gender divides. In J. Heymann & C. Beem (Eds.). *Unfinished work: Building equality and democracy in an era of working families.* New York, NY: The New Press.
Hyde, J., Essex, M., Clark, R., Klein, M., & Byrd, J. (1996). Parental leave: Policy and research. *Journal of Social Issues, 52,* 91-109.
Jordan, L. (1999). *FMLA proposals.* Office of Legislative Research, Hartford, CT: Connecticut General Assembly.
Labor Project for Working Families (2003). *Putting families first: How California won the fight for paid family leave.* Berkeley, CA: Labor Project for Working Families.
MetLife (1997). *MetLife study of employer costs for working caregivers.* Westport, CT: MetLife Mature Market Institute.
MetLife (1999). *MetLife juggling act study.* Westport, CT: MetLife Mature Market Institute.
MetLife (2004). Caregiving in the U.S. Findings from the national caregiver survey. Westport, CT: MetLife Mature Market Institute.
Meyers, M. (1995). Taking pregnancy leaves. Minneapolis, MN: *Star Tribune,* February 6, 1995: A1.
National Partnership for Women and Families (2004). *Get well soon: Americans can't afford to be sick.* Washington, DC: The National Partnership for Women and Families.
National Partnership for Women and Families (2002). *State family leave benefit initiatives in the 2001-2002 state legislature: Making family leave more affordable.* Washington, DC: National Partnership for Women and Families.

President's Commencement Address (1999). Grambling State University, Grambling, LA, May 23. Washington, DC: The White House.

Presidential Memorandum (1999). Memorandum for the heads of executive departments and agencies: New tools to help parents balance work and family. May 24, 1999. Washington, DC: The White House.

Quinn, M. (2005). California's paid family leave act: In its infancy, many fail to take advantage of it. *San Jose Mercury News,* July 1, 2005, 4.

Spalter-Roth, R. & Hartmann, H. (1990). *Unnecessary losses: Costs to Americans of the lack of family and medical leave.* Washington, DC: Institute for Women's Policy Research.

Trzcinski, E. (1994). Pregnancy and parental leave in the United States and Canada. *Journal of Human Resources, 292,* 535-554.

Waldfogel, J. (1999). The impact of the family and medical leave act. *Journal of Policy Analysis and Management, 18,* 281-302.

Weaver, K. (1996).*The family and medical leave act.* Cambridge, MA: Radcliffe Public Policy Institute. Radcliffe College.

Wisensale, S. (2003). Two steps forward, one step back: The family and medical leave act as retrenchment policy. *Review of Policy Research, 20,* 135-151.

Wisensale, S. (2001). *Family leave policy: The political economy of work and family in America.* Armonk, NY: M. E. Sharper.

Birthstrikes?
Agency and Capabilities
in the Reconciliation of Employment
and Family

Barbara Hobson
Livia Sz. Oláh

SUMMARY. The purpose of this article is to analyze women's agency and fertility decisions in the context of policy configurations in welfare states for reconciling employment with having and caring for children and the changing aspirations and expectations for gender equality in

---

Barbara Hobson and Livia Sz. Oláh are affiliated with the Department of Sociology, Stockholm University.

The authors would like to thank Elizabeth Thomson, Michael Shalev, Janet Gornick and Frances Goldscheider for their important insights and suggestions for the first draft of this paper. The authors also want to acknowledge the valuable reviewers comments and those of the guest editors, Linda Haas and Steven Wisensale, who provided us with guidelines for the conceptual revisions made in the final draft. The authors also want to express their gratitude to Teresa Munzi for providing essential information regarding the LIS data, and to Emilia Niskanen for help with locating some errors in the data-file and correcting them. Ann Morrissens had the task of data-preparation in the preliminary analysis. A special thanks goes to Karin Halldén for her help with the ESS data. The authors wish to acknowledge the funding agencies that supported this research: the Swedish Humanistic and Social Science Research Foundation, and for the postdoctoral fellowship of Livia Oláh, the Swedish Council for Working Life and Social Research.

[Haworth co-indexing entry note]: "Birthstrikes? Agency and Capabilities in the Reconciliation of Employment and Family." Hobson, Barbara, and Livia Sz. Oláh. Co-published simultaneously in *Marriage & Family Review* (The Haworth Press, Inc.) Vol. 39, No. 3/4, 2006, pp. 197-227; and: *Families and Social Policy: National and International Perspectives* (ed: Linda Haas, and Steven K. Wisensale) The Haworth Press, Inc., 2006, pp. 197-227. Single or multiple copies of this article are available for a fee from The Haworth Document Delivery Service [1-800-HAWORTH, 9:00 a.m. - 5:00 p.m. (EST). E-mail address: docdelivery@haworthpress.com].

families. Employing the concept of birthstriking, inspired by Amartaya Sen's ideas on capabilities and agency freedom, we consider which individuals and families in the 1990s are delaying or not having children across 12 countries, representing four policy configuration models. Using household level data, we consider differences in education on the likelihood of having a first child. We find the clearest birthstriking effects in societies where there are weak reconciliation policies for motherhood and employment and few protections for families with uncertain economic futures. *[Article copies available for a fee from The Haworth Document Delivery Service: 1-800-HAWORTH. E-mail address: <docdelivery@haworthpress.com> Website: <http://www.HaworthPress.com> © 2006 by The Haworth Press, Inc. All rights reserved.]*

KEYWORDS. Capabilities and agency, fertility, reconciliation of employment and family, policy regimes

INTRODUCTION

Over the last decades, low birthrates and aging populations have been on the policy agenda in many countries. The long-term risks are obvious in terms of the sustainability of welfare states that assume that the productive workforce will provide the resources to shoulder the costs of care for the aged and disabled. Changing patterns of family formation are an important lens from which to view transformations in the construction of gender, work and family, and discussion of these relationships have been prominent in European discourse. Who is having or not having children reflects new risks (unstable and uncertain economic futures) as well as new opportunities and incentives for women to enter employment and ideologies and norms for gender equality and equity.

Institutions are the cornerstone in welfare state research but whereas there has been research on the cost of children, in relation to overall inequality and gender equality, until only recently has the focus turned to fertility itself. Some of the most sophisticated analyses have come from gender research on the welfare state, analyzing the child penalty for women seeking to combine parenting and paid work (see Gornick & Meyers, 2003; Gornick, Meyers & Ross, 1997, for the state of the art in this research). In demographic studies, on the other hand, fertility has been a key topic, yet not until recently have these studies focused on the role of social policies and institutions in shaping fertility. Women's labor force participation was built into demographic models as opportunity costs for women's fertility decisions, but social policy incentives and constraints were not. This has changed over the past few years (Brewster & Rindfuss, 2000; McDonald, 2000; Oláh, 2001).

This article is an attempt to create a bridge across demographic and welfare state research, considering micro-level fertility behaviors in different institutional contexts. Our purpose is to consider women's agency and fertility decisions in the context of policy configurations in welfare states for reconciling employment with having and caring for children and the changing aspirations and expectations for gender equality in families. From this perspective, birthstriking is a concept that is linked to what Amartya Sen refers to as capabilities and agency freedom (Sen, 1992; 2003). For Sen, capabilities involve an individual's real freedom to choose, which goes beyond inequalities in resources, but also embraces capabilities to achieve. In our case, this involves women's decisions around childbearing that exist within specific institutional settings that support or circumscribe the possibilities to combine employment with having a family. In this article, we frame birthstrikes as a question: Can we speak of birthstrike societies in which significant numbers of women lack agency freedom to form families? Are there differences within countries surrounding the variations in capabilities of women (for example, differences by education) to reconcile family and employment? As is true in striking in general, is birthstriking time limited so that when we speak of the 1990s as a birthstrike decade, we are implicitly asking, do we see signs of change, which is discussed in our concluding remarks. In this article, we focus on the 1990s and observe which individuals and families are delaying or not having children across twelve countries that are representative of different policy regimes (Esping-Andersen, 1990) or models of policy configurations for reconciling family and employment (Korpi, 2000).[1]

The article consists of three parts: (1) a presentation of the birthstrike concept and birthstrike decade; (2) a discussion of fertility regimes and welfare regimes; (3) an analysis of the variations across and within our 12 countries considering differences in education on the likelihood of women having a child birth in the 1990s and the likelihood of reconciling having children with employment. We consider how differences in the policy configurations in welfare regimes can mitigate the costs of children through policies that support mothers' employment.

THE BIRTHSTRIKING CONCEPT

The notion of a birthstrike has a legacy in feminism dating back to the early 20th century in which some feminists urged women to undertake a birthstrike as a strategy to campaign for equal treatment (Lewis, 1984). As is obvious, we are not conceptualizing birthstriking as purposeful action, in the sense of mobilized women who refuse to bear children until a condition is met. Rather, in using the term of birthstriking we want to highlight women's agency in the sense of capabilities. First, we assume that women have access to contraception and abortion, that is, they plan fertility. Second, we assume that individual fertility decisions take place within specific institutional contexts with policy configurations that can enhance or weaken capabilities surrounding childbearing.

Taking our inspiration from Amartya Sen's (2003) framework of capabilities and their relation to the institutional environment, we maintain that individual women lack agency freedom who are unable to achieve what is currently considered a conventionally agreed upon norm: that they will be both mothers and earners. Being able to combine employment with childbearing has become part of European discourse, framed as reconciliation of work and family life, with laws, policy and targets to promote it (Hobson, 2003).[2] The male breadwinner model, characterized by a traditional division of unpaid and paid work, is no longer the norm in affluent western states, reflected in survey responses of both men and women (DiPrete, Morgan, Engelhardt & Pacalova, 2003). Currently, there are incentives and pressures for mothers to enter the labor market, including changes in incentive structures for women to be in paid employment (increases in wages for women and decline in the earnings of men as well as insecurity in male jobs) alongside increased costs and higher consumption. Moreover, there are greater risks for mothers who are unable to reconcile employment with family, as economic dependency often translates into poverty after divorce (Hobson & Takahashi, 1997). Finally, gender equality ideologies have increased women's aspirations for greater equity in employment and a fairer division of paid and unpaid work in the household. Birthstriking therefore can be seen as a reflection of the disjuncture between aspirations and expectations and capabilities.

In his analysis of low fertility, Peter McDonald (2000) views this disjuncture between changes in women's economic roles and aspirations and the lack of change in institutions as the incoherence effect. Incoherence is a mechanism that captures the lack of fit in the institutional arrangements for reconciling family and employment, and its impact on gender inequality in the family. According to Turcotte and Gold-scheider (1998), inequality in the family when set against changing cultural norms is a mechanism for explaining low birthrates. We imagine that the incoherence effect is especially strong where there are institutional constraints in societies that inhibit women from combining having employment with having a family. These societies lack policies that allow women to reconcile employment with childbearing and childrearing, including available and affordable daycare, parental leave with adequate compensation, and the right to reduce hours during the early childhood years. Throughout, we refer to these as reconciliation policies.

We also imagine that birthstriking and capabilities can also reflect perceptions of economic uncertainty about the future. Ulrich Beck (1999) has coined the phrase "the risk society" to capture the sense of uncertainty that individuals feel about the instability in their lives (see also Adam, Beck & Van Loon, 2000). Qualitative and quantitative studies confirm that young people are more hesitant to form unions or consider having children in recently economically uncertain times (Santow & Bracher, 2001). Tanner and Yabiku (1999) contend that contemporary youth's transition to adulthood is delayed not because they have different goals than previous generations, but rather because the goal of attaining a stable job remains dominant. Currently, economic realities are frustrating this goal.

Within an institutional and capabilities framework, the perceptions of economic uncertainty in family formation are often conjoined with women's ability to reconcile employment with motherhood. Whereas the postwar settlement in Europe provided adult men in European welfare states with job protections and security, policies that protected male breadwinners from the uncertainties in the market, men's hourly wages and labor force activity decreased in the 1990s (Morissette, 1998; Oppenheimer & Lewin, 1999). From this perspective, women's lost earnings and potential earnings, as a result of childbearing and childrearing, can be very costly for families. Turcotte and Goldscheider (1998) argue that working is increasingly important for entering any kind of union (union formation requires earning power of both partners). A survey in Sweden addressing the precipitous decline in birthrates revealed that young people are less willing to consider childbearing without permanent jobs and housing (SCB, 2001).

Capabilities and economic uncertainties can be understood in terms of changing expectations and patterns in paid and unpaid work in families in the 1990s (Lewis, 2004). They reflect changes in institutional formulas around work and welfare, which call into question household economy models based on higher opportunity costs and static preferences (Becker, 1991; Hakim, 2003), as families cannot predict the future costs of children, and men and women bear these costs differently (Folbre, 1994).

It is important to keep in mind that not only do men and women have different capabilities to combine employment with family life, but also they perceive the risks attached to family formation differently. This is suggested in a study based on Eurobarometer questions on the perceived consequences of family formation (Sjöberg, 2004). Although both men and women viewed having children as enhancing their quality of life and networks, women revealed that having a family had greater consequences for labor market attachment and careers.[3]

In connecting our birthstrike concept to agency and capabilities, we are seeking to link the individual level–a woman's resources, expectations and aspirations–with societal and institutional levels. As we are focusing on the institutional conditions in a specific period, we assume that birthstriking could be time limited so that when we speak of women's agency, we are not just thinking in terms of women consciously deciding not to have children, but also in terms of women delaying them, which can result in childlessness or women having fewer children than they would choose. As questions in the Eurobarometer and the Population Policy Acceptance Study (PPAS) show, in European countries (including our 12 countries), less than 10 percent of women say that they do not want to have any children and nearly 60 percent claim that the optimum number of children is two (Sjöberg, 2004; Tazi-Preve & Dorbritz, 2005). Delay, and its possible impact on childlessness, is a dimension in our conceptual framework of capabilities and the 1990s as a birthstrike decade, in which there was a confluence of changing aspirations and expectations for gender inequality, alongside welfare state restructuring and policy changes.

THE 1990s: A BIRTHSTRIKE DECADE

We focus on the 1990s because it is a decade of dramatic fertility decline in Europe; in Central and Western Europe and in many advanced welfare states, fertility sank below replacement level. It also was a period of welfare state change and increasing global restructuring, undercutting the protections for workers and heightening the economic risks in dependence on a single earner family (Huber & Stephens, 2003). Most dramatically, the 1990s was the decade in which the transition from state-socialist to neo-liberal economies took place. In these societies, the shock therapy of neo-liberalism altered the expectations and capabilities of families who had previously lived under a regime in which employment was guaranteed, stable low prices were maintained through government subsidies, and social policies encouraged early marriages and high birth rates (Standing, 1996). These are societies that experienced some of the most precipitous declines in fertility during the 1990s.

The 1990s is a period in which the ideologies and policies for male breadwinning were on the wane. Pressures both from without and within welfare states to streamline costly benefits led to weakening or end of the marriage subsidy for men in the form of tax supports for single male breadwinner household, to allow women to remain at home as full time carers(Knijn & Kremer, 1997; Taylor-Gooby, 1996). While the demise of the single-earner male breadwinner family has been a gradual process, and still not completed in many countries, the 1990s has been a turning point with the dramatic rises in women's labor force participation in societies with strong male breadwinner ideologies and policies (Lewis, 2002), including Germany, Netherlands, and UK in our analysis.

FERTILITY REGIMES AND WELFARE STATE REGIMES AND POLICY CONFIGURATIONS

Though we focus on the 1990s, we should underscore that fertility decline has been a long process. The demographic trends that we highlight are the results of long-term changes in family patterns in the developed world since the mid-1960s, which is seen as the end of "The Golden Age of the Family" with high marriage and birth rates at relatively young ages, low divorce rates, and the rareness of non-traditional family forms. By the 1990s, marriage rates were low and/or declining, the mean age at first marriage and at first birth increased and fertility declined below the replacement level (i.e., 2.1 children per woman) (Council of Europe, 2002). The rates of family dissolution are rising, even among couples with children; second and higher-order partnerships have become more common, making childbearing decisions even more complex given children from previous relationships.

In the range of below-replacement fertility, demographers distinguish between three levels: (1) *low fertility*, that is below replacement but at least 1.5 children per woman, (2) *very low fertility*, i.e., less than 1.5 but at least 1.3 children per woman, (3) *lowest low fertility*, that is, less than 1.3 children per woman (Billari, 2004; Kohler, Billari & Ortega, 2002). These fertility regimes reflect the patterns of total fertility, age at first birth as well as contraceptive use. In our study of 12 countries, we use two broad categories: medium and low fertility regimes. The former includes France, Netherlands, Norway, Finland, Sweden, the UK and Canada;[4] and the latter comprises Germany, Italy, Spain, Hungary and Czech (see Figure 1).

FIGURE 1. Total Fertility Rates, 1960-2000. Countries Grouped by Their TFR in 2000

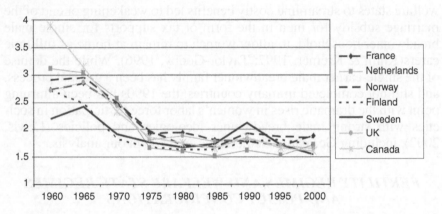

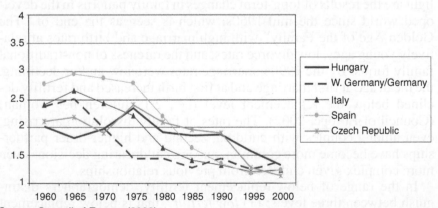

Source: Council of Europe (2002).
Note: The figure for Germany is based on information on West Germany only for the period before the unification.

These fertility clusters have challenged one set of cultural explanations for demographic behavior concerning the role of religion and family values as dimensions of high fertility, as countries scoring high on these dimensions now have the lowest fertility, such as Spain and Italy (Billari, 2004). Furthermore, the discussions around the relationship between women's labor force participation and fertility have raised questions about the simple trade-off between career and childbearing. There has been a dominant assumption in demographic analysis based on rational choice models that women's increased employment opportunities in the labor market will result in low fertility (Becker, 1991). What has been called "the positive turn" describes the following pattern: Beginning in the mid- to late-1980s, the negative correlation between women's labor force participation and fertility shifted to a positive correlation (Ahn & Mira, 2002; Esping-Andersen, 1999). The positive turn has led to a lively debate in the demographic literature (Engelhardt, Kögel & Prskawetz, 2004) but it has also spawned some interest among welfare researchers who have focused on women's labor force participation (Castles, 2003; Esping-Andersen, 1999). The positive turn reflects overall aggregate trends in OECD countries, but the picture appears much more complex when we consider the patterns in specific countries in specific institutional contexts (Hobson & Oláh, 2006).

In contrast to fertility regimes, policy regimes have been constructed around work and welfare variables. They are broad institutional approaches that go beyond specific policies or levels of welfare state spending. Rather, they are based on theorizing around the institutional relationships between states, markets and families and the path dependencies in these relationships. The family had not been well integrated in policy regime theorizing (Lewis, 1992; Orloff, 1993). Gender was a dimension conspicuously absent in the empirical analyses mainly focused on full time (male) workers. However over the last decade gender and family have become central dimensions to welfare state research and integrated into the welfare regime paradigm (Gornick & Meyers, 2003; Korpi, 2000; O'Connor, Orloff & Shaver, 1999).

Welfare regime typologies have been used as a heuristic device for looking at the variations across countries and there is value in using a model that is well recognized. However the Esping-Andersen model based on his (1990) book, *The Three Worlds of Welfare Capitalism,* does not include post-socialist countries. Furthermore, welfare regime typologies assumed welfare state policy constellations around gender and employment before the 1990s, our birthstrike decade. These same critiques can be levelled at the Korpi (2000) gender policy configuration model. Nonetheless, his typology of *Dual Earner, Market Oriented* and *General Family Support* is built from the scoring of different policies that might affect women's ability to combine motherhood and employment and could be adapted (Ferrarini, 2003) to include hybrid models. Our transition, post-socialist economies appear to have characteristics of the dual earner/market oriented types.

Most importantly for our study, Korpi (2000) incorporates gender analytically within a capabilities framework. He argues that variations in different policy configurations, including family allowance, family tax benefits, and public daycare services are highly relevant for variations in gender agency inequalities in women's labor force participation. Given the growing acceptance of the dual earner family norm in European societies, the idea that governments seek to support traditional family models (his General Family Support type) is probably less true of the 1990s. Nevertheless, the path dependencies in these countries, often dominated by Confessional Christian political parties advocating traditional familial values, can influence the policy options governments consider[5] when deciding whether individuals, other family members (grandparents and other relatives), the state or the market should shoulder the responsbility for care. These options shape women's agency and capabilities to have and care for children.

THE PRESENT STUDY

In our comparative analysis, we use the policy configurations in the Korpi model as ideal types and as a heuristic tool for analyzing similarities and differences among our countries and to suggest divergent patterns in the 1990s. Following but modifying his model, we organize our countries into four clusters: Dual Earner, General Support, and Market-Oriented. Our fourth cluster is the Transition Post-Socialist Countries that are a hybrid between the Dual Earner and Market-Oriented types.

In recognizing the 1990s as a pivotal decade in the changes in women's labor force participation among once strong male breadwinner model societies, we expect that the General Family Support cluster of countries will seem less similar than the Korpi model has assumed. For example, other researchers have classified Italy and Spain as a separate model in policy regime literature (Ferrara, 1996) because of the salience and persistence of the family as the form of care provision in Southern Europe, compared to the rest of Europe (Reher, 1998). We expect that France may fit more in the Dual Earner group with Sweden, Finland and Norway. France actually ranks high in Korpi's dual earner category, following the Nordic countries and in Gornick and Meyers' (1997) policy indexes on child care provision and employment index.

Agency and capabilities in Korpi's analysis are embedded in two analytically distinct institutional models for gender inequality and class inequality. Gender inequalities in his model are the result of women's lack of labor force participation and weak reconcilation policies (women who cannot combine employment with motherhood reflect agency inequality); class inequalities are mediated by social insurance programs and are reflected in the low levels of disposable household income. Our approach to gender agency and capabilities seeks to overcome this division of gender and class inequalities into distinct models. Rather we seek to link theoretically how institutional frameworks affect gendered capabilities and family formation through facilitating employment and motherhood and by mitigating the costs of children for families, considering household incomes with and without children. We assume that societies that allow the reconciliation of motherhood and employment make it easier for families to absorb the costs of children. Furthermore, we presume that social protections for workers are important for women workers, who often work in part time or flexible insecure jobs, who are vulnerable in periods of economic downturns and high unemployment as was the case in the 1990s in many countries. Throughout our analysis, we refer to female and overall unemployment levels, which we have gathered for each country for the year before the survey we use in our analysis (see Figure 2). Access to jobs (the job market) as well as security in jobs are connected to capabilities and agency freedom to start a family. Given the countries in this study, Korpi's *Dual Earner, General Family Support,* and *Market Oriented* clusters (gender policy configurations) match his clusters exemplifying his social insurance models, which reflect different types of social insurance coverage for pensions and unemployment (Korpi, 2000; Korpi & Palme, 1998). These policy constellations on reconciliation policies and social insurance coverage pick up aspects of both agency capabilities mechanisms: incoherence and economic uncertainty.

Finally, we assume that variations in reconciliation policies and uncertainties surrounding employment affect different women differently. Our study allows us to consider individual agency: which women in which institutional contexts have more or less agency to combine employment with having children? The capabilities approach we take

FIGURE 2. Total Unemployment Rate and Female Unemployment Rate (%) for the 12 Countries in the Analysis

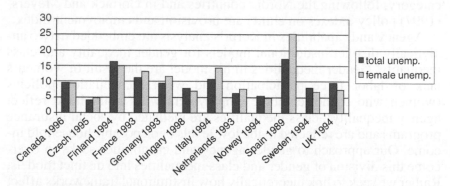

Source: ILO (diff. years)
Note: Both total unemployment rate and female unemployment rate refer to the year before the survey we use from the LIS database.

assumes situated agency; institutional contexts might affect women differently. We consider differences between women across educational levels.

Hypotheses

Highly educated women are generally the most likely to delay or have fewer children (Kravdal, 2001). In societies in which women with a secondary education also tend to delay births, we expect mothers to have less agency to combine having children with employment.

Our capabilities approach suggests that in welfare states with both highly developed reconciliation policies and social provisions that act as a buffer for workers from market downturns, there would be a lower likelihood of birthstriking. We would therefore not find marked differences between highly and lowly educated women. Nordic societies might best exemplify this model.

We hypothesize that in welfare states with weak reconciliation policies and with few protections for workers who face unemployment, we would find significant levels of birthstriking with significant differences across educational groups. Italy and Spain with their high unemployment levels (see Figure 2) and low levels of daycare provisions are the cases that would express these tendencies.

In light of our analysis on agency and capabilities, we must consider norms and expectations in birthstriking. The incoherence effect and uncertainty may be felt strongly in Central Eastern European societies. These are societies in which individuals and families experienced a dramatic change from stable and predictable futures to uncertainties in employment after the transformation to a market economy. They already have dual earner societies in place, but the reconciliation policies and services once provided by the state no longer exist. We should expect pervasive birthstriking effects that cut across educational groups.

Data and Methods

Our empirical analysis is based on data from the Luxembourg Income Study (LIS), which covers a large number of countries including post-socialist states such as the Czech Republic and Hungary, and provides comparable data on income[6] and employment as well as a range of demographic and socio-economic variables for the 1990s. We use data from the fourth wave of LIS surveys, ranging from the mid-1990s to 1999, except for Spain in which the survey year was 1990. (See Tables 1 and 2 in Appendix 1 for the list of surveys and a complete description of the construction of the variables.) We realize the disadvantage in analyzing fertility with this type of cross sectional data, i.e., that we do not know the employment histories before the births, which constrains the choice of the models we can use to explore the mechanisms of the institutional effects on childbearing. Yet LIS has the advantage over other data sets in that it has large sample sizes and includes Eastern European societies, which are countries with some of the lowest birthrates.

In our analysis, we select women aged 25-40, as they are the most likely to have a young child in the household given the relatively high mean age at first birth in European countries in the 1990s (Council of Europe, 2002), as well as in Canada. Single mothers are excluded, as their labor force attachment as well as economic situation are very different than that of women in couples (see Sorensen, 1994). Women in couples may be married or cohabiting.

We use different types of models in our analyses, and in each, the data are analyzed separately for each country to detect within country differences. First, we analyze the likelihood of having a first child using logit regression.[7] Excluding single women, we compare women in couples who have a child under four years of age in the household with women without children to see the variations across educational levels in who did and did not start a family. In this analysis, we are interested in a mother's delaying starting a family in a birthstrike decade. In the model, we control for the woman's age as well as the spouse's (cohabiting partner's) income.

Using OLS-regression, we next focus on the association between number of children and household income (after taxes and transfers), distinguishing between families with no child in the household and those with one, two, three or more young children (i.e., where age of youngest child is below 4) and those with older children only. We control for the woman's educational level and age (as mentioned before, single mothers are excluded).

Finally, using multinomial logit regression analysis, we consider the variations across countries around women's possibilities to combine employment and family responsibilities. Our dependent variable has six categories: (1) employed women with no child; (2) nonemployed women with no child; (3) employed women with a youngest child aged four to eleven years; (4) nonemployed women with a youngest child aged four to eleven years; (5) employed women with a youngest child aged one to three years; and (6) nonemployed women with a youngest child aged one to three years. As most mothers are not working for a portion of the child's first year (in EU countries they are entitled to maternity leave), we excluded those women with a child younger than one year from this analysis. Woman's age and educational attainment are our independent variables in this analysis. In all our models, higher education is our reference category and woman's age is used as a categorical variable with the oldest age range (35-40 years) as our referent.

Family policies can affect different groups of women differently, which is often ignored by research focusing on the effect of policy programs on the propensity to have children (Gauthier & Hatzius, 1997), since aggregate data cannot display differences in entitlements and benefits between different subgroups of a population. In our comparative analysis, we are able to consider how different policy configurations might influence fertility decisions among women with different educational levels.

RESULTS

The Likelihood of Having a First Birth

We would expect that highly educated women are more likely to delay or have fewer children than women with less education. We find this to be true in nearly all our countries (see Table 1). In the Dual-Earner na-

TABLE 1. Relative Odds of Having One Child Below 4 Years of Age in the Household in Different Policy Regime Countries. Logit Regression (S.E. in Parenthesis)

	Woman's educ. primary	Woman's educ. secondary	Woman's educ. high	Husband's income percentile, 0-25	Husband's income percentile, 25-50	Husband's income percentile, 50-75	Husband's income percentile, 75-100	Woman's age 25-29 y.	Woman's age 30-34 y.	Woman's age 35-40 y.	Number of obs.	Pseudo R^2
Sweden	0.89 (0.22)	1.15 (0.16)	1.00	1.19 (0.22)	1.14 (0.22)	0.98 (0.18)	1.00	1.25 (0.23)	1.53** (0.29)	1.00	914	0.007
Norway	1.24 (0.38)	1.30 (0.30)	1.00	1.32 (0.36)	1.58* (0.42)	1.67** (0.43)	1.00	6.46*** (2.00)	5.99*** (1.91)	1.00	501	0.091
Finland	0.79 (0.24)	1.15 (0.19)	1.00	1.57** (0.34)	1.43 (0.32)	1.46** (0.31)	1.00	1.64** (0.36)	2.00*** (0.47)	1.00	771	0.019
France	0.37*** (0.09)	1.15 (0.24)	1.00	1.15 (0.24)	1.69*** (0.34)	1.13 (0.23)	1.00	2.21*** (0.50)	3.02*** (0.75)	1.00	877	0.070
Netherlands	1.44 (0.40)	1.24 (0.30)	1.00	1.82** (0.56)	2.15*** (0.62)	1.40 (0.40)	1.00	1.27 (0.39)	2.16*** (0.68)	1.00	545	0.029
Germany	3.28*** (1.43)	2.25** (0.87)	1.00	1.48 (0.43)	1.17 (0.33)	1.37 (0.37)	1.00	1.62 (0.50)	2.86*** (0.94)	1.00	559	0.035
Italy	1.76** (0.47)	1.65** (0.40)	1.00	5.39*** (1.18)	5.99*** (1.22)	4.63*** (1.54)	1.00	1.11 (0.29)	2.29*** (0.62)	1.00	1046	0.123
Spain	2.33*** (0.31)	1.22 (0.17)	1.00	3.58*** (0.50)	3.08*** (0.42)	3.40*** (0.48)	1.00	1.76*** (0.31)	2.58*** (0.49)	1.00	2056	0.082
UK	1.33 (0.33)	1.60** (0.39)	1.00	1.09 (0.26)	0.94 (0.21)	0.76 (0.20)	1.00	1.30 (0.33)	1.68** (0.44)	1.00	610	0.012
Canada	1.06 (0.18)	1.27** (0.12)	1.00	1.60*** (0.20)	.47*** (0.17)	1.45*** (0.16)	n.a.	1.71*** (0.20)	2.61*** (0.31)	1.00	2912	0.028
Czech	0.88 (0.16)	0.99 (0.17)	1.00	n.a.	n.a.	n.a.	1.00	5.67*** (1.28)	4.78*** (1.20)	1.00	1503	0.055
Hungary	0.93 (0.64)	1.21 (0.85)	1.00	1.83 (0.88)	2.84** (1.42)	#	1.00	1.88 (1.22)	2.48 (1.73)	1.00	128	0.053

*** significant at 1%-level, ** at 5%, * at 10% # too small category, dropped

211

tion group there is no significant difference between higher educated women and those with less education when considering the likelihood of having a first birth in the 1990s. For Sweden and Finland, however, we find an unusual pattern, that women with only a primary school education have the lowest odds for childbearing. These findings, though not significant, are confirmed by other studies (RFV, 2001), and are probably a reflection of the sense of insecurity that arose from the economic crises of the early 1990s in both countries, affecting working class families to a much greater extent than middle class families. The similar pattern for French women can be explained by the fact that lowly educated women have more than one child (Corman, 2001; Hobson & Oláh, 2006).

In the General Family Support group, Germany, Italy and Spain are countries with the lowest fertility rates and weak reconciliation policies. They all show significant educational variations; highly educated women have the lowest odds of having a first birth. The most highly educated seem to opt for no children or delay childbearing (i.e., birthstriking) in institutional settings in which it is extremely difficult to reconcile having children with employment, given few possibilities for part time work as well as limited access to childcare services (Gornick & Meyers, 2003). In Germany, the organization of daycare and even primary school scheduling require a mother at home.

Our Market-Oriented group, Canada and the UK, displayed significantly higher odds for first birth for women with secondary education as compared to the highly educated. In all these countries, the higher educated women are delaying birth. For our Transition Post-Socialist countries, the Czech Republic and Hungary, who have extremely low fertility, we find no significant differences among women across our educational levels. We interpret this as a pervasive birthstriking effect linked to capabilities.

Disposable Household Income and the Effects of Children

In this analysis we focus on the association between children and disposable household income by comparing income for families with different numbers of young children with that of families without children. (We do not report here the results for families with older children.) As women's income tends to decline after birth, this is our indirect way of capturing some of the effects of childbearing and women's employment in different policy constellations.[8]

Since it is well known that most women reduce their employment after a birth, the expectation is that families with young children will be worse off than those without. However we find that in our Dual Earner countries and in France, families with young children have higher household income than the childless; i.e., those who do not have children are the ones who are worse off economically (Table 2). These are countries with strong reconciliation policies so that mothers have the possibility to return to employment after the first year. Families with children in countries of the General Family Support group, other than France, are worse off economically than those without children. In the Netherlands, Spain and Italy the effect is significant independently of the number of children, and in Germany we find significant effects for two-child families. In these countries, women have little chance of combining employment with having a family.

We find a similar pattern in Market-Oriented countries. In both the UK and Canada, children are associated with lower household income when compared to childless families (the effect is not significant for large families in Canada). Also in the transition countries, families with children have lower household income than the childless and this is significant for all Czech families (i.e., with one, two, or more children). In Hungary, it is families with one small child who are significantly worse off economically than those without children, which may reflect greater pressures on young families.

These results suggest that our Dual Earner countries, Sweden, Finland, Norway as well as France (who we suggested might be more similar to the Dual Earner countries in some parts of the analysis), are exceptional in that mothers do not have to interrupt their labor force attachment even in the first years after birth. They are societies with the highest numbers of children in publicly supported daycare. Moreover, among our twelve countries, they have the highest proportions of share of public sector jobs (Hobson & Oláh, 2006). These jobs tend to be more secure and the workplaces are often female dominated and considered to be more family friendly (Hoem, 1995). The positive association between household income and having children in these countries reflects the ways in which institutional settings can reduce the sense of risk and economic uncertainties that might inhibit family formation. Where it is more difficult for women to reconcile childbearing and employment, children have a negative effect on total household income.

TABLE 2. The Effects of Children on Household Income in Different Policy Regime Countries. OLS Regression (S.E. in Parenthesis) #

	1 kid, below 4 years	2 kids, youngest below 4 years	3 or more kids, youngest below 4 years	woman's age 30-34 years	woman's age 25-29 years	primary education	secondary education	cons.	Number of obs.	Adj. R^2
Sweden	8357.04 (6246.69)	28280.19*** (5655.41)	33945.82*** (6672.27)	-19270.35*** (4299.36)	-43808.11*** (5136.67)	-54454.42*** (5886.74)	-34929.85*** (3985.21)	307048.90*** (5698.86)	3038	0.083
Norway	21466.36* (12764.07)	13633.36 (11505.66)	25901.67*** (12221.17)	-28086.97*** (7995.83)	-78384.44*** (9612.51)	-71943.24*** (9383.57)	-33329.64*** (8904.11)	393535.30*** (11879.30)	2034	0.059
Finland	14450.78*** (5343.51)	12812.59*** (4663.26)	31014.20*** (5156.30)	-6991.78** (3588.49)	-23314.14*** (4030.36)	-41122.55*** (4965.59)	-31995.45*** (3392.96)	122549.50*** (6002.31)	2674	0.155
France	7470.01 (5836.91)	6637.23 (5694.10)	18649.86*** (6398.12)	-25005.35*** (3948.97)	-44206.59*** (4600.09)	-122109.00*** (5987.51)	-90646.57*** (5434.34)	212268.40*** (6945.00)	3297	0.211
Netherlands	-3901.18** (1878.26)	-8307.35*** (1607.25)	-3701.29* (1972.59)	-5106.50*** (1245.67)	-8496.14*** (1447.33)	-16147.67*** (1405.48)	-8720.84*** (1294.12)	44214.08*** (1823.81)	1663	0.231
Germany	-799.69 (2709.79)	-7330.27*** (2555.65)	-3319.13 (3497.65)	-5047.29*** (1745.73)	-9357.22*** (1914.35)	-17527.21*** (2784.42)	-10722.89*** (2451.76)	47632.66*** (3266.31)	1963	0.095
Italy	-8058.74*** (1793.18)	-10692.61*** (1692.17)	-9509.78*** (2568.44)	-869.23 (1294.21)	-1322.48 (1409.63)	-23532.58*** (1705.82)	-11805.99*** (1645.60)	46505.06*** (2272.31)	2630	0.119
Spain	-169965.50*** (47390.35)	-205270.00*** (45079.35)	-232062.00*** (55579.15)	-148860.00*** (32264.85)	-167838.30*** (34627.09)	-1569749.00*** (37738.36)	-898154.40*** (42321.81)	3249755.00*** (57539.24)	7485	0.218
UK	-2786.16*** (967.14)	-2872.60*** (905.92)	-3934.47*** (1091.60)	-2072.82*** (693.58)	-4245.76*** (769.56)	-10953.45*** (844.06)	-5698.75*** (880.35)	22341.48*** (1118.16)	1813	0.153
Canada	-2039.63*** (829.96)	-1772.10** (762.30)	-1154.01 (907.64)	-2028.59*** (539.33)	-3478.51*** (599.92)	-19723.85*** (793.75)	-11216.03*** (594.34)	44791.84*** (803.04)	9784	0.108
Czech	-363.01*** (52.87)	-394.86*** (44.68)	-343.50*** (66.00)	-156.73*** (28.35)	-137.43*** (31.30)	-812.09*** (39.77)	-467.17*** (38.90)	1810.05*** (55.65)	6768	0.135
Hungary	-250580.50* (140330.80)	-130570.30 (121834.80)	-163083.30 (155166.40)	47541.74 (83382.06)	-23951.53 (90224.72)	-1327553.00*** (144578.50)	-925199.00*** (150892.80)	2149266.00*** (189228.80)	531	0.160

*** significant at 1%-level, ** at 5%, * at 10%.
# In the model we have controlled for whether the woman is partnered or not. These results are not reported in the table, but are available upon request.

214

Reconciling Employment with Young Children

Finally, we address the reconciliation of work with family responsibilities for women living in couple relationships, using a multinomial logit model. Though we include childless women in the construction of our dependent variable, we are mainly interested in the variations across countries around women's possibilities to combine employment with having children, so we do not display the results for the childless here (see Table 3). We compare women with children of a certain age who are not employed with those employed. The category of having a child aged one to three years is central to our analysis since during these ages the institutional supports for combining employment and childbearing vary significantly. We exclude women with very young children as all our countries have some maternal benefit for children less than one year and a vast majority of women in our twelve countries are not back at work in the first year.

Our results (Table 3) show that women with post-secondary education are much more likely to be employed with small children in nearly all our countries than those with less education. The exceptions are the two post-socialist states in which there is no significant difference across educational levels. In all our other countries, women with the lowest levels of education tend to be out of the labor force when they have young children (the odds ranging from two to thirteen times when compared with our reference category, the highly educated). This is most pronounced in countries with overall high unemployment and high female unemployment (see Figure 2), including France, Spain, and Italy. Mothers with less education are in a weaker position in the labor market, but it is also possible that women in low-skilled and low-paying jobs may be less concerned about continuous employment. However, lowly educated mothers even with children over four years of age tend to have a much higher propensity to be out of the labor force.[9]

We assume that variations in institutional supports for mothers of young children would matter most for those with a middle educational level (secondary education, with a high school degree). Nevertheless, it is hard to find a clear pattern. Among our Dual Earner countries, Sweden is the only country in which mothers with a secondary education do not differ from highly educated women in their labor force attachment during the early years of childrearing. The relative odds are about 2.5 times as great for high school graduates than for highly educated women in Norway and Finland, about the same as in France. One might also expect to find a greater gap between highly and middle educated

TABLE 3. Reconciliation of Employment and Family Life in Different Policy Regime Countries. Multinomial Logistic Regression. Relative Odds (S.E. in Parenthesis)

Country	Education	youngest child 1-3 years old, not employed[1]	youngest child 4-11 years old, not employed[2]	Number of obs.	Pseudo R^2
Sweden	primary	4.99*** (1.31)	4.53*** (1.30)	2516	0.089
	secondary	1.17 (0.26)	1.70** (0.44)		
Norway	primary	6.61*** (2.15)	2.49*** (0.71)	1624	0.061
	secondary	2.64*** (0.84)	1.48 (0.43)		
Finland	primary	6.82*** (2.35)	7.43*** (3.30)	1971	0.082
	secondary	2.22*** (0.47)	3.69*** (1.50)		
France	primary	10.65*** (3.51)	5.75*** (2.20)	2695	0.081
	secondary	2.67*** (0.82)	1.79 (0.67)		
Netherlands	primary	7.95*** (2.87)	2.84*** (0.91)	1422	0.133
	secondary	3.91*** (1.29)	1.31 (0.42)		
Germany	primary	6.53*** (3.76)	2.24*** (0.70)	1529	0.067
	secondary	1.62 (0.87)	0.86 (0.25)		
Italy	primary	13.37*** (5.65)	9.33*** (4.00)	2113	0.113
	secondary	3.34*** (1.38)	2.54** (1.10)		
Spain	primary	9.80*** (1.69)	8.40*** (1.38)	6048	0.110
	secondary	3.67*** (0.71)	3.78*** (0.68)		
UK	primary	1.90** (0.59)	2.21** (0.85)	1496	0.085
	secondary	0.89 (0.29)	1.26 (0.53)		
Canada	primary	5.27*** (0.97)	4.86*** (0.80)	8221	0.064
	secondary	1.85*** (0.26)	1.54*** (0.23)		
Czech Rep.	primary	1.42 (0.41)	2.26*** (0.49)	5262	0.049
	secondary	0.93 (0.25)	1.43* (0.31)		
Hungary	primary	1.92 (1.73)	2.41 (1.96)	420	0.059
	secondary	0.86 (0.82)	0.78 (0.68)		

*** significant at the 1%-level, ** at 5%, * at 10%.
Note: Tertiary education (relative odds = 1) is the reference category.
[1] "Youngest child 1-3 years old, employed" is the comparison group.
[2] "Youngest child 4-11 years old, employed" is the comparison group.

women in countries with market-oriented care services, in which professional women can afford to buy services. But this is not the case. In the UK, a country with one of the lowest levels of publicly supported daycare, there is no significant difference between the highly and middle educated women. In Canada, there are differences but not very great in comparison to other countries: the odds of being out of the labor force are less than twice as high for women with a secondary education than for those with a university education. Considering the General Family Support countries, we find significant differences in Netherlands and France, but not in Germany. Spain and Italy with their strong familialist traditions and lack of reconciliation policies stand out even among the General Family Support Countries.

In Spain and Italy, we find patterns that reveal the linkages between birthstriking and weak capabilities. Both are countries with the characteristics of a low fertility regime with a very low total fertility rate. In both, mothers with secondary education have high propensities to be out of the labor force and this is even true for mothers with children over four. Most striking in these countries is among the lowly educated mothers (who are a very large group in these countries): those with children under four are ten to thirteen times more likely to be among the nonemployed compared to the highly educated; those with older children ages four to eleven years are eight and nine times less likely to be employed.

DISCUSSION

Our birthstriking concept embedded in a capabilities framework suggests that individual decisions around not having or delaying children can be influenced by institutional settings: societies with both weak reconciliation policies and weak protections for workers may operate as constraints for family formation. Italy and Spain provide clear examples. Both countries have high unemployment and among the highest female unemployment among our countries in the early 1990s (Spain at 25 percent and Italy nearly at 15 percent), and both have weak reconciliation policies. Even at the end of the 1990s, there was no compensation for parental leave, low proportions of publicly funded day care (Gornick & Meyers, 2003), and few possibilities for women for part time work (Guillén, 2003). For middle and lowly educated women, who cannot afford to buy services, these represent constraints.

Embedded in the framework of capabilities are aspirations and expectations. Societies in which we can detect a dramatic change in agency to reconcile work and family responsibilities and greater economic uncertainty about the future than in the past are fertile ground for birthstriking. Our transition societies are paradigm societies with these conditions.[10] There has been a remarkable birth decline, resulting in a total fertility rate as low as 1.1 in the Czech Republic and 1.3 in Hungary. We found no significant differences between the highly and lowly educated women in the likelihood of delaying first birth, an indicator of pervasive birthstriking. In contrast to other European countries, these former soviet regime societies show a substantial decrease in women's labor force participation in the 1990s. There are diminishing possibilities for reconciling employment with childbearing, less compensation for parental leave and a nearly complete shift from publicly funded to private daycare (Kocourkova, 2002). Though neither the Czech Republic nor Hungary display the high female unemployment levels of Spain or Italy, we can presume uncertainty in economic futures, in light of the shift from secure jobs for a lifetime to weak protections for workers in neo-liberal market economies and from public sector jobs for women to far fewer public sector jobs.

As we expected, our Dual Earner welfare states, through reconciliation policies, enhance women's capabilities and agency to combine employment with having and caring for children; none fall into the low fertility category. The positive association between having children and household income reflects the importance of high compensation for parental leave and extensive public daycare services, as well as the tendency of mothers in these states to return to their jobs after the first year,[11] contributing to the family economy. Though Nordic countries show no variations between highly and middle educated women in likelihood of having a first birth, in both Sweden and Finland, we found that lowly educated women were not having children compared with women with higher education. This is a surprising result compared to cross-national demographic patterns, but also in light of expectations that Dual Earner societies reduce differences among women in agency and capabilities to reconcile family and work. We interpret the birth delay among lowly educated women within the context of the economic crisis in the 1990s in both countries. In addition, it provides some evidence for our broader argument about capabilities involving aspirations and expectations. In both these societies, the dual earner family norm has been ubiquitous in discourse, policy and practice for decades.

Persistent Trends: A Birthstrike Decade?

We raise the question at the beginning of this article whether we can speak of the 1990s as a birthstrike decade. Whereas striking is a time limited response to specific conditions, our concept of birthstriking occurs in a contextualized period of welfare state change; we are asking whether conditions have changed that might affect agency and capabilities in fertility decisions. It is too soon to have a clear and definite answer about the 1990s, but in the 2000s we can look for continuity in the patterns and trends in the countries where we found patterns of birthstriking in the 1990s. At the outset, we can say that these countries remain low fertility countries, and in the case of the Czech Republic, there is further decline. As the later waves are not yet complete in the LIS for many of our countries, we are unable to do any systematic analysis on whether we find the same patterns. Nevertheless using information from the recent waves of the European Social Survey[12] (from 2002-3), we have some descriptive statistics on whether the patterns of delay of births we observed among women in these countries appeared to be persisting among women between the ages of 30-45; this age range is at least five years beyond the LIS sample years. In Spain it is 10 years. Thus women in Spain who are 30 now would have been 20 in the LIS wave used in this analysis. The patterns we found in Germany, Italy and Spain in the 1990s appear similar in the early 2000s; we find that highly educated women in these countries are still not having children (with high proportions of childlessness; see Appendix 2). In Hungary and the Czech Republic, where we noted pervasive birthstriking across educational levels, only in Hungary do we find some differences in childlessness among the highly and lowly educated, but not nearly as great as in Germany, Italy or Spain. We found almost no difference among educational groups in the Czech Republic, where the already low total fertility rate has declined further to 1.1 by 2001; we suspect that women in these ages are having only one child.

Finally, we have some evidence that the 1990s was an unusual decade for two Dual Earner countries, Finland and Sweden, where we found an unusual pattern. Lowly educated women, who usually do not delay having a family, tended to be ones not having a first birth. By 2003, we find that with the economic recovery in both countries this is no longer the case[13] (see Appendix 2).

FUTURE RESEARCH AGENDAS

Our purpose in this study has not been to test the consistency or inconsistency of welfare regime or models of policy configurations, but rather to highlight the institutional contexts in which childbearing and childrearing decisions take place. However, some of the divergences or lack of clear patterns in these clusters, particularly the General Family Support and Market Oriented groups, suggest that not only are fertility decisions highly complex, but also more generally, that we need institutional models that take into account the multi-layered ways in which gender is embedded in different institutions (Shalev, 2000). Fertility decisions are mediated by a broader set of institutional factors beyond the limited number of reconciliation policies or social insurance programs in welfare regime models. These involve paying attention to differences in labor markets (McCall & Orloff, 2005), job type, rights to reduce hours of work and the social quality of jobs, including both flexibility and security (called "flexicurity" in current EU discourse). Beyond measures of unemployment, there is a need for comparative data with measures on housing markets and youth unemployment; both could offer insights on birthstrike mechanisms of uncertainty and incoherence. Some studies of Southern European countries have analyzed the numbers of young people living at home into their thirties and the low fertility in these societies (Dalla Zuanna, 2001).

We faced many limitations in using cross-sectional data for this analysis. Most importantly, the data set did not permit analyses of the transitions in employment and childbearing. To operationalize an agency and capabilities approach requires longitudinal data in order to examine the period before birth of the child and after birth.[14] A new data set, called Generations and Gender Programme, based on panel surveys of nationally representative samples of the 18-79-year-old resident populations, as well as contextual databases allowing for multi-level analyses, is expected to be completed by 2010. It is coordinated by the United Nations Economic Commissions for Europe; it currently includes ten countries and the number of participating countries is increasing. Complete partnership and birth histories as well as educational and employment histories are gathered for several thousands of women and men in each country. This dataset will enable researchers to examine decisions around the timing and number of births and their relationship to women's transitions in and out of employment, including how these shape and are shaped by a range of factors, including the household economy, the working times of parents, and the previous patterning of paid and unpaid work in families. Another agenda for the future involves reflecting upon childbearing decisions and capabilities in terms of work-life balance and the workplace environment in different welfare states (Haas, Allard & Hwang, 2002).

NOTES

1. Korpi's (2000) models are in effect policy configurations reflecting employment and reconciliation policy formulas. They parallel Esping-Andersen's welfare regime typology: the Dual Earner family model follows the Scandinavian/Social Democratic traditions (Finland, Norway, and Sweden); those referred to as Market-Oriented are called Liberal in the Esping-Andersen typology (UK and Canada); the General Family Support model is equivalent to the Conservative Corporatist in policy regime framework (France, Germany, Netherlands, Italy and Spain). We also add a Post-Socialist Transition category (Czech Republic and Hungary), that consists of features of the Dual earner and Market oriented policy configurations. We discuss these policy configurations in the second section of the article.

2. The EU has set benchmarks for women's labor force participation and for childcare: by 2010, member states should provide childcare to at least 33 percent of all children under three and at least 90 percent of all children between three and mandatory school age.

3. The results show: 23 percent of mothers cut short their education compared to 6 percent of fathers; 25 percent of the women stopped working for good; only 2 percent of men did this; and finally, 15 percent of the women claimed they took a job below their qualifications as a result of having children; 5 percent of the men claimed this.

4. We include Canada in our analysis because it is a case that expresses the market-oriented policy configurations (Korpi, 2000) and because it is similar to our other European societies with below replacement fertility. We do not use the US because of its exceptional fertility pattern. The US is the only country in the developed world where fertility has remained close to the replacement level. This has been explained by a combination of many factors: a high level of religiosity and high rates of unplanned pregnancies and births related to poverty, as well as the more limited access to effective contraceptive methods especially for the poor and less educated, as compared to other industrialized countries (Billari et al. 2004).

5. Korpi (2000) also analyzes different "political tendencies" (p. 148) that drive these policies, which include left parties, confessional parties, and conservative centrist parties. However, these do not fit neatly on the gender policy models.

6. This information is derived from various national income or expenditure surveys. LIS harmonizes most of the income and transfer variables through the process of "lissification" facilitating comparisons across countries.

7. We have also run models on the likelihood of having two children in the household (with the youngest below age four), but we decided not to include them in the article because of the small number of cases in our very low fertility countries.

8. Esping-Andersen (1999) does not take this into account in his analysis of the likelihood of mothers having more than one child. Since most women reduce their labor force participation after they have a child, the causal relation between employment and fertility is going the wrong way.

9. We are not presenting a detailed analysis of mothers with children over four years of age because of the variations in when children start school at four, five or six or the constraints in school scheduling; see Gornick and Meyers (2003) for a discussion of the latter.

10. We might make the same point about East German women who have shown a precipitous decline in fertility and employment, and they have expressed expectations and aspirations to be mothers and earners. Surveys in the mid-1990s have shown having a job was the highest priority for East German women when asked which was more important family or work, even more so than for either East or West German men (Stolle, 1996).

11. We assume that extensive daycare services contributed to the positive association in France, though low levels of parental leave compensation may reflect greater differences between high and low educated women in combining employment and having a family.

12. For more information about the European Social Survey see http://www.europeansocialsurvey.org.

13. For both countries, the mid-1990s was a period of economic crisis. However by the early 2000s, the level of unemployment and of female unemployment decreased. Female unemployment in Finland was at a record high of 15 percent in the mid-1990s; by 2004 it is at 8.9 percent. Similarly in Sweden we see a decline from nearly 7 percent to 5.1 percent.

14. We considered using the European Community Household Panel Study dataset for this study, only our Central Eastern European societies were not in the data set.

REFERENCES

Adam, B., Beck, U., & Van Loon, J. (Eds.) (2000). *The risk society and beyond: Critical issues for social theory.* London, UK: Sage.

Ahn, N. & Mira, P. (2002). A note on the changing relationship between fertility and female employment rates in developed countries. *Journal of Population Economics, 15,* 667-682.

Beck, U. (1999). *World risk society.* Cambridge, UK: Polity Press.

Becker, G. S. (1991). *A treatise on the family.* Cambridge, MA: Harvard University Press.

Billari, F. C. (2004). *Choices, opportunities and constraints of partnership, childbearing and parenting: The patterns of the 1990s.* Background paper for the European Population Forum, Geneva, Switzerland, January 12-14, 2004.

Billari, F., Frejka, T., Hobcraft, J., Macura, M. &Van de Kaa, D. J. (2004). Discussion of paper 'Explanations of the fertility crisis in modern societies: A search for commonalities. (Population Studies, 57 (3): 241-263, by John Caldwell and Thomas Schindlmayr) *Population Studies, 58,* 77-92.

Brewster, K. L. & Rindfuss, R. R. (2000). Fertility and women's employment in industrialized nations. *Annual Review of Sociology, 26,* 271-296.

Castles, F. G. (2003). *The world turned upside down. Below replacement fertility: Changing preferences and family friendly public policy in 21 OECD countries.* University of Edinburgh, Scotland, unpublished manuscript.

Corman, D. (2001). *Success at work and in family life. Studies in selected Western fertility and family dynamics.* Ph.D. Dissertation. Stockholm, Sweden: Demography Unit, Stockholm University.

Council of Europe (2002). *Recent demographic developments in Europe.* Strasbourg, France: Council of Europe Press.

Dalla Zuanna, G. (2001).The banquet of Aeolus. A familistic interpretation of Italy's lowest low fertility. *Demographic Research, 4* (article 5), 131-162. Retrieved May 15, 2005 from http://www.demographic-research.org/

Di Prete, T., Morgan, S. P., Engelhardt, H., & Pacalova, H. (2003). Do cross-national differences in the costs of children generate cross-national differences in fertility rates? *Population Research and Policy Review, 22,* 439-477.

Engelhardt, H., Kögel, T. & Prskawetz, A. (2004). Fertility and women's employment reconsidered: A macro-level time-series analysis for developed countries, 1960-2000. *Population Studies, 58,* 109-120.

Esping-Andersen, G. (1990). *The three worlds of welfare capitalism.* Cambridge, UK: Polity.

Esping-Andersen, G. (1999). *Social foundations of postindustrial economics.* Oxford, UK: Oxford University Press.

Ferrara, M. (1996). The 'Southern Model' of welfare in social Europe. *Journal of European Social Policy, 6,* 17-37.

Ferrarini, T. (2003). *Parental leave institutions in eighteen post-war welfare states.* Swedish Institute for Social Research Dissertation Series no. 58. Stockholm, Sweden: Stockholm University.

Folbre, N. (1994). *Who pays for the kids? Gender and the structures of constraint.* New York and London: Routledge.

Gauthier, A. & Hatzius, J. (1997). Family benefits and fertility: An econometric analysis. *Population Studies, 51,* 295-306.

Gornick, J. C. & Meyers, M. K. (2003). *Families that work: Policies for reconciling parenthood and employment.* New York, NY: Russell Sage Foundation.

Gornick, J. C., Meyers, M. K., & Ross, K. E. (1997). Supporting the employment of mothers: Policy variation across fourteen welfare states. *Journal of European Social Policy, 7,* 45-70.

Guillén. A. (2003). Measuring economic citizenship: A comment on Kessler-Harris. *Social Politics, 10,* 186-196.

Haas, L., Allard, K. & Hwang. P. (2002). The impact of organizational culture on men's use of parental leave in Sweden. *Community, Work & Family, 5,* 319-342.

Hakim, C. (2003). A new approach to explaining fertility patterns: Preference theory. *Population and Development Review, 29,* 349-374.

Hobson, B. (2003). Some reflections and agendas for the future. *Social Politics, 10,* 196-204.

Hobson, B. & Oláh, L. (2006). Tournant positif ou 'greve des ventres'? Formes de résistance au modele de l'homme gagne-pain et a la restructuration de l'Etat-providence [The positive turn or birthstrikes? Sites of resistance to residual male breadwinner societies and to welfare state restructuring]. *Recherches et Prévisions, 83.*

Hobson, B. & Takahashi, M. (1997). The parent-worker model: Lone mothers in Sweden. In J. Lewis (Ed.), *Lone Mothers in European Welfare Regimes: Shifting Policy Logics* (pp. 121-139). London, UK: Jessica Kingsley Publishers.

Hoem, B. (1995). The way to the Swedish gender segregated labor market. In K. O. Mason & A. M. Jensen (Eds.), *Gender and family change in industrialized countries* (pp. 279-296). Oxford, UK: Oxford University Press.

Huber, E., & Stephens, J. D. (2003). *Determinants of welfare state approaches to old and new social risks.* Paper presented at the meetings of the Research Committee 19 of the International Sociological Association, Toronto, Canada, August 21-24.

ILO (International Labour Organisation) (different years). *Database on labour statistics* (Laborsta). Geneva. Switzerland: ILO Bureau of Statistics. Retrieved March 14, 2005 from http://laborsta.ilo.org/

Knijn, T., & Kremer, M. (1997). Gender and the caring dimension of welfare states: Toward inclusive citizenship. *Social Politics, 4,* 328-361.

Kocourkova, J. (2002). Leave arrangements and childcare services in Central Europe: Policies and practices before and after the transition. *Community, Work & Family, 5* (3), 301-318.

Kohler, H. P., Billari, F. C. & Ortega, J. A. (2002). The emergence of lowest-low fertility in Europe during the 1990s. *Population and Development Review, 28,* 641-680.

Korpi, W. (2000). Faces of inequality: Gender, class, and patterns of inequalities in different types of welfare states, *Social Politics, 7,* 127-191.

Korpi, W. & Palme, J. (1998). The paradox of redistribution and strategies of equality and poverty in western countries. *American Sociological Review, 63,* 661-687.

Kravdal, O. (2001). The high fertility of college educated women in Norway: An artefact of the separate modelling of each parity transition. *Demographic Research, 5* (article 6), Retrieved October 30, 2005 from http://www.demographic-research.org

Lewis, J. (1984). *Women in England 1870-1950.* Brighton, UK: Harvester Wheatsheaf.

Lewis, J. (1992). Gender and the development of welfare regimes, *Journal of European Social Policy, 2,* 159-173.

Lewis, J. (2002). Gender and welfare state change, *European Societies, 4,* 331-357.

Lewis, J. (2004). The gender settlement and social provision: The work-welfare relationship at the level of the household. In R. Salias & R. Villeneuve (Eds.), *Europe and the politics of capabilities* (pp. 239-254). Cambridge, UK: Cambridge University Press.

McCall, L. & Orloff, A. (2005). Introduction to special issue: Gender, Class and Capitalism. *Social Politics, 12,* 159-169.

McDonald, P. (2000). Gender equity, social institutions and the future of fertility. *Journal of Population Research, 17,* 1-16.

Morissette, R. (1998). The declining labour market status of young men. In M. Corak (Ed.), *Labour markets, social institutions and the future of Canada's children* (pp. 31-50). Ottawa: Statistics Canada, cat. No. 89-553.

O'Connor, J. S., Orloff, A. S., & Shaver, S. (1999). *States, markets, families: Gender, liberalism and social policy in Australia, Canada, Great Britain and the United States.* Cambridge, UK: Cambridge University Press.

Oláh, L. Sz. (2001). *Gendering family dynamics: The Case of Sweden and Hungary.* Ph.D. Dissertation. Stockholm, Sweden: Demography Unit, Stockholm University.

Oppenheimer, V. & Lewin, A. (1999). Career development and marriage formation in a period of rising inequality: Who is at risk? What are the prospects? In A. Booth, A.

Crouter & M. Shanahan (Eds.) *Transitions to adulthood in a changing economy: No work, no family, no future?* (pp. 189-225) Westport, CT: Praeger.

Orloff, A. S. 1993. Gender and the social rights of citizenship–The comparative analysis of gender relations and welfare states. *American Sociological Review, 58,* 303-328.

Reher, D. S. (1998). Family ties in Western Europe: Persistent contrasts. *Population and Development Review, 24,* 203-234.

RFV (Social Insurance Board) (2001). "När har vi råd att skaffa barn?" (When can we afford to have children?) *RFV 2001:8,* Stockholm, Sweden.

Santow, G. & Bracher, M. (2001). Deferment of the first birth and fluctuating fertility in Sweden, *European Journal of Population, 17,* 343-363.

Sen, A. (1992). *Inequality re-examined.* Oxford, UK: Oxford University Press.

Sen, A. (2003). Capability and well-being. In M. Nussbaum & A. Sen (Eds.) *The quality of life* (pp. 30-53). Oxford, UK: Oxford University Press.

SCB (Statistics Sweden) (2001). Varför föds det så få barn? *Demografiska rapporter 2001:1* (Why so few babies? Demographic reports 2001:1), Örebro, Sweden: SCB.

Shalev, M. (2000). Class meets gender in social policy. *Social Politics, 7,* 220-228.

Sjöberg, O. (2004). *Attitudes related to fertility and childbearing in the EU countries.* Report presented at the Swedish Institute for Futures Studies.

Sorensen, A. (1994). Women's economic risk and the economic position of single mothers. *European Sociological Review,10,* 173-188.

Standing, G. (1996). Social protection in Eastern Central Europe: A tale of slipping anchors and torn safety nets. In G. Esping-Andersen (Ed) *Welfare states in transition: National adaptations in global economies* (pp. 225-255). London, UK: Sage.

Stolle, D. (1996). The impact of German unification on the identity of East German women. *Working Papers. Advanced Research School for Comparative Gender Studies.* Stockholm, Sweden: Stockholm University.

Tanner, J. & Yabiku, S. (1999). Conclusion: The economics of young adulthood–One future or two. In A. Booth, A. Crouter & M. Shanahan (Eds.), *Transitions to adulthood in a changing economy: No work, no family, no future?* (pp. 254-268). Westport, CT: Praeger Publishers.

Taylor-Gooby, P. (1996). The response of government. Fragile convergence? In V. George. (Ed.) *European policy: Squaring the welfare circle* (pp. 199-218). Basingstoke, UK: Macmillan.

Tazi-Preve, I. M. & Dorbritz, J. (2005). *Fatherhood in a new millennium. A country comparison: Austria, Germany, Finland, Hungary and Italy.* Paper presented at the workshop "The Family in the Future–the Future of the Family," Stockholm, Sweden, October 7-9, 2005.

Turcotte, P. & Goldscheider, F. (1998). The evolution of factors influencing first union formation in Canada, *Canadian Studies in Population, 25,* 145-174.

APPENDIX 1

TABLE 1. List of Surveys

Country	Year	Survey
Canada	1997	Survey of Consumer Finances
Czech Republic	1996	Micro-Census
Finland	1995	Income Distribution Survey
France	1994	Family Budget Survey
Germany	1994	German Social Economic Panel Study
Hungary	1999	Hungarian Household Panel
Italy	1995	Bank of Italy Survey
Netherlands	1994	Socio-Economic Panel
Norway	1995	Income and Property Distribution Survey
Spain	1990	Expenditure and Income Survey
Sweden	1995	Income Distribution Survey
United Kingdom	1995	Family Expenditure Survey

TABLE 2. List of Variables

Included in all models:
Woman's age:
Three categories: (1) 35-40 years (our reference category), (2) 30-34 years,
(3) 25-29 years
Woman's educational attainment:
Three categories: (1) the person has not finished secondary school,
(2) high-school diploma, (3) post-secondary education (our reference category)
Included only in the logit models:
Husband's income:
Four quartiles, the highest is our reference category
Included only in the OLS regression models:
Number of children in the household:
Five categories: (1) 0 children (our reference category), (2) one child only, aged
below 4 years, (3) two children and the younger child is below 4 years, (4) three
or more children and the youngest child is below 4 years, (5) one or more
children, all are 4 years or older.
Couple:
Two categories: (1) partnered, (2) single (our reference category).

APPENDIX 2

Proportion of 30-45-Year-Old Women with No Children Across Educational Levels in Germay, Italy, Spain, the Czech Republic and Hungary in the Early 2000s

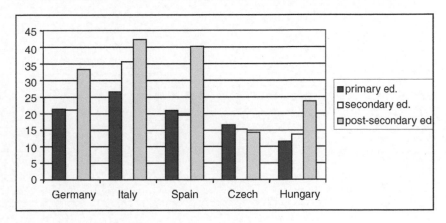

Source: ESS (2002-2003)

Gender Regimes and Cultures of Care:
Public Support for Maternal Employment
in Germany and the United States

Marina A. Adler
April Brayfield

SUMMARY. Our research uses nationally representative survey data to empirically document whether U.S., East German, and West German attitudes toward maternal employment have converged over the last decade. Specifically, our research examines to what extent the gender-related attitude regimes vary and have changed in accordance with policy developments in the United States and the two regions of unified Germany between 1991 and 2002. Data from the *U.S. General Social Survey* (GSS) and *Die Allgemeine Bevölkerungsumfrage der Sozialwissenschaften* (ALLBUS-German General Social Survey) show that the public attitudes toward maternal employment in both regions of Ger-

Marina A. Adler is affiliated with the Department of Sociology and Anthropology, University of Maryland, Baltimore County. April Brayfield is affiliated with the Department of Sociology, Tulane University.

Address correspondence to: Marina A. Adler, Department of Sociology and Anthropology, University of Maryland, Baltimore County, Baltimore, MD 21250 USA (E-mail: adler@umbc.edu).

The authors thank Xiaoxiao Peng, a graduate student in the Department of Sociology at Tulane University, for her technical assistance.

[Haworth co-indexing entry note]: "Gender Regimes and Cultures of Care: Public Support for Maternal Employment in Germany and the United States." Adler, Marina A., and April Brayfield. Co-published simultaneously in *Marriage & Family Review* (The Haworth Press, Inc.) Vol. 39, No. 3/4, 2006, pp. 229-253; and: *Families and Social Policy: National and International Perspectives* (ed: Linda Haas, and Steven K. Wisensale) The Haworth Press, Inc., 2006, pp. 229-253. Single or multiple copies of this article are available for a fee from The Haworth Document Delivery Service [1-800-HAWORTH, 9:00 a.m. - 5:00 p.m. (EST). E-mail address: docdelivery@haworthpress.com].

many are moving in a more supportive direction compared to their respective starting points, but West German attitudes have not caught up with those of the East. Furthermore, we found no evidence of a convergence with attitudes in the U.S. In fact, there was no change in the U.S. in the last decade on the gender arrangement continuum, in its policy regime, or toward more supportive attitudes toward women's employment. *[Article copies available for a fee from The Haworth Document Delivery Service: 1-800-HAWORTH. E-mail address: <docdelivery@haworthpress. com> Website: <http://www.HaworthPress.com> © 2006 by The Haworth Press, Inc. All rights reserved.]*

KEYWORDS. Attitude regime, gender, maternal employment, work-family policy

INTRODUCTION

Some social scientists claim that recent economic, demographic, political, and social developments in Western countries have facilitated a remarkable decline in their national differences and an increasing convergence of cultures, values, and policies, especially with regard to family life (Easter, Halman & de Moor, 1993; Taylor-Gooby, 1996; Voicu &Voicu, 2002; von Wahl, 2005). Likewise, much of sociological research on "welfare state restructuring" predicts growth in cultural diffusion, values convergence, and increasingly egalitarian gender attitudes (Easter et al., 1993; Inglehart & Norris, 2003). Some scholars argue that since the transition from socialism to capitalism, Eastern European countries have changed in terms of "modernity" (see Künzler, Walter, Reichert & Pfister et al., 2001) or "post-modernity" (see Klages, 1993), have increasingly assimilated to the West, or have become more traditional in their division of labor (see Künzler et al., 2001). Other scholars observe a slow pluralization of values as societies have become more heterogeneous (Klages, 1993; Lück, 2004).

Indeed, Europe and the United States have experienced dramatic rises in women's labor force participation, declines in fertility rates, and increases in dual earner couples as normative trends over the past three decades. Consequently, family scholars and policymakers are intrigued by empirical questions about the division of care and market work, the societal position of employed mothers, national cultures of care, and possible transfers of gender arrangements and family values. Overall, based on the prevailing assumption that Western societies are experiencing a general shift in gender arrangements toward greater equality between women and men, the question is whether there is also a shift in gender-related attitude regimes toward more public support for maternal employment.

Despite the proliferation of convergence arguments in the literature, a wide array of empirical evidence also indicates considerable variation in gender equality, family policies, and political cultures among Western countries. Notably, recent scholarship examines the differences in national "packages" of values and policies that structure and reinforce gender relations within and across public and private spheres and encompass the state-family-market triad (see Sainsbury, 1999). These "gender regimes" include (a) the gender cultural system (Pfau-Effinger, 1996; 1998), i.e., the interplay of policies, customs, conventions, and social institutions that guide how women and men relate to one another, and (b) "gender contracts," which refer to a set of unspoken rules about the gendered division of work-family responsibilities (Pfau-Effinger, 1996; 1998). Researchers have documented variation in gender regimes among European nations in general (Crompton, 2001; von Wahl, 2005) and among select countries that represent *different* types of welfare states, such as Austria, the Netherlands, and Sweden (Haas, 2005), as well as *similar* types of welfare states, such as Germany and Japan (Gottfried & O'Reilly, 2002).

While there are dynamic interrelationships among the welfare state policies, political culture, and gender regime promoted within a country, and the gender values shared by its population, the match between public opinion and family policy priorities appears far from perfect (Brayfield, Adler & Luo, 2002; Haas, 2005; Lück, 2004; MacRae, 2005; von Wahl, 2005). There are inconsistencies and lags within and between countries in their gender regimes, including normative gender arrangements, family policies, political cultures, and social values (Haas, 2005; Pfau-Effinger, 1996; 1998). We argue, following Haas (2005), that the analysis of gender regimes and their consequences requires us to consider both structural factors, such as institutional barriers to women's labor force participation (see Lewis, 1992), and cultural factors, such as work-family values (see Pfau-Effinger, 1996). We extend the analysis by insisting that individual attitudes and preferences play an important role in why and how gender regimes change (see Lück, 2004). Hence, we connect national configurations of gender regimes, family policies, and political culture with corresponding attitude regimes to analyze the trajectories of change in public support of women's employment over time.

Specifically, against the background of welfare state restructuring in the 1990s, we use recent gender regime perspectives (Haas, 2005; von Wahl, 2005) and arguments about gender arrangements (Crompton, 1999a; Pfau-Effinger, 1996; 1998; Rosenfeld, Trappe & Gornick, 2004) to analyze trends in public support for maternal employment in three geographic regions with different political-cultural legacies: East Germany, West Germany, and the United States. The restructuring of social policy in unified Germany has moved East Germany from a socialist gender regime to the social conservative regime of West Germany. This type of structural alignment implies general public support for the dominant ideology behind the changes, but the legacies of previous political systems and gender cultures may prevail and individual attitudes may lag behind (Adler, 2002; 2004; Adler & Brayfield, 1997; Dölling, 2003; Pfau-Effinger, 1996; 1998).

Our objective is to investigate to what degree there has been a convergence in the public perception of the value of maternal employment within the context of particular forms of institutional and cultural support for it. How much do changes in family policies and employment policies matter in shaping public support for the gender division of labor? Is it policy *per se* or the legacy of political culture (i.e., cultural lag) that shapes attitude regimes? What is the importance of institutionally supported policy packages in placing nations into particular attitude regimes?

LITERATURE REVIEW

The sociological discourse in comparative research about women's market and care work was originally framed by feminist critics of Esping-Andersen's (1990) welfare state typology, who insisted that the typology should be gendered (Hobson, 1994; Lewis, 1992; Orloff, 1993; O'Connor, 1993; Sainsbury, 1994). These scholars revised the original welfare state regime model to include normative patterns of family arrangements as well as a variety of policies related to gender equality, maternal employment, and work-family concerns, and offered a number of evolving models of gender regimes (Hobson, 1994; Lewis, 1992; O'Connor, 1993; Orloff, 1993; Sainsbury, 1994; Siaroff, 1994). In addition, some scholars have used concepts, such as "family welfare orientation" and "female work desirability" to divide countries into categories like "Protestant liberal," "late female mobilizing," "Protestant social democratic," or "advanced Christian democratic" (Siaroff, 1994). Much of this literature focuses on the patterns of women's ties to the labor market (i.e., degree of decommodification, see Esping-Andersen, 1990) and to the family (i.e., degree of defamilialization, see Orloff, 1993) as well as their private dependence on men (see Konietzka & Kreyenfeld, 2005) within any given welfare state to better understand how governments, markets, families, and local communities serve as key actors in the gendered provision of social policies.

Of prime concern to family researchers and policymakers, the labor force participation rates of women in Western industrialized countries have risen steadily in the last few decades. In the European context this trend has been bolstered by various policy packages designed to facilitate the reconciliation of employment and family responsibilities (Gornick, 2000; Gornick, Meyers & Ross, 1997; 1998; Hofaecker, 2004). Many of these work-family policies have targeted women, not men, thereby leaving the traditional domestic division of labor unchallenged. During the 1990s, new social policies reflected a shift in policy paradigms by recognizing that not only unemployment and work-family reconciliation are of concern, but that the financial burden of state provisions should be curtailed. Accordingly, many Northern and Western European nations, in the process of "Europeanization" and EU supranational developments, have initiated new policies to facilitate the integration of work and family life, especially for women (Haas, 2005; MacRae, 2005; von Wahl, 2005). While the government of unified Germany has resisted some of these changes, East Germans have had to relinquish the many former GDR policies that favored the employment of mothers. In contrast, the United States has not had to respond to these European pressures to enact such social policies (Hofaecker, 2004).

Societal economic conditions (such as unemployment) and institutional arrangements for care and leave (such as the availability of public child care) reflect the extent to which national cultures embrace certain patterns of gender relations. For example, the redistribution of care responsibilities away from the state, such as caring for children, elder relatives, and the sick, is typically associated with an increased burden on women and could signal a lower likelihood that gender values will shift toward greater equality between women and men in the domestic sphere. This is where the political culture and the "culture of care" of a country is relevant–family policy solutions to the question, "who does care work and who pays for it," can be answered with "the state" (public issue), "women" (private issue) or "the market" (economic issue). Depending on the answer, a country can be classified on a continuum of family policy regimes.

Most recently the academic discussion of welfare state typologies revolves around the role of the state-family-market nexus in shaping the complexities of social, family, and employment policy (Haas, 2005; von Wahl, 2005), and terms such as *gender contracts* (Pfau-Effinger, 1996), *gender arrangements* (Pfau-Effinger, 1996), *cultures of care* (Haas, 2005), *work-time regimes* (Gottfried & O'Reilly, 2002), and *work-care balance* (Haas, 2005) have emerged. Within this dialogue, a particularly noteworthy contribution is Haas's (2005) synthesis of structural and cultural classifications into a new typology of gender regimes, which she uses as a heuristic device to capture the dominant constellations of the gender division of labor. Haas (2005) focuses on "the compatibility of work and care in partnerships" (p. 495) and arrives at five ideal types of "work-care balance" for the gendered division of labor: the traditional breadwinner model, the modified breadwinner model, the egalitarian employment model, the universal carer model, and the role reversal model.

We also find the concept of political culture to be especially useful in the analysis of gender and attitude regimes. In general, political culture can be defined as the dominant values, attitudes and beliefs in a particular country, and the related behaviors of the citizenry. It encompasses the national characteristics and cultural identity of a country and the population's attitudes toward the political system and policies (Zimmerman, 1992). Likewise, Ullrich (2003) refers to "cultures of welfare" (*Wohlfahrtskulturen*) or social political culture, which he defines as "the sum total of socially accessible cognitive, evaluative, and normative standards as well as patterns of interpretation, values, norms, and behavioral guidelines" (p. 14, authors' translation). According to Ullrich, the culture of welfare affects institutions directly and indirectly via the social political discourse and interpretations, social political behavioral guidelines, and social policy decisions at the micro level (individual attitudes) and the macro level (public discourse about the policy agenda). Thus, Künzler et al. (2001) argue that the political culture of a country can determine its development by framing its "approach to family and gender relations" via a combination of Catholicism, conservatism, and corporatism (West Germany) or socialism, egalitarianism, and centralism (East Germany). In the United States one could identify a package of Protestantism, economic liberalism, and individualism as undergirding its political culture.

The political cultures associated with various family policy paradigms assign responsibility for family work to either the private sphere (i.e., women) or to the public sphere (i.e., the state, employers, and/or the market). That means that a national culture will include more of an individual orientation or a society-centered orientation to family work, thereby constraining national policy choices. Research shows that the political culture surrounding the symbolic value and meaning of employment is related to the political and economic structure of society (Adler & Brayfield, 1996, 1997; Kalleberg & Stark, 1993). Accordingly, the political culture of a country gives rise to and maintains its particular welfare regime and shapes the broader context for its specific gender policies (Ullrich, 2003). Political culture also contains dominant ideologies that favor a certain gender order and gender-related values, such as gender equity, motherhood, women's independence, work-family balance, and "culture of care" (Haas, 2005). These values can be referred to as a country's "gender culture," which solidifies the gender order and finds expression in public attitudes regarding the gendered division of labor.

The Gender Regimes of the Three Regions

Table 1 summarizes the multidimensional typologies we use in our analysis of East Germany, West Germany, and the United States. According to Inglehart (1989), populations undergoing drastic social changes, such as German unification, can change their values and cognitive structures but this is very difficult. Some research suggests that despite the rapid shift from a socialist, dual earner regime to a social conservative, male-breadwinner regime, East Germans have retained various values and attitudes regarding the intersection of gender, work, and family from socialist GDR (German Democratic Republic) times (Adler, 2002; Adler & Brayfield, 1997). Prior research demonstrated that after unification, as an expression of the GDR's ideological legacy, East German women continued to be highly employment-oriented, even after getting married and having children (Adler, 2002; Rosenfeld et al., 2004). In contrast, West German attitudes reflected the FRG (Federal Republic of Germany) state's historical preference for a male breadwinner family (Adler, 2002; Rosenfeld et al., 2004). As a representative of the liberal welfare state regime, the United States provides an interesting frame of reference because of its lack of paid maternity or parental leave, child allowances, or subsidized public child care in

TABLE 1. A Typology of Gender Regimes: Dimensions Related to Public Support for Maternal Employment

	East Germany Former Socialist Gender Regime	West Germany Conservative Gender Regime	USA Liberal Gender Regime
Normative gender arrangements for the work-family division of labor			
Before 1991	Dual earner/state carer	Male breadwinner/female carer	Dual earner/market carer
2002	Dual earner/female part time (high female unemployment)	Dual earner/female part time (mother care is supported)	Dual earner/market carer
Family policy regime in its support of employed mothers			
Before 1991	High state support (high parental leave, high day care coverage all ages, high child benefits)	Low state support (medium parental leave, low < 3 day care coverage, medium > 3 day care, medium child benefits)	No state support (private issue, market solutions)
2002	Comparatively reduced support (medium parental leave, medium day care coverage, medium child benefits)	Comparatively increased support (medium parental leave, medium day care coverage, medium child benefits)	Comparatively increased support, but still very low (family & medical leave act)
Political culture of care			
Before 1991	Gender equality, women's employment, and work-family reconciliation officially a priority on the public agenda	Gender equality, women's employment, and work-family integration *not* an important issue on the public agenda	Gender equality, women's employment, and work-family integration *not* an important issue on public agenda
2002	Comparatively reduced importance	Comparatively increased importance	Unchanged
Attitude toward maternal employment			
Before 1991	High support	Low support	Medium support
2002	Comparatively increased support	Comparatively increased support	Unchanged support

conjunction with a relatively high rate of maternal labor force participation.

According to von Wahl's (2005) conceptualization of gender regimes, there are three "equal employment regimes": liberal, conservative, and social-democratic. These regimes exemplify "the combined, interdependent ways in which equal opportunity and equal employment are produced and allocated among state, market, and family" (von Wahl, 2005, p. 71). Von Wahl (2005) explains that these regimes go beyond mere welfare state or social policy classifications by including several dimensions that particularly affect women, such as "social dependency, frequently precarious living circumstances, and difficulty accessing the labor market" (p. 70). She argues that the equal employment regimes of the United States and (West) Germany closely correspond to their membership in their respective welfare state typology: liberal and conservative.

Adopting von Wahl's classification system, our description of a *liberal gender regime*, as best exemplified by the United States, is grounded in a political culture of individualism in which inequality is viewed as an individual problem, and is characterized by a "discrimination approach" with low state involvement, anti-discrimination laws, equal opportunity policies, child care as a private or market concern, and private dependence in that lone mothers are not supported by the state. According to von Wahl (2005), "the liberal equal employment regime is especially weak on social policy and minimally supports the integration of mothers into employment" (p. 79). Hence the United States ranks low on measures of economic support for employed mothers and high on measures of "child penalties." For example, U.S. parents were not entitled to any national family-related leave prior to the *Family and Medical Leave Act of 1993* (FMLA), which now requires all public agencies and private-sector companies with 50 or more employees to grant 12 weeks of *unpaid*, job-protected leave to care for a newborn or adopted child or sick family member. This provision only applies after the employee has exhausted all sick and vacation days. Government-sponsored child care benefits are also limited to means-tested programs that assist poor families with early education and child care, such as Head Start and Early Start. While many U.S. employed parents make use of the *Child Care Tax Credit* to help combine employment and childrearing, the *Personal Responsibility and Work Opportunity Act of 1996* (PRWOA) pressures lone mothers to take jobs (i.e., it uses punitive measures such as life-time limits for welfare benefits), despite the lack of affordable child care arrangements in the United States.

In contrast, in the *social conservative gender regime*, as represented by West Germany, the traditional gender division of labor is supported and reinforced by the state, and an exclusive "family phase" employment model predominates (a model in which mothers temporarily withdraw from the labor market for an extended period of time to raise their children), because of the assumption that mothers will care for their young children at home while fathers will provide the necessary financial resources for the family's well-being. Thus, there are few substitute care arrangements for children under age 3, there is low implementation of equality legislation and antidiscrimination laws, and relatively little state support exists for lone mothers. In this gender regime, gender equality is not really on the public agenda– it is regarded as a non-issue because of the formal provision of constitutional equality between women and men (MacRae, 2005). Contemporary German policy encourages women to leave the labor force with various incentives thus reinforcing the male breadwinner family (Konietzka & Kreyenfeld, 2005). It includes a 14-week, paid maternity leave (*Mutterschaftsurlaub*) with job protection, a paid 3-year childrearing leave period (*Elternzeit*) that can be taken by either parent with the provision to return to an equivalent job, the constitutional right of all children aged 3-6 to a place in child care (*Kindergarten*) but not for younger children (*Krippe*) or older ones (*Hort*), child-related tax exemptions (*Kinderleistungsausgleich*) that discourage female employment, and "income splitting" which favors high-income single-earner families (Cooke, 2006).

The *social-democratic gender regime*, as represented by the former socialist German Democratic Republic (East Germany), had a strong tradition of collectivist, redistributive political culture and well-developed egalitarian and affirmative action gender policies, where women have easy access to the labor market, extensive public care for children of all ages, and extensive support for lone mothers. These GDR policies were designed to facilitate the reconciliation of employment and family formation, thereby simultaneously increasing fertility, marriage, and female employment rates (Adler, 1997; 2002; Kreyenfeld, 2001). The former GDR had numerous policies supporting employed mothers in addition to constitutional equal rights and legislation that ensured equal pay and equal opportunity for women. Among the benefits lost to East Germans upon unification in 1990 were (1) interest-free marriage loans and birth grants, (2) a number of special economic provisions for single mothers, (3) housing preferences after marriage and children, (4) the "baby year" with full pay and workplace protection, (5) various other child-related leave benefits, and (6) convenient and free child care for all ages. Hence, from the East German point of view the GDR entitlements were replaced by less generous leaves, tax credits, and less accessible and inconvenient child care (see Kreyenfeld, 2001). Nevertheless, high rates of cohabitation and nonmarital births (Grünheid, 2003), continued high employment orientation of women, and continued egalitarian gender attitudes show that this change in policy framework has failed to re-traditionalize the gender regime in the East (Adler, 2004). This is also confirmed by persistently higher rates of public child care in the East than the West: In 1999, 34% of children aged 3 years and under were in daycare in the East, compared to 1% in the West (Hank, Tillman & Wagner, 2001). Furthermore, while the rates for 4-6-year-olds were comparable in the two regions, 24% of Eastern 7-11-year-olds as compared to only 5% of their Western counterparts were in daycare (Hank et al., 2001).

Other scholars use complementary heuristic devices to characterize the structural and ideological underpinnings of gender regimes. For example, Crompton (1999b) argues that societies can be classified according to a "continuum of gender arrangements." On one extreme end is the traditional male breadwinner/female carer type, followed by the dual earner/female part time carer type (the first modification to the traditional model) and two versions of a second modification, i.e., the dual earner with substitute care provided by either the state (dual earner/state carer type) or the market (dual earner/market carer type), and on the other extreme end is the "ideal" of the dual earner/dual carer type. Policies, using various incentives, reinforce women's carer role as either a full-time or part-time housewife/mother and encourage men's full-time market work. More recently, Rosenfeld et al. (2004) argue that since unification West Germany has moved from a traditional male breadwinner/female carer model to a dual earner/female part-time carer model and East Germany has moved from a dual earner/state carer model to a dual earner/female part-time carer model. Hence, Rosenfeld et al. (2004) arrive at their convergence argument at the analytical level of gender arrangements as supported by the economic and political convergence in the unified German policy package. MacRae (2005), however, argues that while the German gender regime is a male breadwinner regime because mothers have special status under the law, recently Germany also has adopted dual-earner values due to the social forces of "Europeanization." Yet, in social conservative welfare states like West Germany, work-family policies reflect the dominant ideology of patriarchal values with a mixture of equal constitutional rights for women and state provisions to subsidize mothers as unpaid carers or part-time workers. In other words, the male breadwinner family model is reinforced, especially for mothers of very young children.

Nevertheless, the German welfare state, for reasons related to German unification, European integration, and demographic trends, has experienced dramatic changes during the 1990s. The last decade has seen shifts in social policy, especially for the Eastern part of the country. Previous research suggests that the legacy of the socialist political culture persists in shaping East German attitudes about women's labor force participation (Adler, 2004; Adler & Brayfield, 1996; 1997). In fact, some argue that East German women are exhibiting *Eigensinn* (stubbornness) in their adherence to pre-unification values regarding women's employment, and by not converging to West German lower levels of labor force participation (Dölling, 2003). In addition, compared to the United States, West Germany has traditionally lagged behind in women's labor force participation. Although East and West Germans appear to be converging on the dual earner/female part-time carer model (Rosenfeld et al., 2004), East Germany's high level of women's labor force participation, and its high level of public support for women's employment do not converge with those of the West.

Social democratic welfare states and socialist countries, like the former GDR, have a long tradition in which collectivism predominates and responsibility for family well-being belongs to the public sphere, specifically the state. East Germany supported both women's reproductive and productive labor and ideologically promoted the importance of both for women, but not for men. Thus, the state provided a wide array of policies that commodified women as workers and to a certain extent defamilialized women as carers, by giving single mothers and dual earner families access to state-sponsored substitute care arrangements. At the other end of the spectrum, Anglo countries, like the United States, have a long tradition of an individualist ideology, which coupled with the liberal welfare state, has led to very low levels of state involvement in policies that facilitate the integration of employment and family life. Hence, families are left to their own devices in creating patchwork coverage of income-generation (dual earners) and care-giving services via the market. In addition, while the United States has extensive legislation granting women equal employment opportunities, prohibiting gender discrimination, and upholding affirmative action, there are no social provisions that strengthen these laws (Cooke, 2004). In other words, there is no public mandate or agenda to strengthen gender equality in the United States. While the *Family and Medical Leave Act of*

1993 put the integration of employment and family responsibilities on the public policy agenda, little has been done to alter the structural conditions that reinforce a gendered division of labor and women's individual responsibilities for family care.

There is a growing cross-national literature on attitudes and preferences regarding the gendered division of labor in general and public opinion about maternal employment in particular. For example, in his analysis of 22 European and North American countries, Lück (2004) found that gender-related attitudes have remained stable or have become somewhat more supportive in Anglo countries, such as the United States, between 1988 and 2002. Cooke (2006) found that when policymakers rely solely on market forces to shape public attitudes toward maternal employment, traditionalism pervades in the private sphere. Previous research also indicates that East Germans have more positive attitudes toward women's market work than West Germans (Adler & Brayfield, 1996; 1997). Thus, socialism and its legacy have fostered attitudes and preferences that oppose the traditional division of labor. In particular, East German women rate the importance of employment for themselves as higher than West German women, and consequently East German women are much more likely to be employed, even under conditions of high unemployment (Adler, 2004).

The three regions in our analysis occupy different positions in the "benchmarking" of gender relations (Künzler et al., 2001). Table 2 presents data related to women's employment in the three regions. Despite a reduction between 1991 and 2000, the labor force participation rates of women in East Germany remain much higher (over 72%) than those in West Germany and the United States, where rates have climbed in this decade to a little over 60%. In addition, while the rate of full-time employment has dropped from over 90% to about 62% in East Germany, it remained below 60% in West Germany and around 75% in the United States. Likewise, the rate of employment for women with young children declined in East Germany and increased in West Germany and the United States. These patterns support the idea that East Germany has moved to conditions of less dual-earner support (reduced full-time and maternal employment but still high), West Germany has remained in conditions favoring male-breadwinner families (lowest on full-time and maternal employment), and the U.S. has solidified the dual-earner pattern (increased and high full-time and maternal employment).

Proponents of convergence arguments would expect not only a convergence in the gender arrangements, family policy regimes, and gender cultures of the three different gender regime representatives, but

TABLE 2. Percentage of Women, Aged 15 to 64, Employed in East Germany, West Germany, and the United States

	East Germany		West Germany		United States	
	1991	*2000*	*1991*	*2000*	*1990*	*2000*
Employed total [a]	77.2	72.4	58.4	62.2	56.8 [b]	60.2 [b]
Full time (> 36 hrs)[c]	91.0 [d]	62.2	58.0 [d]	58.3	74.8 [e]	75.4 [e]
Mothers total [a]	80.6	71.3	51.5	60.8	66.7 [e]	72.9 [e]
with child < age 3	75.9	52.2	37.3	47.7	53.6 [e]	61.0 [e]
with child age 3-5	82.8	63.7	47.6	55.7	58.2 [e, h]	65.3 [e, h]
Unemployed [f]	12.3	19.4	7.0	7.9	6.4 [g]	5.6 [g]

[a] Engstler and Menning, 2003, Tab A4-1, A4-2 (*"Erwerbsquote"* for all employed in 2000),Table 32, Fig. 64, 65.
[b] U.S. Department of Labor, 2002. Employment status of the civilian population by sex and age, 2001. http://www.dol.gov. (Rate is for women 16 and older).
[c] Winkler, 2000, p. 22 (*"Erwerbsquote,"* includes the currently unemployed, 1999), p. 27.
[d] Bundesanstalt für Arbeit, quoted in Adler 1997 (rates for 1989).
[e] U.S. Department of Labor, 2005. Table 20, http://stats.bls.gov/cps/wlf-table20-2005.pdf
[f] Statistisches Bundesamt, 2002, Tables 2, 3, 9 (*"Erwerbstätigenquote"*).
[g] U.S. Bureau of Labor Statistics, 2003, Employment status, annual averages, household data.
[h] Rate includes all children under age 6.
Note: In German official statistics, "current employment" can take the form of (1) employed (part or full time), (2) employed but temporarily on leave (sick leave, maternity leave, parental leave), or (3) in the labor force but currently unemployed and looking for work. *"Erwerbstätigenquote"* includes only the first two options and *"Erwerbsquote"* adds the unemployed.

also in their attitude regimes. In other words, over the past decade (1) the degree of support for women's employment should have increased in all three regions, and (2) these attitudes should have moved toward a more similar level of support. We argue, however, that regional political cultures continue to exert a powerful influence on public attitudes about women's employment, especially those pertaining to maternal employment. In the United States, the individualist political heritage of the value of family as a private matter stagnated the development of supportive policies for maternal employment. Thus, we do not expect American attitudes to converge with European attitudes. Similarly, the GDR legacy of a collectivist culture and the FRG view of mother care as superior will prevail in shaping the level of support for maternal employment in the two regions of unified Germany. Thus, we do not expect a convergence of East German attitudes with West German attitudes.

DATA SOURCES AND METHODS

We investigate the level of convergence in attitude regimes in the three regions with data from nationally representative samples available for two time periods, 1991 and 2002. The U.S. data come from the *General Social Survey* (GSS), and the German data come from *Die Allgemeine Bevölkerungsumfrage der Sozialwissenschaften* (ALLBUS, the German General Social Survey), both well known, reputable sources. These data give us the opportunity to measure the degree to which public opinion about maternal employment has changed one decade after German reunification. The borders between the GDR and the FRG opened in 1989, and the two regions were officially reunified in 1990. Our baseline data come from the year 1991. Although it is clear that the time period immediately following unification was particularly turbulent and East German perspectives reflect heightened anxieties about the future, deep-seated cognitive structures like gender-related values do not change dramatically in just one year (see Inglehart, 1989). Hence, while we acknowledge the potential impact of the transitional period on attitudes in general, we assume that specific attitudes about women's employment in the year immediately following unification are very similar to those held right before unification. We also acknowledge that the comparison of "snapshots" of cross-sectional data over time does not adequately capture individual-level change in personal attitudes; it is, however, suggestive of aggregate trends in public opinion.

We selected three conventional indicators of attitudes toward maternal employment that were available for both countries in both years. For each of the following statements, respondents reported their level of agreement or disagreement:

- It is much better for everyone involved if the man is the achiever outside the home and the woman takes care of the home and family.
- A preschool child is likely to suffer if his or her mother works.
- A working mother can establish just as warm and secure a relationship with her children as a mother who does not work.

Unfortunately, for the German data, the Likert range of possible response values changed from 1-to-4 in 1991 to 1-to-5 in 2002 in that a middle response category of "neither agree nor disagree" was included in 2002 for German respondents, but not for American respondents. To achieve comparability in value scales between the two years and the two national samples in 2002, we "stretched" the 1991 range for all respondents and the 2002 range for American respondents by reassigning the values of "3 and 4" to "4 and 5" respectively. This "stretching" technique minimizes the possibility that any observed difference in means between the two time periods is not merely an artifact of measurement differences.[1] We also reversed the coding scheme for the third item so that a higher value on that item coincides with a higher level of *agreement* with the statement, and hence, a higher level of support for maternal employment. In contrast, a higher value on the first two items coincides with a higher level of *disagreement* with the two statements, and hence, a higher level of support for maternal employment as well.

After these recoding procedures, we combined responses to the three statements into an additive index to represent each respondent's level of support for maternal employment. This index potentially ranges from 3 to 15. This additive index is reliable for all three geographic regions (East Germany, West Germany, and USA) and in both time periods, with the Cronbach's alpha reliability coefficient ranging from .62 to .76 across the six region-year groups. Table 3 presents Cronbach's alphas and details about sample restrictions and loss of cases for each geographic region in both years, with final analytic sample sizes ranging from 387 to 1,475.

Our analytic strategy proceeds in three stages. First, we examine the degree to which each of the three separate items in our attitude index varies across regions and between the two time periods. This will ensure that when we test for significant differences in the average levels of support for women's employment, a single indicator alone does not drive these differences. Second, we conduct three independent t-tests to measure whether the average level of public support for women's employ-

TABLE 3. Sample Sizes and Reliability Coefficients for Each Region by Year

| | ALLBUS | | | | GSS | |
| | East Germany | | West Germany | | USA | |
	1991	2002	1991	2002	1991	2002
Original sample size	1,544	886	1,514	1,934	1,517	2,765
Skipped cases: Respondents not in this attitude module	0	455	0	998	493	1,857
Respondents with missing values on one or more attitude items	69	44	94	90	56	23
Analytic sample size	1,475	387	1,420	846	968	885
Cronbach's alpha for attitude toward maternal employment scale	.63	.62	.65	.62	.76	.66

ment has increased between 1991 and 2002 within each of the three regions. Third, we conduct a Scheffe's test of the simultaneous comparison of the average level of support for women's employment across all possible region-year pairs. This statistical procedure allows for a more conservative test of significance than a series of separate t-tests of means because it requires the combination of pairings to achieve a higher level of significance than any one separate pairing on its own. Both the t-tests and the Scheffe test evaluate whether the observed differences in mean levels of support are large enough to achieve statistical significance and be interpreted as meaningful differences.

FINDINGS

Table 4 presents the percentage distributions of the constituent items for the attitude toward maternal employment index before listwise deletion of missing values. A comparison of the distribution of the responses in 1991 and 2002 shows that significantly fewer East and West Germans had negative attitudes towards maternal employment in 2002.[2] In addition, Germans in general are voicing either less certain opinions or more positive perceptions of employed mothers. In contrast, there appears to be little change in the distributions of the constituent items for American respondents.

In fact, there was no significant difference in the mean levels of U.S. support for maternal employment between 1991 and 2002 (t ratio = $-.61$, $p = .543$), and the dispersion of the values across the range of the index also remained quite constant (i.e., the U.S. standard deviation was 3.13 in 1991 and 3.06 in 2002). Figure 1 illustrates that, unlike the shift toward more supportive attitudes in Germany, public opinion about maternal employment in the United States appears to be quite stable over the past decade. This figure also shows that the mean levels of German support for maternal employment increased significantly in both regions between 1991 and 2002 (East Germany: t ratio = $-7.57, p < .001$; West Germany: t ratio = $-10.45, p < .001$). The level of attitude dispersion for West Germans is very similar to that of Americans, while the East Germans are much less dispersed, and thus, more cohesive in their support for maternal employment (i.e., the East German standard deviation was 2.89 in 1991 and 2.40 in 2002).

Table 5 presents the details of the Scheffe test of the mean differences in levels of support for maternal employment between all possible region-year pairs. The numbers in the body of the table represent the

TABLE 4. Percentage Distributions of Indicators of Supportive Attitudes Toward Maternal Employment by Geographic Region and Year

	1991						2002					
	1	2	3	4	5	N	1	2	3	4	5	N
Level of disagreement with: *It is much better for everyone involved if the man is the achiever outside the home and the woman takes care of the home and family.*												
East Germany	10.0	22.5	0.0	39.0	28.5	1514	3.8	10.8	10.6	41.1	33.7	416
West Germany	19.7	30.3	0.0	31.8	18.1	1480	7.8	15.5	15.6	36.4	24.7	903
USA	7.6	34.5	0.0	40.7	17.2	996	10.1	28.6	0.0	42.5	18.7	898
Level of disagreement with: *A preschool child is likely to suffer if his or her mother works.*												
East Germany	21.9	35.7	0.0	28.2	14.2	1501	8.6	24.1	11.4	34.7	21.3	395
West Germany	40.1	35.7	0.0	17.0	7.1	1483	14.7	41.1	14.1	21.1	9.0	886
USA	9.1	38.7	0.0	42.3	9.9	996	9.8	35.9	0.0	43.7	10.7	898
Level of agreement with: *A working mother can establish just as warm and secure a relationship with her children as a mother who does not work.*												
East Germany	1.7	8.4	0.0	25.0	64.9	1524	1.0	2.9	1.0	29.3	66.0	420
West Germany	6.4	20.7	0.0	29.8	43.1	1470	3.0	12.4	4.8	35.7	44.2	903
USA	6.3	28.4	0.0	45.3	20.0	1011	9.3	27.1	0.0	39.4	24.2	901

amount of difference between the means of the attitude index for that particular comparison. For example, the first number in the upper left cell signifies the mean level of support in East Germany in 1991 was 1.79 points higher than the mean for West Germany in 1991.

We combine the results in Table 5 with the visual display in Figure 1 to arrive at the following results. While West Germans were less supportive of maternal employment than Americans in 1991, West Germans increased their support to surpass that of Americans in 2002.[3] Nevertheless, West Germans still lag behind East Germans, who remain the most supportive group over time, with significantly higher support in 2002. The gap between the two German regions significantly narrowed over time, mainly because West German support for

FIGURE 1. Mean Level of Support for Maternal Employment in Each Geographic Region by Year

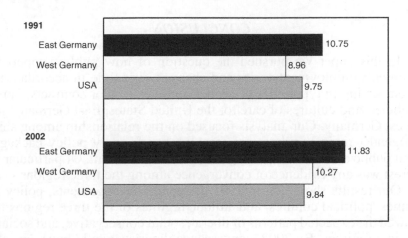

TABLE 5. Scheffe Test of Mean Differences in Level of Support for Maternal Employment Between Region-Year *Comparisons*

	East Germany 1991	West Germany 1991	USA 1991	East Germany 2002	West Germany 2002
West Germany 1991	1.79***				
USA 1991	1.00***	-.79***			
East Germany 2002	-1.09***	-2.87***	-2.08***		
West Germany 2002	.48*	-1.31***	-.51*	1.57***	
USA 2002	.91***	-.88***	-.09	1.99***	.43

*** p < .001, ** p < .01, * p < .05

maternal employment increased at a higher rate than East German support. Whereas West Germans were the least supportive group in 1991, Americans rank the lowest on the index in 2002. Hence, the gap between East Germans and Americans significantly increased over the last decade, mainly because there was no change in American attitudes. Overall, while German attitudes about maternal employment have moved in a more supportive direction, those of Americans have stagnate.

CONCLUSION

In this paper we pursued the question of how public support for women's employment varies and changes over time in accordance to membership in typologies of gender regimes, gender contracts, family policies, and cultures of care for the United States, East Germany, and West Germany. Our analysis focused on the relationship among shifts in gender regime, cultures of care, women-friendly policy packages, and public attitudes supporting maternal employment. Of particular interest was any evidence of convergence among the three regions.

Our results show that in 1991 the gender arrangements, policy regimes, political cultures, and attitude regimes of the three regions followed the expected patterns of liberal, social conservative, and socialist gender regimes. By 2002, convergence theorists would have expected that the attitude gap based on different legacies of political culture in the two regions of Germany and the U.S. to narrow. However, our results show that whereas the public attitudes in both regions of Germany, based on their respective starting points, are moving in a more supportive direction, those in the U.S. have remained unchanged. While West German attitudes toward women's employment have become more positive, they have not caught up with those of East Germans. Furthermore, we found no evidence of a convergence in attitudes between Germans and Americans. In fact, the last decade has seen very little change in the U.S. in terms of its placement on the gender arrangement continuum, family policy regime, culture of care, or toward more supportive attitudes toward maternal employment.

These results point to (a) a continued movement of East German attitudes in line with its previous political culture, (b) a West German political culture shift in terms of increased awareness about the East German gender regime since unification, and (c) a growing divide between German and American attitudes about maternal employment. These findings contradict convergence arguments made about Germany (Rosenfeld et al., 2004) and about advanced industrial countries (Easter et al., 1993; Inglehart & Norris, 2003) at the attitude regime level. It appears that in the case of gender-related attitudes, there is less alignment among countries than proponents of cultural globalization would expect. Thus, it is the legacy of political culture as it relates to the gender regime, not the policy regime *per se* that matters in terms of public attitudes. In fact, the pattern in the U.S. confirms this conclusion; U.S. policy has changed very little, its political culture has not changed at all in the last decade, and neither have attitudes.

We find that the combination of the new gender regime perspectives by Haas (2005) and von Wahl (2005) with conceptualizations of gender contracts (Crompton, 1999a; Pfau-Effinger, 1996; Rosenfeld et al., 2004) is useful in the analysis of the trajectories of national policies and attitudes about the gendered division of labor. Much of previous research has limited itself to the analytical level of one ideal type model, thereby arriving at unidimensional typologies that do not account for the complexity of relationships across an array of countries. We believe future research should continue to explore ways to incorporate ideas from a number of typologies to examine how various gender regimes evolve based on changes in culture, policy, and attitudes. Our findings provoke the next research question: Is East Germany exceptional because of its socialist past or does East Germany lead the way to the future for former socialist and Western industrial countries in continuing its high support for women's employment?

NOTES

1. We also used a standardization procedure, i.e., Z scores, as an alternative to the stretching technique to check the stability of our results. This standardization procedure produced the same substantive results as the stretching procedure. For reasons of easier interpretation we decided to present the results of the stretched range.

2. While skeptics could claim that this finding may be due in part to the inclusion of the middle category of "neither agree nor disagree" in 2002, the fact that the results of the standardization procedure are consistent, discredit this interpretation.

3. Although the difference between the West German mean and the U.S. mean in 2002 did not achieve statistical significance for the attitude index based on the stretching procedure, it was statistically significant for the standardized index. This was the only difference in the results between the two procedures.

REFERENCES

Adler, M. A. (2002). German unification as a turning point in East German women's life course: Biographical changes in work and family roles. *Sex Roles: A Journal of Research, 47,* 83-98.

Adler, M. A. (2004). "Child-free" and unmarried: Changes in the life planning of young East German women. *Journal of Marriage and Family, 66,* 1167-1176.

Adler, M. A., & Brayfield, A. (1996). East-West differences in attitudes about employment and family in Germany. *The Sociological Quarterly, 37*, 401-416.

Adler, M. A., & Brayfield, A. (1997). Women's work values in Unified Germany: Regional differences as remnants of the past. *Work and Occupations, 24*, 245-266.

Brayfield, A., Adler, M. A., & Luo, Y. (2002). Patterns in family policy preferences in the European Union. *Social Thought & Research, 24*, 89-119.

Cooke, L. P. (2004). The gendered division of labor and family outcomes in Germany. *Journal of Marriage and Family, 66*, 1246-1259.

Cooke, L. P. (2006). Policy, preferences and patriarchy: The division of domestic labor in East, West Germany and the United States. *Social Politics: International Studies in Gender, State and Society, 13*(1), 1-27.

Crompton, R. (1999a). The decline of the male breadwinner: Explanations and interpretations. In R. Crompton (Ed.), *Restructuring gender relations and employment: The decline of the male breadwinner* (pp. 1-25). Oxford, UK: Oxford University Press.

Crompton, R. (1999b). Discussion and conclusion. In R. Crompton, (Ed.), *Restructuring gender Relations and Employment: The Decline of Male Breadwinner* (pp. 201-214). Oxford, U.K.: Oxford University Press.

Crompton, R. (2001). Gender restructuring, employment, and caring. *Social Politics, 8*, 266-291.

Dölling, I. (2003). Geschlechtervertrag und Geschlechterarrangements in den neuen Bundesländern [Gender contract and gender arrangements in the new German states]. *Kulturation: Online Journal für Kultur, Wissenschaft und Politik, 26*, 1-17. Retrieved February 26, 2004, from http://www.kulturation.de/frame.php.

Easter, P., Halman, L., & de Moor, R. (1993). Values shift in Western Europe. In P. Easter, L. Halman, R. de Moor (Eds.), *The individualizing society: Values change in Europe and North America* (pp.1-21). Tilburg, The Netherlands: Tilburg University Press.

Engstler, H., & Menning, S. (Eds.). (2003). *Die Familie im Spiegel der amtlichen Statistik.* [The family in view of official statistics]. Berlin, Germany: Bundesministerium für Familie, Senioren, Frauen und Jugend und Statistisches Bundesamt.

Esping-Andersen, G. (1990). *The three worlds of welfare capitalism.* Cambridge, UK: Polity Press.

Gornick, J. C. (2000). Family policy and mothers' employment: Cross-national variations. In T. Boje and A. Leira (Eds.), *Gender, welfare state and the market. Towards a new division of labour* (pp. 111-132). London, UK: Routledge.

Gornick, J. C., Meyers, M. K., & Ross, K. E. (1997). Supporting the employment of mothers: Policy variation across fourteen welfare states. *Journal of European Social Policy, 7*, 45-70.

Gornick, J. C., Meyers, M. K., & Ross, K. E. (1998). Public policies and the employment of mothers: A cross-national study. *Social Science Quarterly, 79*, 35-54.

Gottfried, H., & O'Reilly, J. (2002). Re-regulating breadwinner models in socially conservative welfare states: Comparing Germany and Japan. *Social Politics, 9*, 29-59.

Grünheid, E. (2003). Junge Frauen in Deutschland–Hohe Ausbildung contra Kinder? [Young women in Germany–high qualifications versus children?]. *Bundesinstitut für Bevölkerungsforschung (Bib) Mitteilungen* [Federal Institute for Population Research Bulletin], *24*, 9-15.

Haas, B. (2005). The work-care balance: Is it possible to identify typologies for cross-national comparisons? *Current Sociology, 53*, 487-508.

Hahlen, J. (2003, June 12). *Leben und Arbeiten in Deutschland–Ergebnisse des Mikrozensus 2002.* [Living and working in Germany–Results from the Microzensus 2002]. Pressekonferenz. Wiesbaden, Germany: Statistisches Bundesamt.

Hank, K., Tillmann, K., & Wagner, G. G. (2001). *Außerhäusliche Kinderbetreuung in Ostdeutschland vor und nach der Wiedervereinigung. Ein Vergleich mit Westdeutschland in den Jahren 1990-1999.* [Public daycare in East Germany before and after unification. A comparison with West Germany in the years 1990-1999] (MPIDR Working Paper WP 2000-003). Rostock, Germany: Max Planck Institute for Demographic Research.

Hobson, B. (1994). Solo mothers, social policy regimes and the logics of gender. In D. Sainsbury (Ed.), *Gendering welfare states* (pp.170-187). London, U.K.: Sage.

Hofaecker, D. (2004). The European paragon? European family policy models and their impact on female employment. In P. Amato and N. Gonzales (Eds.), *Vision 2004: What is the future of marriage?* (pp. 60-66). Minneapolis, MN: National Council on Family Relations.

Inglehard, R. (1989). *Culture shift in advanced industrial society.* Princeton, NJ: Princeton University Press.

Inglehart, R., & Norris, P. (2003). *Rising tide: Gender equality and cultural change.* Cambridge, UK: Cambridge University Press.

Kalleberg, A. L. & Stark, D. (1993). Career strategies in capitalism and socialism: Work values and job rewards in the United States and Hungary. *Social Forces, 72*, 181-198.

Klages, H. (1993). *Traditionsbruch als Herausforderung. Perspektiven der Wertewandelsgesellschaft.* [The break with tradition as a challenge. Perspectives on value changes in society] Frankfurt, Germany: Campus Verlag.

Konietzka, D., & Kreyenfeld, M. (2005). Nichteheliche Mutterschaft und soziale Ungleichheit im familialistischen Wohlfahrtsstaat. Zur sozioökonomischen Differenzierung der Familienformen in Ost- und Westdeutschland [Nonmarital motherhood and social inequality in the familiarist welfare state. Socio-economic differentiation of family forms in East and West Germany] *Kölner Zeitschrift für Soziologie und Sozialpsychologie* [Cologne Journal of Sociology and Social Psychology], *57*, 32-61.

Kreyenfeld, M. (2001). *Employment and fertility–East Germany in the 1990s* (Doctoral Dissertation, University of Rostock, November 2001). Rostock, Germany.

Künzler, J., Walter, W., Reichert, E. & Pfister, G. (2001). *Gender division of labour in unified Germany.* European network on policies and the division of unpaid and paid work report. Tilburg University, The Netherlands: Work and Organization Research Center (WORC).

Lewis, J. (1992). Gender and the development of welfare regimes. *Journal of European Social Policy, 2*, 159-173.

Lück, D. (2004). Cultural persistence of traditional gender attitudes over time: Cross-national comparison. In P. Amato and N. Gonzales (Eds.), *Vision 2004: What is the future of marriage?* (pp. 23-31). Minneapolis, MN: National Council on Family Relations.

MacRae, H. (2005). Shifting gender relations in Europe: The influence of European directives on the German gender regime. Paper presented at the Studies in Political Economy conference, York University, Toronto, Canada, February 3-5.

O'Connor, J. (1993). Gender, class and citizenship in the comparative analysis of welfare state regimes: Theoretical and methodological issues. *British Journal of Sociology, 43*, 501-518.

Orloff, A. S. (1993). Gender and the social rights of citizenship. *American Sociological Review, 58*, 303-328.

Pfau-Effinger, B. (1996). Analyse internationaler Differenzen in der Erwerbsbeteiligung von Frauen: Theoretischer Rahmen und empirische Ergebnisse. [Analysis of international differences in the labor force participation of women: Theoretical framework and empirical results.] *Kölner Zeitschrift für Soziologie und Sozialpsychologie* [Cologne Journal of Sociology and Social Psyhology], *48*, 462-492.

Pfau-Effinger, B. (1998). Gender cultures and the gender arrangement–A theoretical framework for cross-national comparisons on gender. *Innovation: The European Journal of Social Science, 11*, 147-166.

Rosenfeld, R., Trappe, H., & Gornick, J. (2004). Gender and work in Germany: Before and after reunification. *Annual Review of Sociology, 30*, 103-124.

Sainsbury, D. (Ed.). (1994). *Gendering welfare states*. London, UK: Sage.

Sainsbury, D. (1999). Gender, policy regimes, and politics. In Diane Sainsbury (Ed.), *Gender and welfare state regimes* (pp. 245-275). Oxford, UK: Oxford University Press.

Siaroff, A. (1994). Work, welfare and gender equality: A new typology. In Diane Sainsbury, (Ed.), *Gendering welfare states* (pp. 82-100). London, UK: Sage.

Statistisches Bundesamt. (2002). *Datenreport 2002* [Data report 2002]. Retrieved [July 5, 2004] from http://www.destatis.de. Wiesbaden, Germany.

Taylor-Gooby, P. (1996). The response of government: Fragile convergence? In V. George and P. Taylor-Gooby (Eds.), *European welfare policy* (pp. 199-219). New York, NY: St. Martin's Press.

Ullrich, C. (2003). Wohlfahrtsstaat und Wohlfahrtskultur. Zu den Perspektiven kultur-und wissenssoziologischer Sozialpolitikforschung. [Welfare state and welfare culture. On the perspectives of the sociology of culture and knowledge] Working paper 67, Mannheimer Zentrum für europäische Sozialforschung. Mannheim, Germany: Universität Mannheim.

U.S. Bureau of Labor Statistics. (2003). Employment status, annual averages, household data. Washington, DC. Retrieved [September 26, 2005] from http://stats.bls.gov/gps/home.htm

U.S. Department of Labor. (2002). Employment status of the civilian population by sex and age, 2001. Retrieved [September 26, 2005] from http://www.dol.gov/.

U.S. Department of Labor. (2005). *Women in the labor force: A databook.* Bureau of Labor Statistics. Retrieved [September 26, 2005] from http://stats.bls.gov/cps/wlf-databook2005.htm.

Voicu, M., & Voicu, B. (2002). Gender values dynamics: Towards a common European pattern? *Romanian Journal of Sociology, 8,* 42-63.

Von Wahl, A. (2005). Liberal, conservative, social, democratic, or . . . European? The European Union as equal employment regime. *Social Politics, 12,* 67-93.

Winkler, G. (Ed.). (2000). *Frauen in Deutschland. 10 Jahre nach der Einheit.* [Women in Germany. 10 years after unification]. Berlin, Germany: Sozialwissenschaftliches Forschungszentrum Berlin-Brandenburg e.V.

Zimmerman, S. L. (1992). *Family policies and family well-being: The role of political culture.* Sage: Newbury Park, CA.

Leave Policies and Research:
A Cross-National Overview

Peter Moss
Fred Deven

SUMMARY. Leave policies for working parents are today widespread among affluent countries, and are required by law in the member states of the European Union. This article reviews leave policies (maternity, paternity, and parental leaves as well as leave to care for sick children) in a wide range of countries, both within and outside the EU, highlighting the main similarities and differences and identifying directions discernible in recent policy developments. It then scopes the knowledge base on the use, practice and impact of leave policies and analyzes why leave policies vary so greatly between countries. The article concludes with a discussion of future challenges and directions for policy and research.

Peter Moss is affiliated with the University of London. Fred Deven is affiliated with the Population and Family Study Center [Centrum voor Bevolknings- en Gezeinsstudie, Markiesstraat 1, 1000 Brussel, Belgium (E-mail: fdeven@pandora.be).

Address correspondence to: Peter Moss, Thomas Coram Research Unit, 27 Woburn Square, London WC1H OAA, United Kingdom (E-mail: peter.moss@ioe.ac.uk).

The authors would like to acknowledge the work of members of the international network on leave policy and research in providing information on leave policy and research in their own countries on which this article has drawn.

[Haworth co-indexing entry note]: "Leave Policies and Research: A Cross-National Overview." Moss, Peter, and Fred Deven. Co-published simultaneously in *Marriage & Family Review* (The Haworth Press, Inc.) Vol. 39, No. 3/4, 2006, pp. 255-285; and: *Families and Social Policy: National and International Perspectives* (ed: Linda Haas, and Steven K. Wisensale) The Haworth Press, Inc., 2006, pp. 255-285. Single or multiple copies of this article are available for a fee from The Haworth Document Delivery Service [1-800-HAWORTH, 9:00 a.m. - 5:00 p.m. (EST). E-mail address: docdelivery@haworthpress.com].

KEYWORDS. Cross-national, maternity leave, parental employment, parental leave

Citizens in most affluent, post-industrial societies today are entitled to interrupt their employment for a period, without losing their jobs, in order to provide care for young children. There are four main types of leave entitlement. Maternity leave is granted to mothers only, and is usually considered to be a measure intended to protect the health and welfare of women and their newborn children around the time of birth. Paternity leave is granted to fathers only, usually at around the time of birth and is intended to enable fathers to provide support to partners at this time and to care for existing children. Parental leave, by contrast, is equally available to mothers and fathers and is a social measure intended to enable parents to provide care for a younger child; it usually starts after the end of maternity leave. Finally, leave may be available in response to unexpected events which require parental care, such as child illness.

Leave policy for workers with young children has been the subject of policy discussion and initiative for many years. As far back as 1919, the International Labour Organisation (ILO) in its Maternity Protection Convention stated that a woman should "not be permitted to work during 6 weeks following her confinement," should be paid benefit during this period and, following this period, should be allowed two half hour breaks from work per day if breastfeeding. National maternity leave policies began to spread from the 1950s (for example, first introduced in Germany in 1952, Belgium in 1954 and Sweden in 1955), to be followed from the 1970s by parental leave (first introduced in Sweden in 1974) and then, from the 1980s, by paternity leave.

International organizations have also become increasingly interested in leave policy. The ILO Workers with Family Responsibilities Recommendation of 1981 proposes that either parent should have access to parental leave and leave to care for a sick child (paragraphs 22 and 23), although it leaves length and other conditions to be decided by individual countries. Over the last decade, there have been a number of reports discussing leave policy from other international organizations, including the Council of Europe (Drew, 2005), the Organisation for Economic Cooperation and Development (OECD, 2002; 2003; 2004; 2005) and UNESCO (Rostgaard, 2003).

The European Union has gone beyond making international comparisons and recommendations, introducing international (i.e., cross-national) law on this policy measure. Council Directive 92/85/EEC of 19th October 1992, on measures to encourage improvements in the safety and health of pregnant workers and workers who have recently given birth or are breastfeeding, lays down minimum conditions for maternity leave among the Union's member states. Council Directive 96/34/EC of 3rd June 1996 gives legal effect to a framework agreement by social partners in 1995 for parental leave. The right to leave has been subsequently incorporated into the Charter of Fundamental Rights of the European Union, adopted in 2000. Article 33 (2) states that "to reconcile family and professional life, everyone shall have the right to protection from dismissal for a reason connected with maternity and the right to paid maternity leave and to parental leave following the birth or adoption of a child."

As we shall discuss, statutory leave policies for parents are widespread today (Gauthier, 2005). However, the form that these policies take varies widely. These variations are revealing, providing an insight into national economic, cultural and social differences concerning dominant views about gender, parenting, childhood, employment and the relationship between social and economic institutions.

National differences in leave policy are also apparent in what departments governments choose to locate leave policy. Different departments have different perspectives, rationalities and objectives; for example, the "logic" of an employment department has very little to do with family and child welfare, typically being more concerned with labor market issues. Location of policy may have implications for the degree of coherence between leave and other policy areas. It is, therefore, significant that leave policy is often located within departments concerned with employment matters and/or the regulation of business. Where this is not the case, leave policy is usually found within social welfare departments, for example in France (Ministry of Social Affairs, Health and Solidarity), Germany (Ministry for Family, Senior Citizens, Women and Youth), Iceland (Ministry of Social Affairs), Norway (Ministry of Children and Family Affairs) and Sweden (Ministry of Social Affairs). An exception is Ireland where responsibility for leave policy is with the Department of Justice, Equality and Law Reform.

In nearly all countries, leave policy is a national responsibility. An exception is Canada, where leave itself is a responsibility of the 10 provinces and territories, while payment to parents taking leave has been a federal responsibility (though from 2006, responsibility for leave payments in Québec will be transferred from the federal to the provincial government). In some countries, notably Germany, Spain and the United States, individual states or regional governments may enhance national entitlements.

In this article, we attempt to provide a state-of-the-art map of the current position on leave policy and research across a wide range of European and non-European English-speaking countries. We compare leave policies, highlighting main differences and similarities, and use the cases of three countries to illustrate different directions discernible in recent policy developments. We then scope the knowledge base concerning the use, practice and impact of leave policies; the aim of this exercise is to establish in what areas there is knowledge about leave policies and their workings and where there are gaps, rather than presenting a detailed review of the findings from the extant literature. We conclude by considering whether and how the large variations in leave policy might be explained; for example, in relation to the interplay of welfare and gender regimes and to "path dependency." We also discuss what lessons we can draw from the evidence on use of leave, as well as future directions for research in the light of the results of our scoping exercise.

We have based much of the article on the first work of an international network on leave policies and research, which builds on earlier collaborative cross-national work (Deven & Moss, 2002; Deven & Moss, 2005; European Commission Childcare Network, 1995; Moss & Deven, 1999). The network at present includes about thirty members (mostly researchers) from more than 20 countries. Among its purposes are the exchange of information about policies, both in individual countries and by international organizations, and research on leave policies; the provision of a forum for the cross-national discussion of issues and trends in policy and research; and providing a source of regularly updated information on policies and research.

This network focuses on policies for parents and others with care responsibilities, including for adult relatives, as well as policies available to the whole population such as life course career breaks and time accounts. But initially, priority has been given to leave policies focused on the care of children. These include maternity, paternity and parental leave and leave to care for sick children as well as entitlements to work reduced hours.

A recent working paper by the network includes 19 "country notes" supplied by network members, in each case covering details of leave policies, an outline of recent policy developments, information on use, and brief details on recent studies and publications in the field (Deven & Moss, 2005). This article mainly draws on information supplied in these country notes. However, because the country notes include only one country from Central and Eastern Europe, Hungary, we have also drawn on recent reports on the countries in this region (Neyer, 2005; Rostgaard, 2003; Stropnik, 2004). This still leaves significant gaps in terms of more affluent countries: for example, of the member states of OECD, this article does not include Greece, Japan, Korea, Luxembourg, Mexico, New Zealand, Switzerland and Turkey.

One other caveat should be made. Leave policies may be statutory entitlements, based on national legislation. But they may be supplemented by or, in some cases, exist only as benefits conferred through collective agreements (therefore covering only those included in the agreements) or by individual employers (therefore covering only their employees). Our focus here is on statutory leave entitlements (for a fuller discussion of supplementation, see Math & Meiland, 2004).

CURRENT LEAVE POLICIES

Table 1 provides a summary of statutory leave policies across the 19 countries featured in this article.

Maternity Leave

Of these 19 countries, three have no statutory maternity leave. In the case of the United States, there is a general leave entitlement–Family and Medical Leave–that can be used for a range of purposes including *de facto* as maternity leave (though coverage is not universal, about 40 percent of workers being excluded because they work in smaller organizations). In Australia and Sweden, leave is available around the time of childbirth but is not restricted to women, being subsumed into parental leave. While such leave is paid at a high level in Sweden, it is unpaid in Australia and the United States.

In the remaining countries with statutory maternity leave, the period is mostly between 14 and 20 weeks, with earnings-related payment (be-

TABLE 1. Provision of Statutory Leave Entitlements in Selected Countries

	Type and length of leave (in months)					
	Maternity	Paternity	Parental	Post-natal leave Total	Paid	Sick children
Australia	×	×	✓ 12 F	12	0	×
Austria	✓✓✓ 3.5	×	✓✓ 22* F	24	24*	✓✓✓ 0.5
Belgium	✓✓✓ 3.5	✓✓✓ 0.5	✓✓ 6 I	9.5	9.5	✓ 0.5
Canada(a)	✓✓✓ 3.5	✓ < 0.5	✓✓✓ 8.5 F	12	11.5	×
Denmark	✓✓✓ 4	✓✓✓ 0.5	✓✓✓ 7.5 F	10.5	10.5	×
Finland	✓✓✓ 4	✓✓✓ 1	✓✓✓ 6 F	36	36	×
France	✓✓✓ 3.5	✓✓✓ 0.5	✓✓ 33* F	36	36*(b)	✓ < 0.5
Germany	✓✓ 3.5	×	✓✓ 34* F	36	24*(c)	✓✓✓ 1
Hungary	✓✓✓ 5.5	×	✓✓✓ 31.5(d)	36	36	✓✓✓ (d)
Iceland	✓✓✓ 4	✓✓✓ 3	✓✓✓ 3 F	9	9	×
Ireland	✓✓ 6	×	✓ 6.5 I	12	4	✓✓✓ < 0.5
Italy	✓✓✓ 4.5	×	✓✓ 10(e)I	12.5	12.5	✓ (e)
Netherlands	✓✓✓ 3.5	✓✓✓ < 0.5	✓ 6 I	8.5	2.5	✓✓✓ 0.5
Norway	✓✓✓ 2	✓ 0.5	✓✓✓ 10 F/I	11.5	11.5	✓✓✓ (f)
Portugal	✓✓✓ 5.5	✓✓✓ 1	✓ 6 I	11.5	5.5	✓✓✓ 1.5
Spain	✓✓✓ 3.5	✓✓✓ < 0.5	✓ 32.5 I	36	3.5	✓✓✓ < 0.5
Sweden	×	✓✓✓ 0.5	✓✓✓ (g) F/I	(g)		✓✓✓ (g)

	Type and length of leave (in months)				
	Maternity	Paternity	Parental	Post-natal leave Total Paid	Sick children
U.Kingdom	✓✓ 12	✓✓ 0.5	✓ 6 I	18 6	✓ ?
U.S.	✕ (h)	✕	✕	0	✕

✕ -no statutory entitlement
✓ -statutory entitlement but unpaid; ✓✓ -statutory entitlement, paid but *either* at low flat rate *or* earnings-related at less than 50 percent of earnings *or* not universal *or* for less than the full period of leave; ✓✓✓ -statutory entitlement, paid to all parents at more than 50 percent of earnings (in most cases up to a maximum ceiling).
* -payment is made to all parents with a young child whether or not they are taking leave.
? -length of leave unstated.
Unbracketed numbers for each leave column indicate total length of leave *in months* (to nearest month); *bracketed* numbers in 'total post-natal leave' column indicate length of leave which receives some payment.
Parental Leave: F = family entitlement; I = individual entitlement; F/I = some period of family entitlement and some period of individual entitlement.
(a) There are differences in length of leave between provinces and territories; three provinces allow 3-5 days of unpaid leave to care for members of immediate family.
(b) Only paid to parents with one child until 6 months after the end of maternity leave.
(c) Payment after maternity leave until child is 2 years and means tested.
(d) For insured parents, leave is paid at 70 percent of earnings until child's 3rd birthday, then at flat rate; only mother is entitled to use in child's first year. Leave for sick children varies according to child's age from unlimited (child under 1) to 14 days for a child aged 6 to 12 years.
(e) 6 months per parent, but total leave per family cannot exceed 10 months. Leave for a sick child is unlimited for a child under 3 years, 5 days per parent for a child aged 3 to 8 years.
(f) 10 days per parent if one child under 12 years; 15 days if 2 or more children. Extended rights to leave if chronically sick child.
(g) 480 days of paid leave per family (divided between individual entitlements and family entitlement), 390 days at 90 percent of earnings and 90 days at a low flat rate; each parent also entitled to 18 months unpaid leave; 60 days leave per year per child to care for a sick child.
(h) Parents may take up to 12 weeks unpaid leave for childbirth or the care of a child up to 12 months as part of the federal Family and Medical Leave Act; employers with less than 50 employees are exempt. Five states and Puerto Rico provide some benefit payments to parents missing work at around the time of childbirth.

tween 70 and 100 percent) throughout; in some cases, leave may be extended where there are multiple births. There are three main exceptions, all of which are countries with extended maternity leave. Maternity leave in Ireland is 26 weeks and 52 weeks in the UK; in neither case is leave paid for the full period, and in the UK earnings-related payments last for only 6 weeks (i.e., most of the leave period is paid at a low flat rate or unpaid). Though maternity leave in Hungary is 24 weeks (with earnings-related payment throughout), part of parental leave–until the child reaches 12 months old–can only be taken by the mother (or a single father), in effect an extended maternity leave.

There is not much flexibility in maternity leave, indeed taking leave is obligatory in some countries. Where it occurs, flexibility mainly takes the form of some choice about when women can start to take leave and how much time they may take before and after birth. Portugal and Spain, however, have introduced another dimension of flexibility: mothers may transfer or share part of the maternity leave period with fathers. Portuguese mothers may also choose between two periods of leave, one shorter but paid at 100 percent of earnings, the other longer but paid at 80 percent.

All other Central and Eastern European (CEE) countries provide maternity leave, either 16-18 weeks (e.g., Bulgaria, Estonia, Latvia, Poland, Romania, Ukraine) or 24-28 weeks, with earnings-related benefits (Rostgaard, 2003).

Paternity Leave

The distinction between paternity leave and parental leave is blurring in some countries where a portion of parental leave is only usable by fathers (i.e., a "fathers" quota). Here, we have confined paternity leave to denote a short period of leave to be taken immediately after the birth, concurrently with maternity leave; parental leave can usually only be taken after maternity leave. On this basis, a majority of the 19 countries have paternity leave, which mostly varies from 2 to 10 days and is usually (though not always) paid on the same basis as maternity leave. There are three exceptions: Finland, which provides 18 days of paternity leave, with a further 12 "bonus" days for fathers who take the last two weeks of parental leave; Portugal, which now provides 20 days paternity leave, 5 days of which are obligatory, i.e., fathers must take leave; and Iceland (discussed further below), where 9 months of post-natal leave available per family is divided into 3 months maternity leave, 3 months paternity leave and 3 months parental leave to be shared between parents as they choose. (In Iceland, the line between paternity and parental leave is extremely blurred, since paternity leave is usually taken after mothers have taken 6 months of maternity and parental leave.)

Among CEE countries, only Slovenia offers paid paternity leave, which at 90 days is far longer than any of the countries in Table 1 (Rostgaard, 2003). Moreover, though 15 days of paternity leave must be used during maternity leave, the remainder can be used at any time until a child's 8th birthday. Only the first 15 days are paid at full wage replacement; during the remaining period, fathers are paid only social security contributions based on the minimum wage.

Parental Leave

All EU member states must provide at least 3 months leave per parent for childcare purposes. Four of the non-EU countries in this overview also provide a statutory parental leave entitlement, the exception being the United States (which as already noted has only a generic and unpaid leave, which does not apply to all employees).

Statutory parental leave varies on four main dimensions: length; whether it is an individual or family entitlement; payment; and flexibility. Broadly, countries divide up into those where parental leave, when added to maternity leave, comes to around 9-15 months, and those where maternity and parental leave together run for around 3 years. In the former camp are Australia, Belgium, Canada, Denmark, Iceland, Ireland, Italy, the Netherlands, Norway, Portugal and the United Kingdom. In the latter camp are Finland, France, Germany, Hungary and Spain. In the case of Finland, a parent taking three years leave would need to draw on maternity and parental leave (which together last for about 39 weeks after the birth) and an additional leave referred to as home care leave. Two countries fall in between. In Austria, parental leave, on a full-time basis, can be taken until a child's 2nd birthday (or until the 4th birthday if part-time leave is taken). In Sweden, paid leave is expressed in days—480—to emphasise that it can be taken very flexibly; moreover, each parent is also entitled to take unpaid leave until a child is 18 months.

Parental leave is an entirely family entitlement in eight countries, to be divided between parents as they choose (Austria, Australia, Canada, Denmark, Finland, France, Germany, Hungary and Iceland); an entirely individual entitlement in another seven countries (Belgium, Ireland, Italy, the Netherlands, Portugal, Spain, United Kingdom); and mixed (part family, part individual entitlement) in two countries (Norway and Sweden) (Moss, 2005).

A majority of countries (12) provide some element of payment. However, in five cases, payment is flat-rate or means-tested or paid for only part of the leave period, or a combination of these. Only six out of the 19 countries pay an earnings-related benefit equivalent to more than half of normal earnings. The twelfth country, Finland, combines a relatively high level earnings-related benefit during parental leave, with a low flat-rate benefit for home care leave which has supplements for users with additional children and lower incomes.

The most generous payments are in the Nordic countries, especially Iceland, Norway and Sweden. Here, most or all of the leave period is paid at 80 percent of earnings or higher (up to a maximum "ceiling" amount, a principle applied in all countries paying earnings-related benefits). Hungary, too, is relatively generous, paying a benefit of 70 percent of earnings to parents on leave until a child's 2nd birthday, then a lower flat-rate payment until the child is 3 years old.

Flexibility takes three main forms. First, the possibility to use all or part of leave when parents choose until their child reaches a certain age (e.g., Austria, Belgium, Germany, Portugal, Sweden); second, the possibility of taking leave in one continuous block or several shorter blocks (e.g., Sweden); and third, the possibility to take leave on a full-time or part-time basis (i.e., so parents can combine part-time employment with part-time leave) (e.g., France, Germany, Portugal, Québec, Sweden). Other forms of flexibility include options to take longer periods of leave with lower benefits or shorter periods with higher benefits (e.g., Germany, Norway).

Various measures have been introduced to encourage fathers to use parental leave. Mostly these take the form of wholly or partly individualized entitlements, whereby fathers not using their leave lose it, since unused leave cannot be transferred to a partner. Examples of these "fathers' quotas" include Norway and Sweden, while as already noted Iceland has a long paternity leave that shares many similarities with a parental leave father's quota.

Central and Eastern European countries mostly offer, like Hungary, parental leave until a child is 2 or 3 years of age, with either earnings-related or flat-rate benefit payments. In two cases, the Czech Republic and Estonia, leave can last longer. In countries such as the Czech Republic, Poland and Slovakia, benefit payment is means-tested, so it is only paid to lower income families. Once again, the main exception is Slovenia, which offers a shorter period of leave (260 days), in effect until the end of the child's first year, but a high (100 percent) earnings-related benefit (Rostgaard, 2003).

Childcare Leave or Career Breaks

In five countries, parents can take additional leave after parental leave finishes. In three cases the leave is unpaid: 3 months per parent per year until a child is 8 years in Iceland; a year in Norway; and 2-3 years in

Portugal. Parents with three or more children in Hungary can take leave until their youngest child is 8 years old, with a flat-rate benefit. Finland, already mentioned, is exceptional in that its home care leave is both available to all parents and paid, albeit with a relatively low flat-rate allowance (so blurring the distinction with parental leave) (Moss, 2005).

Three countries provide some form of career break from employment not necessarily tied to childbearing and childcare. Employees in Austria can take 6 to12 months; in Sweden, 3 to 12 months; in Belgium 1 to 5 years. Leave is unpaid and dependent on employer agreement in Austria, while in Sweden there is some payment but there is a quota on how many people in the country can take leave at any one time. In Belgium, there is a flat rate payment but no more than 5 percent of employees in a company may take this "time credit" at the same time.

Other Employment-Related Measures

The EU parental leave directive gives all workers an entitlement to "time off from work on grounds of *force majeure* for urgent family reasons in cases of sickness or accident making their immediate presence indispensable," without specifying minimum requirements for length of time or payment. Among EU member states reviewed here, six (Austria, Germany, Hungary, Italy, Portugal and Sweden) specify an entitlement to leave of 10 days or more to care for sick children, though the age range of children covered varies. The most generous leave is in Sweden, where there is earnings-related paid leave of 60 days per year per child under the age of 12 years. For all others, except Italy, leave is paid. In some cases, the length of leave decreases as children get older; for example, in Hungary, leave ranges from being unlimited for a child under 12 months to 14 days a year for children from 6 to 12 years old.

Leave is short or unspecified and unpaid in the other member states. Of the non-EU countries, only Norway has an entitlement to paid sick leave specifically to care for sick child. In Australia, all employees have the right to use up to 5 days of personal or sick leave per year to care for a sick family member.

Five countries (Hungary, Italy, Norway, Portugal and Spain) enable women to reduce their working hours in the first 9 to12 months after birth, usually related to breast-feeding. Four countries (Austria, Norway, Spain and Sweden) give parents the right to work part-time hours until their child reaches a certain age (between 6 and 8 years). In Italy, the Netherlands and the UK, parents do not have a right to work part time but they can request flexible working hours from their employers, who must consider their request and may only refuse them if there is a clear business case for doing so.

MAJOR CHANGES IN LEAVE POLICY AND OTHER RELATED DEVELOPMENTS

Leave policy is frequently changing. Table 2 summarizes the changes that have occurred among the 19 countries between 1999 and 2004. These changes mainly involve enhancement of leave entitlements, in the form of new and/or longer periods and greater flexibility. Not only is leave a very active policy area, but it is also an area where the welfare state is developing rather than retrenching. One trend has been a growing emphasis on fatherhood, for example the introduction or extension of paternity leave in Belgium, Finland, France, Portugal and the UK or the improvement of men's parental leave rights (Iceland, Sweden). On the other hand, a major reform of the leave system in Denmark in 2002 increased benefit payments (to equivalence with maternity leave payment throughout, when before half the period of parental leave was paid at 60 percent of maternity leave benefit), while at the same time reducing leave duration and removing a two-week father's quota.

In addition to Denmark, three other countries have made major changes to their leave policies since 1999, and represent the divergent approaches to leave policy that are apparent from cross-national comparison. Canada added 25 weeks of paid parental leave in 2000, a substantial extension to the existing 10 weeks; paid maternity and parental leave were effectively increased from 6 to 12 months. Canada now has 15 weeks paid maternity leave followed by 35 weeks paid parental leave, a family entitlement to be divided between parents as they choose, both paid at 55 percent of average earnings up to a maximum "ceiling."

In the same year, Iceland undertook a radical reform of its parental leave system. Previously, this had been complicated and differentiated, with different rights for different groups, including men being less favorably treated; for example, men working in the public sector had no rights and men working in the private sector had rights dependent on their spouses. In 2000, the overall leave period was extended to 9 months, divided into three equal parts: 3 months for mothers, 3 months for fathers and 3 months per family for parents to divide as they choose; the whole period is to be paid at 80 percent of earnings. In addition, each

TABLE 2. Changes in Leave Policy 1999-2004

	Maternity Leave	Paternity Leave	Parental Leave	Leave to care for sick children
Australia				
Austria			↑ flexibility	✓ (serious illness)
Belgium	✓ eligibility	✓ ↑ length		
Canada(a)			↑ length & eligibility	✓ (serious illness)
Denmark			↑ payment ↓ length ✗ father's quota	
Finland	↑ payment	↑ length & payment	↑ flexibility & payment	
France		✓	↑ payment	
Germany			↑ flexibility ↓ payment	
Hungary			↑ flexibility	
Iceland		✓	↑ length ✓ unpaid childcare leave	
Ireland				
Italy			↑ father's quota	
Netherlands				
Norway				
Portugal	↑ flexibility & protection	✓ ↑ length & part obligatory	↑ flexibility	↑ length
Spain				
Sweden			↑ father's & mother's quota	
U.Kingdom	↑ length and payment	✓	✓	✓
U.S.				

Key: ✓ = entitlement introduced; ✗ = entitlement removed; ↑ = entitlement improved; ↓ = entitlement reduced.

parent can now take 13 weeks a year of unpaid leave until a child is 8 years old.

The UK was the last EU member state to adopt the Directive on parental leave, introducing the measure in 1999 (25 years after Sweden, the first country to introduce parental leave). However, the entitlement introduced was the minimum required meeting the Directive–13 weeks unpaid leave per parent. In 2003, maternity leave was extended from 40 weeks (already the longest in Europe) to 52 weeks, with payment (mostly a low flat rate) increased from 18 to 26 weeks. The government is committed to extending payment to 52 weeks, and has been considering a proposal to make part of this extended paid maternity leave transferable to fathers. Lastly, also in 2003, a period of 2 weeks of paternity leave was implemented, but paid (like most of maternity leave) only at a low flat-rate.

As can be seen, levels of payment vary: from leave that is largely unpaid or paid at a low flat-rate in the UK, to leave that attracts earnings-related benefits at a moderate rate (Canada) or a high rate (Iceland). The UK measures allow no flexibility in use; indeed, the 13 weeks of parental leave cannot be taken in one block (as is the case with all other leave schemes), but only in three 4-week blocks spread over 3 years. By contrast, the Icelandic scheme allows parents to take parental leave in one block or several blocks over time. None of these schemes, however, include part-time options, which are possible in a number of countries (e.g., France, Germany).

All three countries have improved previous leave policies, but in very different ways. Canada has enhanced parental leave as a family entitlement, adopting a gender neutral approach. Iceland has introduced a mix of family and individual entitlements, in which fathers and mothers have equal individual rights; with this move, Iceland has joined a small group of countries (including Norway and Sweden) that are seeking to promote gender equality through leave policies that actively encourage paternal use by combining well paid leave and a substantial period of leave that only fathers can use. By contrast, the UK has introduced an individual but unpaid entitlement to parental leave and a short and low paid paternity leave, both overshadowed by the extension of a partly paid maternity leave for women only, in effect supporting a gendered approach to childcare.

These different policies produce very different results in terms of parental use. Although a substantial number of Canadian mothers are not eligible for leave, use of this option among those who are eligible has increased substantially since the extension of leave; the overall proportion of all new mothers receiving maternity or parental benefits rose from 54 percent in 2000 to 61 percent in 2001. Fathers' participation rate has trebled, though from a low base (from 3 percent in 2000 to 10 percent in 2001). The change has been even more striking in Iceland following the major reform of leave policy, including 3 months of paternity leave. By 2003, 84 fathers took a period of leave for every 100 mothers taking leave, and fathers took an average of 94 days leave compared to 182 for mothers. In the UK, most women return to work before the end of the long and mostly low paid or unpaid maternity leave period, commonly citing financial reasons, and there is no information on the use of unpaid parental leave; it is, however, thought to be very low among both women and men. The minister responsible for parental leave in 2004 acknowledged that "the right to take three months unpaid parental leave . . . is little known or used and needs to be reviewed to make it more helpful to families" (Hewitt, 2004, p. 18).

RESEARCH ON LEAVE ARRANGEMENTS FOR PARENTS

This section covers the knowledge base on leave arrangements for parents, especially parental leave, identifying areas which have been most subject to research with a particular focus on work since the beginning of 2000. It builds upon previous review work (see Deven & Carrette, 2005; Deven & Moss, 2002; Moss & Deven, 1999). It also draws on other overviews and benefits as well as from the information on recent research projects and publications provided by network members in their country notes (Deven & Moss, 2005).

Overall, this domain of research enjoys growing interest from policymakers and academics alike (including a growing number of doctoral dissertations), both in its own right and as part of a wider research domain concerned with the relationship between work and family. Four major areas in the leave policy research domain are apparent: (1) cross-national comparisons; (2) evaluation studies or impact analyses of leave policies; (3) use of paternity leave or/and of parental leave by fathers; and (4) the importance of workplace culture and practices, especially for fathers. Work on the first two appears to have been increasing rapidly over the last few years, while the last two show a continuation of earlier research interest.

Cross-National Comparative Work

At present, there are no regularly updated, large-scale data sets enabling comparison of the use of leave policies across countries, as well as between different socio-demographic groups. The ongoing monitoring of the attitudes, opinions and preferences of the EU adult population provided by Eurobarometer, a survey conducted at least two times a year in all EU member states on behalf of the European Commission, occasionally provides relevant data. In Spring 2003, for example, the survey questioned approximately 12,000 men in the member states about their knowledge of and intention to use parental leave (Eurobarometer, 2004).

A number of intergovernmental organizations have reviewed and compared national legislation and monitor developments. At the level of the European Union, databases such as MISSOC (social protection systems) or EIRR (industrial relations indicators) monitor overall developments; occasionally some comparative information is provided on eligibility, duration, and compensation of some types of leave or related arrangements such as birth grants or family allowances (e.g., EIRR, 2001). Math and Meiland (2004) provide a comparative study in 19 EU member states, largely based on contributions from members of the European Industrial Relations Observatory. They pay particular attention to the role of collective bargaining in four types of family-related leaves.

A report by Rostgaard (2003), commissioned by the Council of Europe and the UNESCO Department of Education, focuses on the situation in Central and Eastern European countries, while Kokourkova (2002) compares leave policies and their recent development in four countries in Central Europe. Drew (2005) takes the widest European perspective reviewing leave in all 45 member states of the Council of Europe, providing comparative information on legal rights and entitlements, time limits and flexibility, as well as payments to leave takers, availability and job security. There is here at least some information for a number of countries in Eastern Europe or formerly part of the Soviet Union that are often excluded in other comparative reports (Stropnik, 2004).

Looking more widely than Europe, large-scale projects such as the OECD thematic review of national early childhood education and care (1998-2004) provide relevant information on leave and related policies in the 20 countries covered (see OECD, 2001 for the first report covering 12 countries, with a second report covering all countries reviewed in preparation). The OECD also provides overall data on "family-friendly" policies and more detailed cross-national analyses for 13 countries through its *Babies and Bosses* project (OECD, 2002; 2003; 2004, 2005).

Ferrarini (2003) analyzed the role of paid parental leave policies in 18 welfare states. By considering parental leave policies from an institutional approach, he showed that the differences at the turn of the 20th century were substantial, and that the institutional structures of parental leave benefits entail different choice capacities of parents, for the participation of mothers in paid work as well as for the involvement of fathers in care work. He also observed that the cross-national patterns of paid parental leave largely follow the lines of broader family policy strategies, and that left party incumbency and women's share of ministerial posts are the most important explanatory factors behind the development of paid parental leave in support of the dual earner family.

Gornick and Meyers (2003) analyze "family leave" policies on the basis of five key principles such as the provision of periods of leave for mothers and fathers throughout their children's preschool years, with both job security and wage replacement or the embedding of gender equality in all family leave policies. Their analysis pays particular attention to how current policy in the U.S. fares against these principles, concluding that it does badly on nearly every one of the principles. The consequences are weakened labor market attachment for women, which in turn worsens gender inequality; economic insecurity for families, especially for those headed by low-educated and low-income workers; and constraints on parental time for caring for the youngest children. They conclude that "the family leave system in the United States ensures American working parents remarkably little time for caregiving during their children's earliest years and imposes the costs of caregiving on women, parents, and, to a lesser extent, employers" (Gornick & Meyers, 2003, pp. 143-144).

Other American scholars have also sought to inform a U.S. audience about European policies, mostly by contrasting policies and practices in the United States and the European Union (e.g., Haas, 2002; Hernanz, Malherbet & Pellizzari, 2004; Waldfogel, 2001, 2003), with Sheila Kamerman and the Institute for Child and Family Policy at Columbia University continuing their program of research comparing the main child-related leave policies in highly industrialized and developing countries (Kamerman, Neuman, Waldfogel & Brooks-Gunn, 2003; see also www.childpolicyintl.org).

Evaluation and Impact Studies

Increasingly, the various types of leave are used as a major tool by policymakers (public authorities, employers) to facilitate the combination of work and family life. This has led to increasing numbers of studies commissioned by policymakers and implementers. Three types of studies are briefly considered here. First, analyses of the implementation of the 1996 EC Directive; second, analyses of national legislation;

and finally, various types of impact studies analyzing the consequences or effects on one or more stakeholders of the leave policies.

The EC Directive on Parental Leave (96/34/EC). On the basis of a collaborative research project, Falkner, Hartlapp, Leiber and Treib (2002) took parental leave as a case to study the national implementation, enforcement and application of EU labor law Directives. They especially considered the degree of mismatch between European policy and domestic structures. The existence of considerable external pressure, supplied by the Directive, to adapt national regulations was under certain conditions conducive to smooth implementation, and several member states not only brought domestic standards up to the new EU requirements but went beyond.

Hardy and Adnett (2002) assessed the social, economic and legal implementations of the parental leave Directive and identified differing national strategies for implementation. They consider the Directive an inadequate legal framework, a limited measure which increases rather than reduces gender inequalities in the labor market. They suggest that the design of minimum standards, such as the Directive provides, needs to reconcile family-friendly practices with greater gender equality.

Evaluation of national legislation. Examples of such national assessments can be found in Austria (ÖIF, 2005), Germany (Empirica, 2004), the Netherlands (van Luijn & Keuzenkamp, 2004) and the U.S. (Breidenbach, 2003; Han & Waldfogel, 2003). The following research questions are usually at the heart of those studies: What is the need for various leave schemes (and other measures)? What is the extent of the "need" and of use? What is the profile of the users? Why are some categories of employees more or less likely to use leave schemes? Are schemes effective in meeting the needs of working parents? What kind of problems do potential users encounter?

Van Luijn and Keuzenkamp (2004), for example, investigated the use of leave schemes in the Netherlands. They surveyed 3100 employees aged between 20 and 61 years, with a subgroup who had stopped working to care for a family member. The largest discrepancy between need and use arose when urgent family incidents required almost immediate solutions. Or to take another example, Breidenbach (2003) studied the 1993 U.S. Family and Medical Leave Act (FMLA) from a family perspective, highlighting both positive and negative consequences as well as pointing to possibilities for improving its ability to assist American families in times of need.

Effects on particular stakeholders. These overall evaluation studies are complemented by more specific studies which analyze impact of leave policies on particular actors. Until recently, such analyses focused almost exclusively on mothers, their employment status and the probability of their re-entry to work after childbirth and a period of leave. Such research has been conducted in the U.S. and for most Nordic countries. Hofferth and Curtin (2003), for example, examined changes in the U.S. between the late 1980s and the mid-1990s in four areas: (1) how soon mothers were employed following childbirth; (2) whether they returned to the same employer; (3) whether their post-return earnings were higher than before they took leave; and (4) whether any of these changes are linked to changes in the FMLA and/or state leave policies over the period.

Some scholars provide comparative data for two or more Nordic countries. Rønsen (1999) examined the female employment rates after childbirth in Finland, Norway and Sweden, focusing on the impact of parental leave and childcare programs on the transitions to full-time and part-time work. Rønsen (2001) also assessed the short-term effects of the Norwegian cash-for-care reform, a scheme introduced in 1998 that gives cash to parents of 1- and 2-year-olds who do not use publicly funded childcare services. She noted a small decline in the work probability of most mothers after the reform, except among those at the highest educational level. Career interruptions due to parental leave have been compared between Danish and Swedish mothers (Pylkannen & Smith, 2003).

Indirect evidence on the impact and effects of leave policies on children comes from studies of parental employment (often, somewhat misleadingly, presented as studies of *maternal* employment on children). These studies (most often British or American) are sometimes based on longitudinal studies (e.g., Berger, Hill & Waldfogel, 2005; Waldfogel, Han & Brooks-Gunn, 2003). Increasingly, attention is being drawn to the need to introduce more variables into analyses, such as more details of the mother's employment, father's occupational status, family income during children's infancy, and especially the quality of non-parental childcare (e.g., Ram, Abada & Hou, 2004).

More direct study of the impact of leave arrangements on children is getting some attention from researchers and policymakers alike. At first, the focus has mainly been on the effects of periods of maternity leave on the health of newborns and infants (Ruhm, 2000; Tanaka, 2005). Galtry and Callister (2005) updated previous work on assessing the optimal length of leave for child and parental well-being. They note that such policies need to take account of seemingly contradictory policy objectives: protecting biological maternity (i.e., pregnancy, childbirth, post-birth recovery and breastfeeding); promoting gender equity in childrearing; optimizing women's economic and labor market outcomes; and protecting and enhancing children's health and development. They observe that "if only [based] on research on labour markets and on gender equity, then short leaves seem the best policy option. But once biomedical research is considered the design of leave becomes far more complex" (p. 244).

Other dimensions of child development receive scant attention (e.g., Kamerman, 2003; Lero, 2003). Deven and Carrette (2005) point to the methodological issues for research from the perspective of children and observe that the majority of studies suffer from important methodological limitations. The concept of child development, for example, is treated in a rather narrow way, with studies of the impact of parental leave arrangements focusing predominantly on children's health and on cognitive outcomes, e.g., verbal and mathematical skills.

A Luxembourg study asked parents (mostly mothers) what they perceived as the advantages for their infants of using their 3 months of parental leave. Among the main reasons given, 35 percent of the users referred to the well-being of the child by referring to "providing more security and stability," "respecting the biological rhythm of the child," and "facilitating a period of breastfeeding" (KPMG, 2002).

Fathers and Father Involvement

Recent years have seen a growing interest in fathers and their involvement in the household and in care work, with reviews of this work becoming available. Burgess and Russell (2004), for example, recently reviewed the predominantly U.S.-based research literature on father involvement. Overall, a picture emerges of a growing interest and practice both at the individual and at the societal level, although important differences remain related to social class and education.

Within this broad context, an increasing number of studies focus on fathers' attitudes and behaviors in the (non-)use of paternity leave and parental leave. It was striking, for example, that most articles in a special journal issue on leave arrangements for parents, related to fathers (see *Community, Work & Family*, 2002, 5/3). Studies continue on this subject. Brandth and Kvande (2003) revealed various factors which impact on the use of parental leave by Norwegian fathers (e.g., women working part-time and differences in earnings between parents). Chronholm (2004) combined survey-based data with more focused interviews in his doctoral thesis on the parental leave experiences of

Swedish fathers, bringing into his study a comparison between Swedish-born and immigrant fathers. Also in Sweden, Duvander and Andersson (2005) document a positive relationship between a father taking a moderately long period of leave and a couple's propensity to have a second and third child, but no such effect of taking very long paternal leave. Einarsdottir and Petursdottir (2004) report on a comparative study of issues of time and gender in modern German, Icelandic, Norwegian and Spanish families with young children. Special attention is paid to how cultural traditions, attitudes and norms facilitate or hinder men's use of their parental rights. One of their conclusions is that flexibility within a universal but gender-biased system does not have a large potential for change.

Deven (2005) has developed a framework incorporating the various dimensions at play to understand the use or non-use of parental leave by fathers, taking the perspective of various stakeholders into account.

Workplace Culture

Workplace or organizational culture refers to the basic pattern of shared assumptions, values and beliefs. Workplaces are considered with regard to the behavior of the management, the amount of workgroup support and the (often unwritten) rules reflecting ways of thinking about and acting, all of which can influence whether and how fathers and mothers use various work-life balance policies. Russell and Hwang (2004) comprehensively reviewed the impact of workplace practices on overall father involvement, covering parental leave as one of four workplace practices and policies. They note that most of the research to date has focused on examining assumed direct links between workplace policies such as parental leave or work demands (e.g., work hours) and father involvement.

Yet, it may be that the workplace, by providing alternative career options and alternative role models of success (that include work-family balance), could function to increase the level of motivation for a father to be involved with his children. On the other hand, the workplace could provide self-development opportunities that enhance communication and interpersonal skills that will increase a father's self-confidence as a parent (Russell & Hwang, 2004, p. 500).

Research by den Dulk (2001) and by Haas, Allard and Hwang (2002) provides relevant data as well as a better understanding of factors associated with workplace culture. Haas et al. (2002) point to several aspects of organizational culture having independent effects on the likelihood of Swedish fathers taking parental leave. But they conclude that "the amount of variance explained by organizational culture variables, was, however, surprisingly low, in comparison to that explained by individual- and family-level attributes" (p. 338), though adding that this may be specific to the Swedish context where fathers have strong legal entitlements to take leave. The Dutch government recently commissioned a study among a representative sample of Dutch companies and organizations in order to highlight their "joys and sorrows" related to various leave policies (Duyvendak & Stavenuiter, 2004).

DISCUSSION AND RECOMMENDATIONS

The great diversity in leave policies should by now be apparent. What can explain this diversity? Is it possible to discern some pattern in the diversity? The threefold typology of welfare state regimes (liberal, conservative, social democratic) proposed by Esping-Andersen (1990, 1999) provides one starting point for cross-national comparison of welfare policies. In this case it has explanatory power, though limited, grouping together countries with considerable variations in leave policy. Certainly, taken overall, the five Nordic countries (with their "social democratic" welfare regimes) provide the most generous leave policies and these policies are complemented by high levels of publicly funded childcare services. Denmark, Finland and Sweden, for example, offer an entitlement to children from at least 12 months of age to such services ensuring a smooth transition from parental to non-parental care. But there are also major differences between them, both in overall policy terms (Deven & Moss, 2005) and in particular aspects of policy. Rostgaard (2002), for example, has analyzed the considerable differences between Denmark, Norway and Sweden when it comes to policy towards fathers; while Finland has adopted a 3-year leave period, the other four countries have focused on shorter periods.

Taken overall, Anglo-Saxon or liberal welfare regimes have the least developed leave policies, but again there are considerable variations. Australia and the U.S. remain the only affluent countries to have no universal entitlement to any form of paid leave at or after childbirth. But, as we have shown, both the UK and Canada have in recent years developed their leave policies, albeit in different ways. The UK seems to exemplify the dilemmas facing these countries, struggling to reconcile divergent policy imperatives: to support working parents while maintaining a deregulated and "flexible" labor market.

The remaining Western European states, mostly with "conservative" welfare regimes, show considerable diversity, with common features hard to find. Compare, for example, the very different leave policies in Belgium and France, Italy and Germany, or Portugal and Spain (see Table 1, also Deven & Moss, 2005). The greatest consistency is to be found in Central and Eastern Europe, where leave entitlements survived transition relatively unscathed, and indeed have come to assume greater significance in the wake of the cut-backs in nursery provision and the decline in employment that has followed regime change. The 1990s saw in many parts of this region a shift from nursery care to parental leave (UNICEF, 1999). Yet even here there is the exception of Slovenia, which has gone for a highly paid but relatively short leave period rather than the lowly paid and longer term leave found elsewhere.

Divergent leave arrangements can also be understood in terms of, and as reflecting, the values or norms relating to gender and parenting that permeate national social policy. What Connell (1990) has termed "gender regimes," that is the way in which the state embodies a set of power relationships between men and women, do not necessarily correspond with the welfare regimes defined by Esping-Andersen.

Neyer (2005) argues that the pattern of welfare state regimes becomes more diverse if we place emphasis on the way in which family policies such as leave arrangements structure gender relations in the family and in society. An attention to gender and care has led some feminist welfare state researchers to group countries in different ways. Fux (2002), for example, clusters European countries into three types of family policy regimes according to their emphasis on state-, family-, or individual-centered approaches.

The interplay between Esping-Andersen's welfare regimes and gender regimes may help explain the differences in leave policy apparent within the Nordic states. Iceland, Norway and Sweden have introduced policies characterized by high benefit payments and substantial "father only" leave periods, that explicitly assume that women with children should work and that men with children should play an active part in their care. The results can be seen in rising proportions of fathers taking leave. By contrast, another Nordic country, Denmark, has lower levels of benefit payment and has recently dropped "fathers only" leave provision. A fifth country, Finland, is one of several countries providing long periods of poorly paid or unpaid parental or childcare leave (others include France, Germany, Spain and many CEE countries) or long periods of maternity leave (such as Ireland and the UK). Finland finds itself in company with countries that appear to embody the "maternalist" assumption "that the mother's primary and natural duty is to look after her child, and that as an extension childcare is and should be a 'women's issue'" (Connell, 1990, p. 183). The consequence is highly gendered use of leave schemes that operate in practice as extended forms of maternity leave.

Leave policies result from the interplay of broad political, economic and cultural influences, exemplified above by reference to welfare regimes, labor market policies and gender and parenting values. But they also bear the imprint of singular national conditions and decisions that further shape the distinct form that leave policies take in each country. What has been termed "path dependency," which emphasizes the significance of specific timing, the large consequences that can flow from contingent events, and the near impossibility of reversing a particular course of action once introduced (Pierson, 2001), can be illustrated in the case of the United Kingdom. The UK came late to maternity leave, in 1976, and for various political reasons specific to that timing settled on a form unusual in its length and low level of payment. At that time, too, employment among women with young children was at a low level and even fewer women resumed work soon after childbirth. In 1979, the UK entered its period of Thatcherite government with a strong turn to neo-liberal economic and welfare policies, inimical to the extension of statutory leave entitlements. Indeed, the UK government throughout this period vetoed the attempts of the European Commission to introduce a European-wide directive on parental leave. Government hostility and media indifference sustained widespread ignorance about different forms of leave, in particular parental leave.

The Labor government, returned to power in 1997, recognized parental employment as a high profile policy issue. Employment rates among women with young children, and women's return to work soon after childbirth, had risen rapidly since the late 1980s (Brannen & Moss, 1998). Yet, at the same time, the new government espoused the Thatcherite legacy of a deregulated labor market and retained a liberal approach to the welfare state, exemplified by low benefit levels, targeted policies and an emphasis on private responsibility. Faced by balancing these policy concerns, and after nearly two decades in which leave policy had been little discussed, it decided to build on the long-established extended maternity leave rather than change course. Required to introduce parental leave after having adopted the 1996 EU directive, it opted for a minimalist entitlement that has been of little further interest to government and parents alike. The current highly distinctive UK leave policy can, therefore, be understood in terms of a liberal welfare regime, strongly market-oriented economic policy and a particular sequence of policy development in which a decision made in 1976 has formed the basis for policy decisions occurring more than 20 years later.

Given these variations in policy, what can be said about the use of the various types of leave, and the relationship between policy and use? This field is only partially mapped; only in the Nordic countries are there regular, consistent statistical accounts of the use of leave, according to gender, and occasionally also according to occupation and education of the parent (Rostgaard, 2005). Lack of comprehensive and comparable basic statistics on use are compounded by even less adequate information about the proportion of parents who are not eligible. That proportion can be far from negligible, at least for countries such as Australia, Canada, and the United States, but this may also hold for a number of European countries.

With all these caveats, we can only hazard some broad generalities about use. Generally speaking, maternity leave that is paid, as it mostly is, appears to be extensively, and often fully, used by mothers who are eligible. Where figures are available for paternity leave, they show a relatively significant rate of use. Use of parental leave schemes varies considerably, depending in particular on whether they are unpaid or paid and, if paid, at what level. Where parental leave is unpaid, as in Spain, there are no regular statistics on use but it is thought to be low by both mothers and fathers. Where leave is a family entitlement only, fathers' use is low. However, where parental leave has both an individual entitlement element *and* is relatively well paid, fathers' use is higher. We have already mentioned the case of Iceland, where making use of leave under the new policy is rather high. Over 80 percent of fathers in Norway and Sweden, too, take parental leave, though they take fewer days on average than Icelandic fathers (Deven & Moss, 2005; Math & Meiland, 2004).

A combination of poor statistical information and the uneven spread of research means that we have even more limited knowledge about diversity issues in the use and experience of using leave policies. While there is a growing body of information on gender, and the relative use of leave by women and men, other dimensions of diversity–at individual, family or employment levels–have been poorly served, which is of concern at a time of increasing diversity in all societies covered by this overview. As Rostgaard (2005) observes:

> Overall, we now have gained some basic knowledge about the difference in national, institutional arrangements of parental leave.

We know that there is great national variation in the conditions for leave, in terms of eligibility criteria, payment, and length of leave. Still, our knowledge at best concerns the average situation: how parental leave policies accommodate the middle-class, middle-income, two-parent family in full-time employment. There is a serious lacuna in the lack of focus on the specific circumstances and needs of different family types and population groups, particularly part-time and "flexible" workers, single parents, people with disabled children, and ethnic minorities. (p. 29)

Failure to include accurate monitoring of leave policies from the start and to commission thoroughly designed research before policy measures are implemented, which would highlight the profile, the dynamics (e.g., parental decision-making) and the experiences of leave takers, not only makes it difficult to evaluate leave policies in relation to diversity; it also prevents light being thrown both on parents who do not use leave though eligible and on parents who are unable to use leave because they are not eligible or otherwise excluded from such entitlements or services. Self-employed parents represent an obvious case of non-eligibility as most leave arrangements initially result from a trade-off between employers and representatives of the employees. Beyond this *de jure* non-eligibility, various subgroups of parents may also face *de facto* access problems: the unemployed, the poorly educated, ethnic minorities and immigrants–all those occupying precarious positions in the labor market, reflected often in poor social security rights or lack of protection from collective agreements, contributing to a substantial risk of social exclusion and poorer conditions for effective parenting.

Future research, therefore, seems to require a number of streams: the creation and interrogation of large-scale national and cross-national data sets that can throw light on eligibility for, use of and impact of leave policies among different groups and across different countries; as well as more qualitative studies that can throw light on how and why different groups use or do not use leave, and how this fits within their broader strategies for employment and family life. Policymakers need to pay more attention to defining clear objectives for leave policies in their countries, and to undertaking strong evaluations of whether national leave policies further these objectives and to what extent these objectives are in fact contradictory.

REFERENCES

Berger, M.L., Hill, J., & Waldfogel, J. (2005). Maternity leave, early maternal employment and child health and development in the U.S. *The Economic Journal, 115* (501), 29-47.

Brandt B. & Kvande, E. (2003). *Fleksible fedre (Flexible fathers)*. Oslo, Norway: Universitetsforlaget

Brannen, J. & Moss, P. (1998). The polarisation and intensification of parental employment in Britain: Consequences for children, families and the community. *Community, Work & Family, 1*, 229-247.

Breidenbach, M. (2003). *A family impact analysis of the Family and Medical Leave Act of 1993 (Wisconsin Family Impact Analysis Series)*. Madison, WI: University of Wisconsin Center for Excellence in Family Studies.

Burgess, A. & Russell G. (2004). Fatherhood and public policy. In *Supporting fathers, Contributions from the international fatherhood summit* (pp. 109-145). The Hague, Brussels: Bernard van Leer Foundation.+

Chronholm, A. (2004). *Föräldraledig pappa: Mäns erfarenheter av delad föräldralighet (Fathers on parental leave–Men's experiences of shared parental leave)*. Göteborg, Sweden: Doctoral Dissertation at the Department of Sociology, Göteborg University.

Connell, J. (1990). The state, gender and sexual politics. *Theory and Society, 19*, 507-544.

den Dulk, L. (2001). *Work-family arrangements in organisations: A cross-national study in the Netherlands, Italy, UK and Sweden.* Rotterdam, The Netherlands: Rozenberg.

Deven, F. (2005). A review of research on leave arrangements for parents. In F. Deven & P. Moss (Eds.) (2005). *Leave policies and research: Reviews and country notes* (CBGS Working Papers 2005/3). Brussels, Belgium: CBGS.

Deven, F. (2005b). Assessing the use of parental leave by fathers: Towards a conceptual framework. In B. Peper, A. van Dooren & L. den Dulk (Eds.) *Flexible working and organisational change: The integration of work and personal life* (pp. 247-267). Cheltenham, UK: Edward Elgar Publishing.

Deven, F. & Carrette, V. (2005). A review of the impact on children of leave arrangements for parents. In L. Hantrais et al. (Eds.). *European cross-national research and policy: Cross-national research papers, 7th series (special issue)* (pp. 59-66). Loughborough, UK: European Research Centre, Loughborough University.

Deven, F. & Moss, P. (2002). Leave arrangements for parents: Overview and future outlook. *Community, Work & Family, 5*, 237-255.

Deven, F. & Moss, P. (Eds.) (2005). *Leave policies and research: A review and country notes (CBGS Working Papers 2005/3)*. Brussels, Belgium: CBGS.

Drew, E. (2005). *Parental leave in Council of Europe member states*. Strasbourg, France: Council of Europe, Equality Division / Directorate General of Human Rights CDEG.

Duvander A-Z. & Andersson, G. (2005). *Gender equality and fertility in Sweden: A study on the impact of the father's uptake of parental leave on continued childbear-*

ing. MPIDR Working Paper WP 2005-013. Retrieved 10/25/05 from htpp://www. demogr.mpg.de/papers/working/wp-2005-013.pdf.

Duyvendak, J.K. & Stavenuiter M. (Eds.) (2004). *Working fathers, caring men. Reconciliation of working life and family life.* The Hague/Utrecht: SZW/ Verwey-Jonker Institute.

Einarsdottir, P. & Petursdottir, G.A. (2004). *Culture, custom and caring: Men's and women's possibilities to parental leave.* Akureyri, Iceland: Centre for Gender Studies.

EIRR (2001). Maternity, paternity, and parental benefits across Europe. *European Industrial Relations Review*, No. 329: 21-27, No. 330: 15-17, No. 331: 13-18.

Empirica (2003). *Bericht über die Auswirkungen der §§ 15 und 16. Bundeserziehungsgeldgesetz (Research report on the effects of paragraphs 15 and 16 of the parental leave legislation).* Berlin, Germany: Empirica Institut.

Esping-Andersen, G. (1990). *The three worlds of welfare capitalism.* Cambridge, UK: Polity Press.

Esping-Andersen, G. (1999). *Social foundations of postindustrial economies.* Oxford, UK: Oxford University Press.

Eurobarometer (2004). *European attitudes to parental leave* (Special Eurobarometer No. 189). Brussels, Belgium: European Commission.

European Commission Childcare Network (1995). *Leave arrangements for workers with children.* Brussels, Belgium: European Commission Equal Opportunities Unit.

Falkner, G., Hartlapp, M., Leiber, S., & Treib, O. (2002). *Transforming social policy in Europe? The EC's parental leave directive and misfit in the 15 Member states (MPIFG Working Paper 02/11).* Köln, Germany: Max-Planck-Institut für Gesellschaftsforschung.

Ferrarini, T. (2003). *Parental leave institutions in eighteen post-war welfare states.* Stockholm, Sweden: Swedish Institute for Social Research

Fux, B. (2002). Which models of the family are encouraged or discouraged by different family policies? In F-X. Kaufmann, A. Kuijsten, H-J. Schulze & K.P. Strohmeier (Eds.), *Family Life and Family Policies in Europe–Volume 2* (pp. 363-418). Oxford, UK: Oxford University Press.

Galtry, J. & Callister, P. (2005). Assessing the optimal length of parental leave for child and parental well-being: How can research inform policy? *Journal of Family Issues, 26,* 219-246.

Gauthier, A.H. (2005). Trends in policies for family-friendly societies. In M. Macura, A.L. MacDonald & W. Haug (Eds.), *The new demographic regime: Population challenges and policy responses* (pp. 95-110). New York/Geneva: United Nations (UNECE/UNFPA).

Gornick, J.C. & Meyers, M.K. (2003). *Families that work. Policies for reconciling parenthood and employment.* New York, NY: Russell Sage Foundation.

Haas, L. (2002). Parental leave and gender equality: What can the U.S. learn from the European Union? *Review of Policy Research, 20,* 89-114.

Haas, L. Allard, K., & Hwang, P. (2002). The impact of organizational culture on men's use of parental leave in Sweden. *Community, Work & Family, 5,* 319-342.

Han, W-J., & Waldfogel, J. (2003). Parental leave: The impact of recent legislation on parents' leave taking. *Demography, 40,* 191-200.

Hantrais, L. (2004). *Family policy matters*. Bristol, UK: Policy Press.

Hardy, S. & Adnett, N. (2002). The parental leave Directive: Towards a 'family-friendly' social Europe? *European Journal of Industrial Relations*, 8, 157-172.

Hernanz, V., Malherbet F., & Pellizzari, M. (2004). *Take-up of welfare benefits in OECD countries: A review of the evidence (OECD Social, Employment and Migration Working Papers No. 17)*. Paris, France: OECD.

Hewitt, P. (2004). *Unfinished business: The new agenda for the workplace*. London, UK: Institute for Public Policy Research.

Hofferth, S.L. & Curtin, S.C. (2003). *The impact of parental leave statutes on maternal return to work after childbirth in the United States (OECD Social, Employment and Migration Working Papers No. 7)*. Paris, France: OECD.

Kamerman, S.B., Neuman, M., Waldfogel, J., & Brooks-Gunn, J. (2003). *Social policies, family types and child outcomes in selected OECD Countries (OECD Social, Employment and Migration Working Paper No. 6)*. Paris, France: OECD.

Kokourkova, J. (2002). Leave arrangements and childcare services in Central Europe: policies and practices before and after transition. *Community, Work & Family, 5*, 301-318.

KPMG (2002). *Etude d'évaluation de l'impact du congé parental au Grand-Duché de Luxembourg (Evaluation of the impact of parental leave in the Grand duchy of Luxembourg)*. (Rapport final, mimeo).

Lero, D.S. (2003). Research on parental leave policies and children's development: Implications for policy makers and service providers. In R.E. Tremblay, R.G.Barr & R. deV Peters. (Eds.), *Encyclopaedia on early childhood development*. Retrieved 10/25/05 from www.excellence-earlychildhood.ca/documents/LeroANGxp.pdf.

Math, A. & C. Meiland (2004). *Family-related leave and industrial relations*. Dublin, Ireland: European Foundation for the Improvement of Living and Working Conditions (EIROnline).

Moss, P. (2005). A review of leave policies. In F. Deven and P. Moss (Eds.), *Leave policies and research: Reviews and country notes (CBGS Working Papers 2005/3)* (pp. 3-15). Brussels, Belgium: CBGS.

Moss, P. & Deven, F. (Eds.) (1999). *Parental leave: Progress or pitfall? Research and policy issues in Europe*. The Hague / Brussels, Belgium: NIDI /CBGS Publications, volume 35.

Neyer, G. (2005). Family policies in Europe: Fertility policies at the intersection of gender policies, employment policies and care policies. *Österreichische Zeitschrift für Politikwissenschaft, 34*, 91-102.

ÖIF (2005). Evaluation kinderbetreuungsgeld: Eine Zwischenbilanz nach 3 Jahren Laufzeit (Evaluation of the childcare benefit. An interim report after three years of implementation). Wien, Austria: Östereichisches Institut für Familienforschung.

Organisation for Economic Cooperation and Development (2001). *Starting strong: Early childhood education and care*. Paris, France: OECD.

Organisation for Economic Cooperation and Development (2002). *Babies and bosses: Reconciling work and family life* (Volume 1: *Australia, Denmark and The Netherlands*). Paris, France: OECD.

Organisation for Economic Cooperation and Development (2003). *Babies and bosses: Reconciling work and family life (Volume 2: Austria, Ireland and Japan).* Paris, France: OECD.

Organisation for Economic Cooperation and Development (2004). *Babies and bosses: Reconciling work and family life (Volume 3: New Zealand, Portugal and Switzerland).* Paris, France: OECD.

Organisation for Economic Cooperation and Development (forthcoming). *Babies and bosses: Reconciling work and family life (Volume 4: Canada, Finland, Sweden and the United Kingdom).* Paris, France: OECD.

Pierson, P. (2001) Post-industrial pressures on the mature welfare state. In P. Pierson (Ed.), *The new politics of the welfare state* (pp. 80-104). Oxford, UK: Oxford University Press.

Pylkkanen, E. & Smith, N. (2003). *Career interruptions due to parental leave: A comparative study of Denmark and* Sweden (OECD Social, Employment and Migration Working Papers No. 1). Paris, France: OECD.

Ram, B., Abada, T., & Hou, F. (2004). The effects of early maternal employment on children's cognitive outcomes: The Canadian experience. *Paper presented at the Population Association of America annual meeting,* available at http://paa2004. princeton.edu.

Rønsen, M. (1999). Assessing the impact of parental leave: Effects on fertility and female employment. In P. Moss and F. Deven (Eds.). *Parental leave: Progress or pitfall? Research and policy issues in Europe* (pp. 193-225). The Hague/Brussels, Belgium: NIDI/CBGS Publications, vol. 35.

Rønsen, M. (2001). *Market work, child care and the division of household labour. Adaptations of Norwegian mothers before and after the cash-for-care reform (RAPP 2001/3).* Oslo, Norway: Statistics Norway.

Rostgaard, T. (2002). Setting time aside for the father: Father's leave in Scandinavia. *Community, Work & Family, 5(3),* 343-364.

Rostgaard, T. (2003) *Family support policy in Central and Eastern Europe–A decade and a half of transition (Early Childhood and Family Policy series No. 8).* Paris, France: UNESCO. http://unesdoc.unesco.org/images/0013/001337/133733e.pdf.

Rostgaard, T. (2005). Diversity and parental leave. In F. Deven & P. Moss (Eds.). *Leave policies and research: Reviews and country notes (CBGS Working Papers 2005/3)* (pp. 29-39). Brussels, Belgium: CBGS.

Ruhm, C. (2000). Parental leave and child health. *Journal of Health Economics, 19,* 931-960.

Russell, G. & Hwang, P. (2004). The impact of workplace practices on father involvement. In M. Lamb (Ed.), *The role of the father in child development* (4th edition), pp. 476-503. Hoboken, NJ: Wiley.

Stropnik, N. (2004). Family policy in European post-socialist countries. Paper presented at the 20th International Federation of Home Economics World Congress (Kyoto, Japan, 1-7 August).

Tanaka, S. (2005). Parental leave and child health across OECD countries. *The Economic Journal, 115* (501), 7-28.

UNICEF (United Nations Children's Fund) (1999). *Women in transition (MONEE Project, Regional Monitoring Report 6).* UNICEF Innocenti Research Centre: Florence, Italy.

Van Luijn, H. & Keuzenkamp, S. (2004). *Werkt verlof? (Does leave work?).* Den Haag: Sociaal Cultureel Planbureau.

Waldfogel, J. (2001). International policies towards parental leave and child care. *The Future of Children, 11,* 99-111.

Waldfogel, J. (2002). Child care, women's employment, and child outcomes. *Journal of Population Economics, 15,* 527-548.

Waldfogel, J., Han, W.J., & Brooks-Gunn, J. (2003). The effects of early maternal employment on child cognitive development. *Demography, 39,* 369-392.

Seeking the Balance Between Work and Family After Communism

Steven Saxonberg
Tomáš Sirovátka

SUMMARY. During the 1990s the Central-European governments all took steps in varying degrees toward implementing more conservative, re-familization policies, which support women in their roles as mothers and make it more difficult for them to remain in the labor market. This article discusses the relationship between gender attitudes and gender policy in Central Europe and the latest changes in both. We focus on two countries, Catholic Poland, and the secular Czech Republic, in order to control for the role of Catholicism as an explanatory factor of familism. Beside statistical sources, administrative data and information from interviews with policy makers, we use data from the International Social Survey Programme (ISSP) 1994 and 2002 on gender and family, analyzing them at both the micro and macro levels. Our study shows that post-communist re-familization policies are coming increasingly into

Steven Saxonberg is affiliated with Dalarna University, Sweden. Tomáš Sirovátka is in the Department of Social Policy and Social Work, Masaryk University, Jostova 10, 60200 Brno, Czech Republic (E-mail: Sirovatk@fss.muni.cz).

Address correspondence to: Steven Saxonberg, Department of Government, Uppsala University, 74120 Uppsala, Sweden (E-mail: sax@post.utfors.se).

This study was supported by the Czech Ministry of Education (project MSM 0021622408 "Reproduction and Integration of the Society").

[Haworth co-indexing entry note]: "Seeking the Balance Between Work and Family After Communism." Saxonberg, Steven, and Tomáš Sirovátka. Co-published simultaneously in *Marriage & Family Review* (The Haworth Press, Inc.) Vol. 39, No. 3/4, 2006, pp. 287-313; and: *Families and Social Policy: National and International Perspectives* (ed: Linda Haas, and Steven K. Wisensale) The Haworth Press, Inc., 2006, pp. 287-313. Single or multiple copies of this article are available for a fee from The Haworth Document Delivery Service [1-800-HAWORTH, 9:00 a.m. - 5:00 p.m. (EST). E-mail address: docdelivery@haworthpress.com].

© 2006 by The Haworth Press, Inc. All rights reserved.
doi:10.1300/J002v39n03_04

contradiction with the needs and aspirations of the populace, which is becoming more positive towards gender equality. *[Article copies available for a fee from The Haworth Document Delivery Service: 1-800-HAWORTH. E-mail address: <docdelivery@haworthpress.com> Website: <http://www.HaworthPress.com> © 2006 by The Haworth Press, Inc. All rights reserved.]*

KEYWORDS. Aspirations, Catholic Church, communist legacy, defamilization, family policy, fertility rates, gender equality, re-familization

During the communist era, a new model of gender relations emerged, which combined aspects of both "de-familist" (Esping-Andersen, 1999) family policies that promoted gender equality and conservative, "familist" policies that supported traditional gender roles. On the one hand, all women were expected to work and female labor market participation rates were among the highest in the world. Policies, such as easy access to daycare, facilitated the ability of women to work even when they had children. On the other hand, no measures were undertaken to encourage fathers to share in the child-raising and household responsibilities and parental leaves were designed to strengthen the mother's role as the sole carer. With this unusual mixture of policies, it was not clear what direction post-communist family policies would take. Since women were used to working and having access to daycare, we might expect them to resist conservative "re-familization" policies that encourage women to return to their homes. Yet, since their labor market participation was something that many women felt forced into, rather than a right that they fought for, they might be less likely than Western women to perceive their work as part of a "liberation" process.

Research on post-communist family policy shows that during the 1990s the Central-European governments all took steps in varying degrees toward implementing more conservative, re-familization policies, which support women in their roles as mothers and make it more difficult for them to remain in the labor market (Castle-Kanerova, 1992; Ferge, 1997a, 1997b; Fodor, Glass, Kawachi & Popescu, 2002; Fultz, Ruck & Steinhilber, 2003; Pascall & Manning, 2000; Saxonberg, 2002; 2003). So far, little has been written about the development of post-communist family policy during the first half of this new decade.

Furthermore, very little has been written about the relationship between these policies and the attitudes of post-communist citizens toward gender relations. Indeed, many authors have claimed that an anti-feminist atmosphere arose out of the communist era, which can explain the relative weakness of the women's movement in post-communist countries (i.e., Funk, 1993; Heitlinger, 1996; Renne, 1997; Robinson, 1995; Rueschemeyer, 1995; Wolchik, 1995). However, it has been quite rare to base these claims on a detailed analysis of attitudes based on survey data. When researchers actually use survey data, they tend to rely on aggregated descriptive data rather than using any statistical methods to analyze the data at the micro-level and do not use any scaling techniques to create measurement models of attitudes (see, for example, Čermáková, Mařiková & Tuček, 1995; Crompton & Harris, 1997; Maříková, 1997; Mirody & Giza-Poleszczuk, 2000; Raabe, 1998, 1999); for an exception, see Panayotova and Brayfield (1997), but they only discuss Hungary.

Thus, our study will add to the discourse on post-communist gender relations by bringing up to date the latest changes in family policy as well as providing a more sophisticated discussion of gender attitudes and the relationship between gender attitudes and gender policy in Central Europe. We focus on two countries, Poland and the Czech Republic, to control for the common hypothesis that Poland provides a special case because of the Catholic Church. The International Social Survey Programme (ISSP) on the "Role of Government III" from 1996 shows that while the Czech Republic is a rather secular country (with only 19.9% of its citizens claiming to attend religious services at least once a month), Poland is one of the most Catholic countries in the world (with over 90% claiming to belong to the Church and 73.6% claiming to attend services at least once a month). According to the Catholic argument, by promoting traditional gender roles the Church has influenced policy makers to introduce conservative-familist policies and the Church has succeeded in promoting conservative gender attitudes (Bystydzienski, 1995; Fuszara, 1994; Nowakowska, 1997; Siemienska, 1994). Cichomski, Morawski, Zawadzki and Boski (1999) confirm this result based on the 1994 ISSP survey on gender and the family.

THEORETICAL DISCUSSION

The communist ideological legacy provides the most common hypothesis for explaining the development of post-communist family policy, gender relations and gender attitudes. The basic argument has been that the ideological legacy is anti-feminist, for two opposing reasons: the communists were themselves anti-feminists, and because much of the populace considered them to represent feminism.

As anti-feminists, the communist regimes ridiculed the western feminist movement and claimed it was "petty bourgeois." In addition, although they forced women to work, as anti-feminists they did not consider it important at all to give working women the same career opportunities as men or have them represented at the highest levels of society (except in the symbolic and powerless parliaments). Neither did the communist regimes encourage men to share in the household and child-raising duties. In addition, to preserve their monopoly of power, they prevented open discussions of feminist issues and did not allow independent women's groups to organize. In fact, given the repressive nature of the communist regimes, the household had greater status than in the West and women often did not mind having the extra responsibility for this sphere (cf. Heitlinger, 1996).

Thus, women have not protested much against having the double burden of paid work and being the main person responsible for unpaid work. As Čermáková (1997, p. 391) observes, a "gender contract" emerged during the communist era, in which virtually all women worked, but only men had careers. Instead, women accepted lower positions and lower salaries than men, so that they could balance work and family. Raabe (1998, p. 57) adds, "Czech women and men continue to endorse such gender differentiation."

Even though the communist leaders persecuted feminists and rejected feminist ideas, much of the populace associated the regimes with feminism, since they claimed to support gender equality, which makes it easy for post-communist citizens to associate feminist arguments with the former regime (Fuszara, 1991, 1994; Robinson, 1995; Siemenska, 1999). This association became even stronger when western feminists starting visiting Central Europe after the collapse of communism and sometimes used phrases like "liberation" and "oppression" that reminded people of Marxist-Leninist rhetoric (cf. Funk, 1993; Renne, 1997; Šiklová, 1998; Wolchik, 1995). Nevertheless, since the regimes claimed they supported equality, "the emancipation of women is associated with the overthrown regime; many people consider it a relic of the Communist system" (Janowska & Goral quoted in Robinson, 1995, p. 215). Not only did the communist regimes give feminism a bad name because citizens began to associate equality with communism, the regimes also gave feminism a bad name, because they themselves harshly criticized and ridiculed it.

According to this argument, in the absence of a feminist discourse, post-communist women have rather conservative attitudes toward gender relations (Crompton & Harris, 1997; Saxonberg, 2000). Given the absence of political mobilization around feminist issues and the general conservative, anti-feminist climate in post-communist countries, policy makers did not feel any pressure to pursue de-familization policies, nor did they themselves believe in such policies. Thus, it is not surprising that the post-communist regimes basically followed re-familization policies (cf. Ferge, 1997a, 1997b; Saxonberg 2003).

Although we admit that the communist ideological legacy has played a major role in shaping family policy, we argue that a more nuanced view of ideology is necessary to fully understand post-communist dynamics. We find it fruitful to differentiate between attitudes toward "abstract" and "concrete" feminism. Our notion of abstract and concrete feminism comes from Havelková's (1996) distinction between "abstract" and "concrete" citizenship. She defines abstract citizenship as "an image of the system into which certain ideals are projected" (Havelková, 1996, p. 248). Meanwhile, concrete citizenship is "the attitudes that are rooted in the concrete knowledge and experiences of the individual within a particular social or political system" (Havelková, 1996, p. 248).

In the context of gender roles, we use abstract feminism to denote the more theoretical feminist criticism of patriarchal power relations in society and the criticism of traditional ideal roles for men and women (based on the notion of male breadwinners and female housekeepers). Concrete feminism concerns attitudes toward gender issues faced at the practical, daily level, based on everyday experiences of balancing work and family. In analyzing gender attitudes, we differentiate between abstract and concrete feminism to see if Havelková is correct that Czech (and in our case also Polish) women are more interested in their citizenship rights at the concrete, daily level, than at the abstract, theoretical level. If this is the case and women support greater gender equality at the concrete level, while opposing it at the abstract level, then this contradiction can help explain why women have tended to remain in the labor market, but have not organized much politically around their interests. Instead, if aspirations to work remain high, we might expect women in such a situation to remain politically passive, but react to their double burden of paid and unpaid work by having fewer children, rather than withdrawing from the labor market.

As already noted, in addition to the communist legacy thesis, authors writing on Poland have claimed that gender attitudes and family policies there are especially conservative because of the role of the Catholic Church in promoting traditional family values. If the Catholic hypothesis is correct, we would expect Poland to have more conservative family policies than the Czech Republic and we would also expect Poles to have less positive attitudes toward gender equality than Czechs.

DATA

Our analysis of family policies is mostly based on national and international statistics coming from yearbooks and survey data bases, as well as on secondary literature and interviews that we have conducted with ministry officials in both Poland and the Czech Republic (mostly conducted in 1999).

Our analysis of gender attitudes comes mostly from the International Social Survey Programme's data bases "Family and Changing Gender Roles II" (from 1994) and "Family and Changing Gender Roles III" (from 2002). The ISSP data bases provide the most comprehensive surveys on gender attitudes and include 34 countries in the 2002 edition. In the Czech Republic the 2002 survey includes 471 men and 818 women, while in Poland it includes 529 men and 723 women. The 1994 survey includes 503 men and 521 women in the Czech Republic; for Poland the totals are 725 men and 872 women. The wording of the items used is given in Table 1 and Table 2.

Since every participating country is responsible for conducting the survey in its country and since the questionnaire is worked out together with all the participating countries, we can be rather certain that the questions are translated quite well. In addition, although language problems could theoretically arise because either the institutional arrangements are much different or because some terms do not translate well to other languages, these problems are not likely to arise in our present case, because Poland and the Czech Republic have rather similar systems (such as the division of daycare into kindergartens for 3-6-year-olds and nursery schools for 0-3-year-olds) and the languages have relatively similar structures, being both Slavic. Even if one sometimes can criticize the exact wording of some questions, the ISSP surveys provide the best available international data sets on gender issues.

In order to determine which questions best measure gender attitudes or career aspirations, we have used either confirmatory factor analysis or exploratory factor analysis. In order to analyze the socio-economic factors that influence gender attitudes and the relationship between

TABLE 1. Career Aspirations of Czech and Polish Women (ISSP 1994 and 2004)

	Czech Republic		Poland	
	1994	2002	1994	2002
Factor 1: Work Aspirations				
% believing mothers should work full- or part-time if they have pre-school children	49.5	64.9	26.6	46.1
% believing mothers should work full-time or part-time if their children are in school	81.6	84	62.8	78.4
Factor 2: Economic Independence				
% believing that having a job is the best way for a woman to be an independent person	55.1	65.9	73.2	80.9
% agreeing that both the man and the woman should contribute to the household income	83	90	63.5	76.9
Factor 3: Housewife Satisfaction				
% disagreeing that being a housewife is just as fulfilling as working for pay	51.6	45.6	28.4	30.7

attitudes and voting preferences, we have applied structural equation modeling (SEM). SEM allows us to create path models, in which independent socio-economic variables influence intermediary variables (attitudes), which in turn influence party preferences. SEM also allows us to have several intermediary variables and/or dependent variables in the same equation. A final advantage of using SEM is that it allows us to easily use non-observable latent variables, that are based on the combination of several questions.

In one case, we only look at the answer to one question, which is based on a 5-point scale. There we apply ordinal logit regression analysis, because this method is especially geared for analyzing ordinal dependent variables.

FINDINGS

State-Socialist Family Policy

During the four decades of communist rule in Eastern and Central Europe a "state socialist" model of family policy emerged (Saxonberg, 2003). According to this model, women were encouraged to both work for pay and have children, but men were not encouraged to share in

TABLE 2. The Percentage of All Respondents Favoring Concrete Feminism (ISSP 1994 and 2004)

	Czech Republic		Poland	
	1994	2002	1994	2002
Factor 1: Household Equality				
Men ought to do a larger share of household work than they do now (percentage agreeing)		61.3		64.5
Men ought to do a larger share of childcare than they do now (percentage agreeing)		67.1		72.6
Average		64.5		68.6
Factor 2: Child Relations				
A working mother can establish just as warm and secure a relationship with her children as a mother who does not work (percentage agreeing)	47.3	71.2	49.2	58.2
A pre-school child is likely to suffer if his or her mother works (percentage disagreeing)	31.6	35.7	22.0	30.8
A job is all right, but what most women really want is a home and children (percentage disagreeing)	19.1	16.6	17.8	26.7
Average	32.7	41.2	29.7	38.6
Change from 1994		+8.5		+8.9
Factor 3: State Support to Families				
Working women should receive paid maternity leave when they have a baby (percentage agreeing)	96.0	85.7	92.1	91.4
Families should receive financial benefits for childcare when both parents work (percentage agreeing)	93.5	80.6	47.0	46.5
Average	94.8	83.2	69.6	69
Change from 1994		−11.6		−0.6

housework. Women had considerable incentives to enter the labor market because it became increasingly difficult for a family to survive on one income as real wages declined. Consequently, virtually all women worked if they were not on maternity leave or extended maternity leave.

Since it is difficult for women to have children and also work for pay full time, the communist regimes began investing in inexpensive public daycare, which allowed women to quickly re-enter the work force. In addition, maternity leave schemes were enacted to alleviate the loss of income during the period the mother was out of the labor market. As a result of these policies, the communist countries enjoyed the world's highest female labor market participation rates (Saxonberg, 2003).

Despite these similarities among countries, some differences emerged. Poland generally gave less support to families than Czechoslovakia and generally followed a more "liberal" type of state-socialist policy. Thus, the Polish communists gave less support to daycare than the Czechoslovak regime. For example, during the last year of communist rule in 1989, 20.3% of Czech children under 3 attended daycare facilities (mostly nursery schools), while only 9.1% of Polish children did so.[1] The difference was also great for 3-6-year-olds, with 78.9% of Czech children attending kindergartens compared to 48.2% of Polish children. One reason for this difference could be the role that Polish grandparents played (cf. Siemienska, 1994, p. 19). Being a rural country where several generations of a family lived together or near each other, made it easier for grandparents to take care of children than in the more urbanized Czechoslovakia. However, even if the demand for daycare might have been lower in Poland than in Czechoslovakia, this radical difference in numbers of children attending daycare was also certainly a result of state policy.

Another difference was in parental leave. In the 1980s both Poland and Czechoslovakia provided rather generous rates of pay for maternity leaves (100% of the mother's salary in Poland and 90% in Czechoslovakia), but the leave was much longer in Czechoslovakia than in Poland (28 weeks versus 16); see, for example, Fultz, Ruck and Steinhilber (2003). In addition, although both countries provided for an additional 3-year "extended" maternity leave, in Poland it was means-tested (Balcerzak-Paradowska, 1991). These leaves were very "familist," as they were only available for mothers; this therefore preserved the father's role as the main breadwinner.

In summary, the state-socialist model combined elements of both familism and de-familism. It was familist in the sense of providing relatively long child-caring leaves that were only available for mothers, thus reinforcing a gendered division of household labor. However, it was de-familist in the sense of providing for cheap and readily available daycare, which enabled mothers to work. In addition, income and labor market policies made it extremely difficult for women to stay out of the labor market, as it was difficult for families to survive on one income.

Post-Communist Family Policy and the Move Toward Re-Familization

After the fall of the communist-led regimes in 1989, Poland and the Czech Republic have generally pursued re-familist policies, which bring the families back to a more traditional, familist strategy, based on the male-breadwinner model. These policies reinforce traditional gender roles by giving mothers incentives to return to the home, while leaving out incentives for fathers to share in child-raising responsibilities. Polish governments have pursued more implicit re-familist policies based on market-liberal ideas of means-testing and minimal public family support. Meanwhile, Czech governments have pursued more explicit re-familist policies, based on more openly conservative measures that directly encourage mothers to spend more time at home.

Maternity leave benefits have remained relatively generous after the fall of the communist governments. The lengths remain the same in both countries: 26 weeks in the Czech Republic (28 weeks in case of a second child) and 16 weeks in Poland (18 weeks for all successive births), although it should be noted that in the late 1990s the period briefly increased up to 26 weeks (Nowakowska & Swedrowska, 2000), before the social democratic coalition government lowered it once again to the original 16-week level. While successive Polish governments have kept the wage replacement rate up at 100% (Balcerzak-Paradowska, 2002), a center-right Czech government lowered it from 90% of one's gross wage to 69% of the net wage (MISSCEEC II).

This is the only area in which Poland has a more generous policy than the Czech Republic, although the higher rate is counterbalanced by the much shorter period of the leave. In both cases, these leaves reinforce traditional gender roles, because this period is designed for the mother. In Poland, fathers were not given the right to any of these maternity leave days until 2001, when they received the right to utilize two weeks of 16 weeks maternity leave and four weeks in case of a longer 18 week leave. Even in a country with full gender equality, few men would go on leave during the first 4-6 months of childbirth, since mothers normally breastfeed their babies during this period. Thus, the fact that the maternity leave is for such a short period encourages the continuation of traditional gender roles.

This means that the most important policy for encouraging men to share in the child-raising chores is the further period of "extended parental leave," as men could be persuaded to share in these leaves if the conditions are generous enough or a portion of the leave period is reserved for the father (as in Sweden and Norway). Since 1989, the Czech government has increased the leave by half a year, making it up to 3 1/2 years in the Czech Republic, while it remains 3 years in Poland (EIRO, 2003). In both countries the benefits level for the extended leave is so low that given the fact that fathers usually have higher incomes than the mothers few men can afford to take advantage of their right to a leave.

For example, the 2002 ISSP survey shows that 63.9% of Czech women and 64.2% of Polish women claim that their spouse's earn more than themselves, while only 16% of Czech women and 22.3% of Polish women claim that they have higher incomes than their spouses.[2]

In Poland, moreover, the extended parental leave remains means-tested, which further reduces the incentive for men to utilize their right to stay at home. In addition, the cut-off level for receiving means-tested benefits was so low that Wiktorow and Mierzewski (1991) note that "only a few" families were able to qualify for these benefits. Although possibilities for women to balance work and family have worsened in both countries, Poland's reliance on means-testing shows that the country is following a more market-liberal policy than the Czech Republic. Thus, our results go against the Catholic hypothesis that would predict that Catholic Poland would follow more conservative policies of giving economic support to mothers, who stay at home for long periods in order to strengthen the "traditional family." Instead, the secular Czech Republic has pursued more conservative policies in supporting the traditional family, even though a market-liberal prime minister, Václav Klaus, ruled the country from 1992-97.

While extended parental leaves have been developed in the Czech Republic and remained in Poland, state aid to nursery schools for 0-3-year-olds has been radically reduced as the responsibility for running them has been transferred to the locally municipalities (Baclzerzak-Paradowska,1997; Golinowska, 1996). The number of nursery schools for 0-3-year-olds in the Czech Republic decreased from 1,313 facilities and nearly 53 thousand places to a mere 65 facilities and slightly more than 1,800 places in 2000. This corresponds to a large drop from 13.2% to about 0.6 % of the relevant age cohort in the Czech Republic (calculations based on data by Zdravotnická, 1990, 2001 and ČSÚ, 2002). On the other hand, 2-year-olds may attend kindergarten if capacity is available after meeting the demand for children above 3. Thus, about one quarter of all three-year-olds attend kindergarten (Matějková & Palonczyová, 2004). Nowadays nurseries only exist in big cities and the parents pay between 25 to 75% of the costs, depending on their incomes. For an average family nursery school costs are about four times higher than kindergarten.

Despite the reduced access to nursery schools, enrollment in kindergartens for 3-6-year-olds remains quite high in the Czech Republic. In 2002, 87% of all 3-6-year-olds attended kindergartens, which is actually 6.5% higher than in 1989 (own calculations based on the MONEE database, 2004). Nevertheless, the outcome is clear: mothers are expected to leave the labor market for three years for each child, as they have little or no access to child care for children under three and the extended parental leaves have such low benefit levels that fathers rarely share in parental leave. Thus, policies have become more familist and based on the traditional male-breadwinner model.

In Poland the number of places in kindergarten was always well below existing demand, while there was much less parental demand for nurseries for children under 3 years. In 1989 only 8.7 % of children 0-3 attended nursery schools and 48.2 % of children 3-6 attended kindergarten. By 2002 the percentage of children attending nursery schools dropped further to 4.2%, while the percentage of 3-6-year-olds attending kindergarten actually increased slightly to 49.9% (our calculations based on MONEE database, 2004). Since 1989, parents have been forced to pay an increasingly high portion of the operating costs for using preschool facilities. This is especially the case for kindergartens, where parents now pay 30-40% of these costs. Balcerzak-Paradowska and colleagues (2003) calculate that in 2000 parents paid about 6% of a woman's average wage for each child in a nursery school and about 19% per child in kindergarten; only about 20% of children from low-income families benefited from special fee reductions. Thus, kindergartens are actually more expensive than nursery schools, but they are also more readily available.

In a situation in which parents have much less access to daycare and extended parental leaves do not give fathers incentives to utilize their right to participate in child-rearing responsibilities, women face great incentives to leave the labor market when they have children. If they have difficulty finding daycare for children under 3, then they are likely to leave the labor market for three years if they have a child and can leave the labor market for as much as 6 years if they have two children. This obviously hurts their chances of pursuing a career if they choose to have children.

Once again, Poland's policies refute the Catholic hypothesis. Poland's policies are more market liberal than in the secular Czech Republic, as Poland gives much less support to daycare (in the form of kindergartens) than the Czech Republic, its maternity leave period is shorter than the Czech Republic, and its extended parental leave is means-tested.

Even though both Polish and Czech policies give women incentives to leave the labor market, evidence indicates that most women believe that they must work for economic reasons. For example, data from the

1994 International Social Survey Programme (ISSP) "Family and Changing Gender Roles II" shows that an incredible 93-94% in both countries claim that women must work to support their families! Although this question was not repeated in the 2002 survey, 76.9% of Polish women and 90% of Czech women believe that "both the man and woman should contribute to the family income." Another survey undertaken in 1995 shows that only 16% of all Czech women would want to stay at home if their husbands "earned sufficient income for the family" (Raabe, 1999, p. 224), although the largest group (63%) would prefer to work part-time or intermittently. In yet another study during that year, 78% of Czech women responded that they would not like to leave their jobs for a year to do housework (Maříková, 1997, p. 10).

Policies Against Aspirations

So far we have shown that in Poland and the Czech Republic the governments have pursued implicit or explicit re-familization policies that encourage women to leave the labor market. Now we will investigate whether these policies coincide with the aspirations of the women living in these countries.

We have applied confirmatory factor analysis to questions dealing with career aspirations (contact the authors for the results). Since we are interested here in needs and aspirations of women, we have filtered out male respondents. We have recoded the answers, so that the tables always show the percentage having career aspirations. Consequently, Table 1 shows the percentage disagreeing or strongly disagreeing with statements that imply that women desire traditional roles, while it shows the percentage of those agreeing with statements that indicate they have career aspirations.

Table 1 shows that Polish and Czech women generally aspire to work and to have careers and their aspirations are rising. Under the first factor, *work aspirations*, a very large majority of women think that they should work if their children are in school. Meanwhile, nearly two-thirds of Czech women and close to half of Polish women think that they should work full-time or part-time if they have pre-school children. For the second factor, *economic independence*, again large majorities (65.9% of Czech women and 80.9% of Polish women) agree or strongly agree that having a job increases a woman's independence, while as already noted, 76.9% of Polish women and 90% of Czech women believe that "both the man and woman should contribute to the family income."

Despite the high degree of work aspirations when having children and the high degree of aspirations for economic independence, the results are less clear for the *housewife satisfaction* factor. Only in the Czech Republic does the majority of respondents disagree that "being a housewife is just as fulfilling as working for pay" and this is only true in the 1994 survey. Despite the large gap between the Czech Republic and Poland, the differences in attitudes between the two countries is decreasing, as aspirations have decreased in the Czech Republic, while they have increased in Poland.

We should also note that finding housework satisfying does not necessarily imply a lack of interest in having a job. It matters what kinds of jobs are available. Although Polish women were the most likely to answer that housework is as satisfying as having a job, a survey in 1992 shows that 72% of married mothers in Poland found having professional work to be "very important" for their lives (Firlit-Fesnat, 1997, p. 22). However, if the choice is between a monotonous, low skilled job with long hours or being a housewife, then some women might find being a housewife to be at least as satisfying as having a paid job. Moreover, as already noted, almost all Czech and Polish women feel they must work whether they want to or not. So even if some Czech and Polish women find household work fulfilling, we can assume that the vast majority of women still feel they must work and probably a clear majority want to work. Thus, we can extrapolate that a majority would also favor policies that make it easier for them to balance work and family.

Finally, it is important to note that with the exception of Czech women's attitudes toward *housewife satisfaction*, the results show that the career aspirations of Czech and Polish women have clearly increased. Thus, it is clear that post-communist family policies in these countries have been running contrary to the aspirations of women.

The Concrete Attitudes of the Entire Society

Now that we have examined the aspirations of women, we look at attitudes toward gender relations among the entire population. We begin by examining attitudes toward gender equality at the concrete, daily level and then move on to the abstract, theoretical level. Using confirmatory factor analysis, we observe three dimensions of concrete feminist values: (1) attitudes toward *household equality* (that is, whether men should share in the household responsibilities of child-raising and doing household chores, such as cleaning and cooking), (2) *child rela-*

tions (that is whether one believes that children suffer if the mother works), and (3) whether the *state should support families*. This last factor enables us to more clearly investigate whether state policies are in line with attitudes. In addition, questions about state support are important because if women are forced to work, then their ability to balance their careers with their families is strongly influenced by state policies.

Our measurement model shows that support for concrete feminism is rather high. On the issue of *household equality*, a large majority in both countries believe that men should do a larger share of the housework and child caring (see Table 2), despite the communist legacy which emphasizes women's full responsibility for the household. It is interesting to note that already in 1994, a survey taken by the Institute of Sociology of the Czech Academy of Sciences showed that 40.9% of the men give their family more priority than their work (Čermáková et al., 1995). Although this was lower than among women (63.3%), the results show that many men feel responsible for family life and might be willing to share more in household responsibilities if they were given a greater incentive. Nevertheless, Čermáková et al. (1995) conclude that most families practice a partnership on financial matters but are still basically patriarchal when it comes to domestic work. Our results indicate that patriarchal family relations do not necessarily correspond to the desires of most families, but rather might be the result of familist family policies.

In contrast to *household equality*, attitudes toward *child relations* are less feminist, as only a minority in both countries believes that child relations do not suffer when the mother works. This does not necessarily reflect anti-feminist attitudes, though. Instead, it might reflect negative attitudes toward daycare. Observers note that communist era nurseries did not offer high quality care (see, for example, Götting, 1998; Heitlinger, 1996) as the child to carer ratio was very high and little effort was made to apply modern pedagogical methods. Thus, post-communist citizens are not likely to trust the government to be able to provide quality daycare. This lack of trust is enhanced by the fact that the personnel qualification and performance standards of nursery schools continue to be under the jurisdiction of the health ministry [!], which shows parents that the state considers their young children to be health problems, rather than people, who are in need of psychological and pedagogical support for their development. So it is not surprising that parents do not trust the public sector to provide nursery schools that use modern pedagogical methods. A previous study of Czech attitudes reflects this skepticism, showing that Czechs are much more skeptical of state subsidies toward nurseries than for kindergartens, elementary school and high school (Raabe, 1999).

When it comes to *state support to families*, the Czech and Polish respondents are extremely positive. We interpret this finding as a positive attitude toward concrete feminism or at least showing a potentially positive attitude. The existence of readily available and affordable daycare alternatives make it much easier for women to stay in the labor market when they have children, as do generous parental leaves that encourage men to share in early childcare. Both measures require the state to support families. Unfortunately, the wording of the questions makes the results a bit difficult to interpret, since the question does not make more precise what kinds of aid for families the respondent supports (even though the question asks "when *both* parents work," emphasis here). Nor does the other question indicate whether men should be allowed to receive payment for parental leave. Nevertheless, at the very least, the responses to these questions show that Poles and Czechs would be critical of market liberal reforms that cut back on aid to families.

We use structural equation modeling to determine whether we can expect support for concrete feminism to continue growing. Thus, we analyze the impact of these variables for indication whether this support is likely to continue:

- age (which shows whether younger generations are becoming more favorable toward gender equality),
- educational level (which shows whether we can expect the increasing educational levels to contribute to a re-evaluation of traditional gender roles, as citizens become more tolerant and critical thinkers),
- sex (which could indicate that differences over gender attitudes could lead to increasing conflict and perhaps political mobilization if women are becoming more favorable toward gender equality at the same time as a gender gap in attitudes exists).
- Finally, we add the degree of Catholicism, to test at the micro-level the hypothesis that the Catholic Church has influenced Poles to become more conservative toward gender roles. We have created this variable by first ascertaining whether or not the respondent is Catholic.

Age and educational level have been found to be robust predictors of gender attitudes in Western Europe (Banaszak & Plutzer, 1993; Morgan &

Wilcox, 1992; Wilcox, 1991a; 1991b) and in Poland (Saxonberg, 2000; Siemieńska, 1999). Western studies have generally neglected to ask whether a gender gap exists in gender attitudes, but Saxonberg (2000) found that a very strong gender gap exists in Poland, as women tend to be much more in favor of gender equality than men. Although studies of Western Europe have tended to use a general measure of religiosity, since the literature on welfare state regimes in the West (i.e., Esping-Andersen, 1990) and in Poland (Bystydzienski, 1995; Fuszara, 1994; Nowakowska, 1997; Siemienska, 1994) emphasizes so strongly the role of the Catholic Church, we examine the degree of Catholicism instead. We code the variable by considering how often professed Catholics attend services (with 1 = never and 8 = several times a week).

As Table 3 shows, educational level is positively correlated with attitudes toward *household equality* and *child relations* in both countries. Since educational levels are increasing in both countries, we can expect a growing number of Czechs and Poles to believe that men should share household and child-raising responsibilities more equally. Support will also continue to increase for the belief that women can work without hurting their children's development and their family life. For the Polish case, we have even more reason to suppose that support will continue to increase for the belief that women can work without hurting their relationships to their children, because age is also statistically significant. Thus, a generation gap exists, as the younger generations are more likely than older generations to believe that women can work and still have good relationships with their children.

When it comes to the government financing family programs, however, we might expect Czechs and Poles to become a bit more negative in the future as age is positively correlated with attitudes toward *state support to families* for the Czech Republic, while education is negatively correlated for Poland. Thus, younger generations in the Czech Republic are likely to be more negative to state support than the older ones, which implies that a generational shift in attitudes is going on. Similarly, since Poles are becoming more highly educated with the rapid expansion of new colleges and universities, we might expect Poles to become increasingly negative toward state support for families. Nevertheless, since the starting point is an extremely high level of support for state aid to families, it should be noted that the majority of citizens in both countries are still likely to continue to support state aid to families in the foreseeable future.

TABLE 3. Structural Models of Concrete Feminism and Party Support (ISSP 2002). Standardized Correlations

	Czech Republic		Poland	
	Full Model	Better Fit	Full Model	Better Fit
Correlation with *Household equality*				
a) age	−.02		0.08**	.08**
b) educational level	.06*	.06**	.06*	.06**
c) degree of Catholicism	−.13**	−.10*	.04	
d) sex (women = 2, men = 1)	.32***	.32***	.16***	.17***
Correlation with *Child relations*				
a) age	−.04		−.25***	−.26***
b) educational level	.06*	.08**	.16***	.26***
c) degree of Catholicism	.01		−.06	
d) sex (women = 2, men = 1)	.07*	.08**	.11**	.10**
Correlation with *State support*				
a) age	.14***	.14**	.06	
b) educational level	.02		−.23**	−.25**
c) degree of Catholicism	−.12		.04	
d) sex (women = 2, men = 1)	.09*	.09*	.00	
Correlation with *Leftist party*				
a) Household equality	−.22		−.05	
b) Child relation	−.07		.97	1.00
c) State support	.98*	1.00	.33	
Test Statistics				
Chi-square p-value	.000	.000	.000	.000
RMSEA	.063	.058	.072	.066

Note: *** = significant at .001 level, ** = significant at .01 level, and * = significant at .05 level.

Our analysis once again contradicts the hypothesis about the role of the Catholic Church. The degree of Catholicism is not a significant predictor of attitudes concerning concrete feminism for any issue in Catholic Poland. In the comparatively secular Czech Republic, the degree of Catholicism is only significant for explaining attitudes toward *household equality*, but is insignificant for the remaining two factors.

Two other interesting results arise from our structural analysis. First, sex is a highly significant determinant of concrete feminist attitudes for all factors except for *state support to families* in the Polish case. Since it is significant for 5 of the 6 cases, then it is possible to predict that women might eventually come into more open conflict with men over gender roles. However, this is not likely to happen until women become supportive of abstract, theoretical feminism and put their concrete, daily experiences in a more general structural framework of power relations within society. Second, preferences for political parties are not significantly related to concrete feminist attitudes except for *state support to families* and then only among Czech respondents. This indicates that women are still not mobilizing to put gender issues on the political agenda. If no party stresses gender issues, then it is not likely that voters will take into account gender issues when voting. Similarly, if the communist ideological legacy continues to influence post-communist citizens into having a negative attitude toward abstract, theoretical notions of feminism and gender relations, then it is not likely that voters will organize to press political parties into taking up gender issues during election campaigns.

In summary, our results show that although Czechs and Poles do not seem to consider gender issues when voting, they are generally extremely positive to concrete feminism for the factors *household equality* and *state support to families* and their support is rising. In addition, our structural analysis indicates that we can expect their support to continue to rise. Furthermore, although a majority believes that children suffer if the mother works, the percentage disagreeing is increasing. Moreover, the fear that children suffer might reflect the memories of poor quality nursery schools from the communist era rather than an aversion to gender equality. These memories make parents mistrustful as to whether their governments will really be capable of providing high quality daycare.

Abstract Feminist Values

The best question in the ISSP survey for analyzing support for abstract, theoretical feminism is whether one agrees or disagrees that "A man's job is to earn money; a woman's job is to look after the home and family." This question raises the more abstract theoretical issue as to what men's and women's role should be in society in general. It implies that men should continue to dominate the public sphere, while women should retire to the private sphere.

It turns out that the communist legacy still looms large at this abstract level, as only a minority in each country disagrees or strongly disagrees with this statement that implies that societal power relations should be based on traditional patriarchal gender arrangements. However, the communist legacy also appears to be losing its influence, as opposition to traditional gender roles at this abstract level is growing in both countries, especially among women. Thus, among women, the percentage disagreeing that "a man's job is to earn money; a woman's job is to look after the home and family" has increased from 27.5% to 32.8% among Czech women and from 23.9% to 40.2% among Polish women. Meanwhile, it has increased from 21.8% to 24.9% among Czech men and from 15.3% to 28% among Polish men. Interestingly, at the micro level the Catholic legacy no longer seems valid, as Polish men and women are more positive to abstract feminism than their Czech counterparts.

Thus, we see that the anti-feminist stance at the abstract, theoretical level of society goes against the largely pro-feminist stance at the concrete daily level and against the career aspirations of the majority of women. Here we see how the communist legacy continues to influence women, even if this legacy is declining with time. Since women still lack a feminist consciousness at the abstract theoretical level and they tend to see feminism as a "dirty word," they are rather reluctant to become politically involved in women's organizations and organize around their interests. They have not actively campaigned for the types of reforms in family policy that would support their career aspirations and greater gender equality at the concrete level. Rather than utilizing the voice option of political action, they often chose the exit option of leaving the reproduction market. This could help explain the sharp drop in fertility rates in both countries. In the Czech Republic, fertility rates fell from 1.87 children per woman in 1989 to 1.14 in 2002, while in Poland they fell from 2.05 children per woman to 1.34 (Eurostat, 2004). While fertility rates radically declined, female labor market participation only declined modestly, as females still comprise 43.6% of the Czech labor force and 45.4% of the Polish in 2002 (own calculations based on Eurostat, 2003).

Our ordinal logic regression also shows that we can expect support for abstract, theoretical feminism to continue to increase, as age, educational level and sex are all significantly correlated with support for abstract feminism (contact the authors for the results). Thus, the younger generations are becoming increasingly positive toward theoretical feminism (hence the negative correlation), while those with a greater education are more positive. Again, since educational levels are increasing in both countries, we can expect support for theoretical ideas of more equal gender roles to increase. Since sex is also significantly correlated, we might eventually see the emergence of open conflict as women feel the need to push for changes in gender roles, which many men oppose. Finally, the degree of Catholicism turns out to not be significant for Poland, although it is significant for the Czech Republic. This ambivalent result once again sheds doubt on the Catholic legacy.

The Communist Legacy and the Push Toward Re-Familization

Again, as with our discussion on attitudes, the communist legacy goes a long way in explaining post-communist family dynamics. In a situation in which feminism was considered a "dirty word," both because no discourse about patriarchy was allowed to emerge during communist rule and because western feminist terminology often reminded post-communist citizens of Marxist-Leninist jargon, policy makers never really considered following de-familization policies. It became clear in discussions with ministry officials and policy makers conducted in Poland and the Czech Republic in 1999 (including the former minister of labor and social affairs in Poland, Jacek Kuron) that policy makers had not even considered the Swedish-type of individual earner-carer model, which aims at promoting gender equality.

Not only did policy makers never consider de-familization policies, given the lack of support among the population for abstract feminist ideals, women's organizations did not pressure governments into introducing measures promoting gender equality. The argument was that under communism many women had been forced against their will to work, when they really would have preferred to stay at home. For example, in 1995, 6 of the 31 organizations listed in the Czech handbook of women's organizations openly argued for the need for women to be able to become housewives if they desire, while not one group argued for the need for men to share in child-raising responsibilities (Saxonberg, 2003).

Serious discussions of family policies have only emerged in recent years, as post-communist governments are beginning to realize that the dramatic drop in fertility rates are not a temporary reaction to the insecurity of the first years of the transition to a market economy. Either because of work aspirations or out of economic necessity, the vast majority of women have tried to remain in the labor market. Instead of exiting the labor market, they have exited the reproductive market to a large extent.

Serious economic problems have also influenced the move toward re-familization. Both countries faced problems in raising funds to finance the public sector during the first years of the transition and Poland faced the additional burden of a looming debt crisis (Saxonberg, 2001; 2003). The ensuing budgetary pressures convinced the governments that it was necessary to cut social spending (cf. Pestoff, 1995; Standing, 1996). Thus, policy makers enacted some measures, such as transferring the responsibility for running nursery schools (for 0-3-year-olds) from the state and state enterprises to local municipal governments, partially to save money (for the Czech case, see Potůček, 1999). Since national governments did not give the local municipalities funds to continue subsidizing nursery schools, this reform caused a sharp drop in access to daycare (Heinen, 2002). The decision to offer mothers extended parental leave rather than access to nursery schools saves even more money in the Polish case, because parental leaves are means- tested and most parents do not receive any economic support for their child-caring leaves.

However, the economic conditions by themselves cannot fully account for the policy preferences in the Czech Republic to support long paid extended parental leaves rather than a shorter but more generous parental leave as existing in Norway and Sweden. Moreover, measures promoting gender equality, such as reserving some months for the fathers, as done in these Scandinavian countries, do not cost any extra money at all. Given the anti-feminist communist legacy, policy makers never seriously considered de-familization policies and did not face the active opposition of organized women when implementing these policies.

CONCLUSION

Post-communist family policies are coming increasingly into contradiction with the needs and aspirations of the population. The Polish and Czech governments have basically followed re-familization strategies because of the anti-feminist communist ideological legacy, which have prevented them from seriously considering de-familization policies that would promote gender equality. Economic pressures have also played a role, as these governments thought that re-familization policies would save them money.

In addition, our analysis of gender attitudes indicates that de-familization policies that promote gender equality would be more likely to meet the needs and rising aspirations of post-communist women than today's policies. Such policies could encourage women to have more children, since they would make it easier for them to balance work and family. Today's policies, in contrast, have encouraged women to leave the reproduction market in order to be able to remain in the labor market.

NOTES

1. Own calculations based on MONEE database 2004, own calculations, and for the Czech Republic, *Vývojová ročenka školství v ČR 2003, Zdravotnická ročenka České republiky-ÚZIS 2003*. Children of 0-3 (3-6) attending pre-school facilities as a fraction of children in age 0-3 (3-6), only half of children 0-1 year of age counted as almost all children of 0-6 months are in care of mothers (maternity leave), children attending kindergarten in age over 6 excluded.

2. In those cases, in which the respondent answers that they have no income, we code it as meaning that their spouse has a higher income, while in those cases in which they respond that their spouse has no income, we count them as meaning that they have a higher income than their spouse.

REFERENCES

Balcerzak-Paradowska, B. (1991). Urlop wychowawczy w Polsce. Kontekst socjalny i demograficzny [Child-raising leaves in Poland. The social and demographic context]. In D. Graniewska, B. Balcerzak-Paradowska & D. Staszewska (Eds.), *Okresowa dezaktywizacja kobiet wychowujacych dzieci jako element polityki rodzinnej* [The temporary de-activation of women in child-raising as an element of family policy] (pp. 46-63). IPISS: Warszawa, Poland.

Balcerzak-Paradowska, B. (1997). Publiczne instytucje usług społeczhych a rodzina. In H. Żeglicka [Public institutions, social service and families] (Ed.), *Partnerstwo w rodzinie i na rzecz rodziny* [Partnership in families and family themes] (pp. 55-69). Warsaw, Poland: Instytut Pracy I Spraw Socjalnych.

Balcerzak-Paradowska, B. (2002). Świadczania rodzinne. Zmiany okresu transformacjia, stan obecny i perspektywy [Family benefits in Poland. Changes in the 1990s and prospects for the future]. *Polityka Spoleczna, 29*, 35-40.

Balcerzak-Paradowska, B., Chloń-Domińczak, A., Kotowska I.E., Olejniczuk-Merta, A. & Topińska, I. (2003). The gender dimension of social security reform in Poland. In E. Fultz, M. Ruck, & S. Steinhilber (Eds.), *The gender dimension of social security reform in Central and Eastern Europe* (pp. 187-314). ILO: Budapest, Hungary.

Banaszak, L.A. & Plutzer, E. (1993). The social bases of feminism in the European Community. *Public Opinion Quarterly, 57*, 29-53.

Bystydzienski, J. M. (1995). Women and families in Poland: Pressing problems and possible solutions. In B. Łobodzińska (Ed.), *Family, women and employment in Central-Eastern Europe* (pp. 193-203). Westport, CT: Greenwood Press.

Castle-Kanerova, M. (1992). Social policy in Czechoslovakia. In B. Deacon (Ed.), *The new Eastern Europe. Social policy past, present and future* (pp. 91-117). London, UK: Sage.

Čermáková, M. (1997). Postavení žen na trhu práce [The position of women in the labor market]. *Sociologický časopis, 33*, 389-404.

Čermáková, M., Mařiková, H. & Tuček, M. (1995). Role mužů a žen v rodině a ve společnosti 1 [The role of men and women in the family and in society 1]. *Data & Fakta, 2*.

Cichomski, B., Morawski, P., Zawadzki, W., & Boski, P. (1999). Konserwatyzm-liberalizm w społecnej ideologii ról kobiet [Conservatism-liberialism in social ideology and the role of women]. In J. Miluska & P. Boski (Eds.) *Męskość w perspektyvwie indywidualnej i kulturowej* [Masculinity in an individual and cultural perspective] (pp. 98-111). Warsaw, Poland: Wydawnicktwo instytutu psychologii PAN.

Crompton, R. & Harris, F. (1997). Women's employment and gender attitudes: A comparative analysis of Britain, Norway and the Czech Republic. *Acta Sociologica, 40,* 183-202.

ČSÚ (Český statistický úřad) (2002). *Statistická ročenka České republiky [Statistical yearbook of the Czech Republic].* Praha, The Czech Republic: ČSÚ.

EIRO (2003). National centres answers to study questionnaire on "family and parental leave provision and collective bargaining." Retrieved March 15, 2004 from http://www.eiro.eurofound.eu.int/2004/03/word/cs_parental_annex.doc.

Esping-Andersen, G. (1990). *The three worlds of welfare capitalism.* Cambridge, UK: Polity Press.

Esping-Andersen, G. (1999). *Social foundations of postindustrial economies.* Oxford, UK: Oxford University Press.

Eurostat (2003). *Employment and labour market in CEC.* Brussels, Belgium: European Community.

Eurostat (2004). Database. Retrieved November 17, 2004 from http://epp.eurostat. cec.eu.int/portal/page?_pageid=1996,39140985&_dad=portal&_schema=PORTAL& screen=detailref&language=en&product=Yearlies_new_population&root=Yearlies_ new_population/C/C1/C12/cab12048

Ferge, Z. (1997a). The changed welfare paradigm: The individualization of the social. *Social Policy and Administration, 31,* 20-44.

Ferge, Z. (1997b.) Women and social transformation in Central-Eastern Europe. *Czech Sociological Review, 5,* 159-178.

Firlit-Fesnat, G. (1997). Kobiety i meżczyźw rolach rodzinnych i zawodowych: marzenia o partnerstwie a Żywotność [Women and men in family and professional roles: Dreams about partnership and the strength of tradition]. In H. Żeglicka (Ed.), *Partnerstwo w rodzinie i na rzecz rodziny* [Partnership in the family and for the family] (pp. 21-31). Warsaw, Poland: Instytut Pracy i Spraw Socjalnych.

Fodor, E., Glass C., Kawachi, J. & Popescu, L. (2002). Family policies and gender in Hungary, Poland and Romania. *Communism and Post-Communist Studies (35),* 475-490.

Fultz, E., M. Ruck. & S. Steinhilber (Eds.) (2003). *The gender dimension of social security reform in Central and Eastern Europe.* Budapest, The Czech Republic: International Labour Organization.

Funk, N. (1993). Introduction. In Nanette Funk & Magda Mueller (Eds.), *Gender politics and post-communism: Reflections from Eastern Europe and the former Soviet Union* (pp. 1-14). New York & London: Routledge.

Fuszara, M. (1991). Will the abortion issue give birth to feminism in Poland? In M. Maclean and D. Groves (Eds.),*Women's issues in social policy* (pp. 205-228). London, UK: Routledge.

Fuszara, M. (1994). Market economy and consumer rights: The impact on women's everyday lives and employment. *Economics and Industrial Democracy, 15*, 75-87.

Golinowska, S. (1996). Zawodowa i domowa praca kobiet. Polska i kraje Europy Srodkowej i Wschodniej [Professional work and housework of women: Poland and countries of Central and Eastern Europe]. *Polityka Społeczna 23*,16-22.

Götting, U. (1998). *Transformation der wohlfahrtsstaaten in Mittel- und Osteuropa [Transformation of the welfare state in middle and eastern Europe]*. Opladen, Germany: Leske & Budrich.

Havelková, H. (1996). Abstract citizenship? Women and power in the Czech Republic. *Social Politics, 6*, 243-260.

Heinen J. (2002). Ideology, economics, and the politics of child care in Poland before and after the transition. In S. Michel & R. Mahon (Eds.) *Child care policy at the crossroads, gender and welfare state restructuring* (pp. 71-92). London, UK: Routledge.

Heitlinger, A. (1996). Framing feminism in post-communist Czech Republic. *Communist and Post-Communist Studies, 29*, 77-93.

Maříková, H. (1997). Žena v zaměstání a muž v rodině [Woman in employment and man in the family]. *Sociální politika, 22*, 9-11.

Matějková, B. & Palonczyová, J. (2004). *Rodinné politiky ve vybraných zemích II* [Family policy in chosen countries II]. Praha, The Czech Republic: Výzkumný ústav práce a sociálních vecí.

Mirody, M. & Giza-Poleszczuk, A. (2000). Changing images of identity in Poland: From the self-sacrificing to the self-investing woman? In G. Kligman and S. Gal (Eds.), *Reproducing gender: Politics, publics, and everyday life after socialism* (pp. 151-175). Princeton, NJ: Princeton University Press.

MISSCEEC II. (n.d.). *Mutual information system on social protection in the Central and Eastern European countries*. Bulgaria, Czech Republic, Estonia, Hungary, Latvia, Lithuania, Poland, Romania, Slovak Republic and Slovenia. *Situation at 1 January 2002*. Retrieved November 19, 2004 from http://europa.eu.int/comm/employment_social/missceec/index_en.html.

MONEE database (2004). TransMONEE database. Florence, Italy: UNICEF ICDC.

Morgan, A. & Wilcox, C. (1992). Anti-feminism in Western Europe 1975-1987. *West European Politics, 15*, 151-169.

Nowakowska, R. (1997). The new right and fundamentalism. In T. Renne (Ed.), *Ana's land: Sisterhood in Eastern Europe* (pp. 26-41). Boulder, CO: Westview Press.

Nowakowska, U. & Swedrowska, A. (2000). Women in the labor market. In U. Nowakowska (Ed.), *Polish women in the 1990s* (pp. 41-75). Warsaw, Poland: Women's Rights Center.

Panayotova, E. & Brayfield, A. (1997). National context and gender ideology: Attitudes toward women's employment in Hungary and the United States. *Gender and Society, 11*, 627-655.

Pascall, G. & Manning, N. (2000). Gender and social policy: Comparing welfare states in Central and Eastern Europe and the former Soviet Union. *Journal of European Social Policy 10*, 240-266.

Pestoff, V. A. (1995). Citizens as co-producers of social services: From the welfare state to the welfare mix. In V.A. Pestoff (Ed.), *Reforming social services in Central and Eastern Europe–eleven nation overview* (pp. 11-28). Kracow, Poland: Kracow Academy of Economics.

Potůček, M. (1999). *Křižovatky české sociální reformy* [The crisis of Czech social reforms]. Prague. The Czech Republic: Slon.

Raabe, P.H. (1998). Women, work, and family in the Czech Republic–and comparisons with the West. *Community, Work & Family, 1,* 51-63.

Raabe, P.H. (1999). Women and gender in the Czech Republic and cross-national comparisons. *Czech Sociological Review, 7,* 223-230.

Renne, T. (1997). Disparaging digressions: Sisterhood in East-Central Europe. In T. Renne (Ed.). *Ana's land: Sisterhood in Eastern Europe* (pp. 1-21). Boulder, CO: Westview Press.

Robinson, J. (1995). Women, the state, and the need for civil society. In D. M. Stetson & A. Mazur (Eds.), *Comparative state feminism* (pp. 203-220). Thousand Oaks, CA: Sage.

Rueschemeyer, M. (Ed.). (1995). *Women in the politics of post-communist Eastern Europe.* Armonk, NY: M.E. Sharpe.

Saxonberg, S. (2000). Polish women in the mid 1990s. *Czech Sociological Review, 8,* 233-253.

Saxonberg, S. (2001). *The fall: A comparative study of the end of Communism in Czechoslovakia, East Germany, Hungary and Poland.* Amsterdam, The Netherlands: Harwood Academic.

Saxonberg, S. (2002). Kryzys polityki rodzinnej w postkommunistycznej [The crisis of post-communist familiy policy]. *Przeglad europejski, 1,* 248-264.

Saxonberg, S. (2003). *The Czech Republic before the new millennium: Politics, parties and gender.* New York, Boulder: Columbia University Press, East European Monographs.

Siemienska, R. (1994). The contemporary dilemma of the Polish family and its genealogy. *The European Journal of Women's Studies, 1,* 207-225.

Siemienska, R. (1999). Rola rodziny w sferze życia prywatnego i publicznego. Akceptowane modele i czynniki je kształtujące [The role of the family in the private and public sphere. Acceptence of models and factors influencing it]. In J. Miluska & P. Boski (Eds.), *Męskość-kobiecość w perspektyvwie indywidualnej i kulturowej [Maleness-Femalness in an individual and cutlural perspective]* (pp. 208-223). Warsaw, Poland: Wydawnicktwo instytutu psychologii PAN.

Šiklová, J. (1998). Why Western feminism isn't working. *The new presence: The Prague Journal of Central European Affairs* (January), 8-10.

Sirovátka, T. & Rákoczyová, M. (2002). Aktivní politika zaměstnanosti v druhé polovině devadesátých let [Active labor policy in the second half of the 1990s]. *Sociální politika, 27,* 17-20.

Standing, G. (1996). Social protection in Central and Eastern Europe: A tale of slipping anchors and torn safety nets. In G. Esping-Andersen (Ed.), *Welfare states in transition. national adaptations in global economies* (pp. 225-255). London, UK: Sage Publications.

Wiktorow, A. & Mierzewski, P. (1991). Promise or peril? Social policy for children during the transition to the market economy in Poland. In G. A. Cornia & S. Sipos (Eds.), *Children and the transition to the market economy* (pp. 207-233). Aldershot, UK: Avebury.

Wilcox, C. (1991a). The causes and consequences of feminist consciousness among western European women. *Comparative Political Studies, 23* (4), 519-36.

Wilcox, C. (1991b). Support for gender equality in West Europe. *European Journal of Political Research, 20,* 127-147.

Wolchik, S. L. (1995). Women and the politics of transition in the Czech and Slovak Republics. In Marilyn Rueschemeyer (Ed.), *Women in the politics of post-communist Eastern Europe* (pp. 3-27). Armonk, NY: M.E. Sharpe.

Zdravotnická ročenka České republiky [Health Yearbook of the Czech Republic] (1990). (2000). Praha, The Czech Republic: ÚZIS.

Trading Well-Being
for Economic Efficiency:
The 1990 Shift in EU Childcare Policies

Inge Bleijenbergh

Jet Bussemaker

Jeanne de Bruijn

SUMMARY. In 1992, the European Union (EU) adopted the Recommendation on Childcare and became involved in childcare policy. For the first time, care services and domestic care were acknowledged as the common responsibility of all the European and national political units. The article shows the interaction between childcare policy at the European level and in three welfare states with strong male breadwinner policy logics: Germany, the Netherlands, and the United Kingdom (UK). At the European and national levels, arguments prioritizing economic efficiency and equal opportunities gained ground at the expense

Inge Bleijenbergh can be contacted at Radboud University, Nijmegen School of Management, P.O. Box 9108, 6500 HK Nijmegen, The Netherlands (E-mail: i.bleijenbergh@fm.ru.nl). Jet Bussemaker is in the Department of Social Science, Vrije Universiteit, Amsterdam, and a member of Dutch Parliament, The Netherlands (E-mail: M.Bussemaker@ fsw.vu.nl). Jeanne de Bruijn is in the Department of Social Science, Vrije Universiteit, Amsterdam, The Netherlands (E-mail: JGM.de.Bruijn@ fsw.vu.nl).

[Haworth co-indexing entry note]: "Trading Well-Being for Economic Efficiency: The 1990 Shift in EU Childcare Policies." Bleijenbergh, Inge, Jet Bussemaker, and Jeanne de Bruijn. Co-published simultaneously in *Marriage & Family Review* (The Haworth Press, Inc.) Vol. 39, No. 3/4, 2006, pp. 315-336; and: *Families and Social Policy: National and International Perspectives* (ed: Linda Haas, and Steven K. Wisensale) The Haworth Press, Inc., 2006, pp. 315-336. Single or multiple copies of this article are available for a fee from The Haworth Document Delivery Service [1-800-HAWORTH, 9:00 a.m. - 5:00 p.m. (EST). E-mail address: docdelivery@haworthpress.com].

315

of arguments prioritizing the well-being of children. Formerly male breadwinner states reached a consensus on the policy goal of shared responsibility for caregiving by emphasizing common economic interests and the principle of equal opportunities while still allowing for nation variability in how this policy goal will be carried out. *[Article copies available for a fee from The Haworth Document Delivery Service: 1-800-HAWORTH. E-mail address: <docdelivery@haworthpress.com> Website: <http://www. HaworthPress.com> © 2006 by The Haworth Press, Inc. All rights reserved.]*

KEYWORDS. Childcare policies, European Union, gender equality, Germany, Netherlands, United Kingdom

In 1992, the Council of Ministers of the European Union (EU) introduced the Recommendation on Childcare, committing itself to stimulating the development of childcare services in its member states.[1] It "recommended that Member States should take and/or progressively encourage initiatives to enable women and men to reconcile their occupational, family and upbringing responsibilities arising from the care of children" (Official Journal of the European Communities, 1992a, p. 17). The Recommendation consists of seven articles that formulate common goals on the affordability and accessibility of the services, the introduction of care leaves, the organization of work and the sharing of care responsibilities between men and women. Thought at first glance to be a measure of mere symbolic value, the Recommendation on Childcare illustrated an important conceptual change pertaining to the responsibility of the EU. With this Recommendation, childcare policy (formal day care and out-of-school care and care by recognized host parents) became a topic of EU concern. Still emphasizing the common responsibility of governments, employers, trade unions and families for childcare services, it was the first time European social policy crossed the paid employment nexus and became involved in unpaid as well as paid care.

At the same time in various European welfare states, public childcare became a topic of political concern. This was especially striking in countries with strong male breadwinner policy logics like Germany, the Netherlands, and the UK. Here services were traditionally limited and childcare was considered a private responsibility (Bussemaker, 1998; Lewis, 1997). In this article, we analyze the European policy debates leading to the Childcare Recommendation and the simultaneous debates in Germany, the Netherlands, and the UK. We selected these three countries with strong traditional gender values (male policy logics) and low levels of childcare provision, because we expected the biggest shift to be made in these countries.

In 1989, in the Netherlands and the UK 2% of the children in the 0-3 age group went to public day care; in West-Germany this was 3%. This contrasted with countries with less traditional gender values (moderate or weak breadwinner policy logics) like Denmark and France, that provided public childcare for 44% and 25% of the same age group (Phillips & Moss, 1989). In this article, we examine the arguments used by various political actors in the EU, Germany, the Netherlands, and the UK to support or impede new initiatives on childcare and the political factors that created opportunities for a shift in childcare policy. Did the emerging policy logic at the EU level resemble national policy logics or were there clear differences between the national and supranational levels? What were the contributions of the different countries to the debates leading to the Childcare Recommendation? And how did they implement the Recommendation?

THEORY

The aim of this article is to demonstrate how assumptions concerning gender relations play a role in the development of European social policy and how social policy at the European and national level interacts. To analyze gender assumptions in national and European social policy, we use the analytical concept of "policy logics." Policy logics are the assumptions, principles and premises of welfare regimes, here especially related to gender (Lewis & Hobson, 1997, p. 6; Sainsbury, 1999). The concept of policy logics emerged from the theoretical pursuit of a welfare typology that does justice to the role of gender assumptions in social policy. Mainstream classifications like Esping-Andersen's (1990) triad of corporatist, liberal and social democrat welfare regimes conceal gender differences within welfare states (Bussemaker & van Kersbergen, 1994; Lewis, 1992; Orloff, 1993). Lewis (1992) and Ostner and Lewis (1995) note that differences in gender assumptions historically cut across mainstream typologies of welfare states. They developed a gender classification focusing on strong, moderate and weak male breadwinner regimes, later redefined as "gender policy logics" (Lewis & Hobson, 1997, p. 2). One of the indicators used in their classification is the level of social services, particularly with regard to childcare.

Male Breadwinner Policy Logic

There are "strong" male breadwinner policy logics in Germany, the Netherlands, and the UK, the nations considered here. Ireland is another strong male breadwinner policy state. In these nations, a lack of public childcare services leads to low (mainly part-time) female labor market participation and longstanding inequality between men and women in regard to social security. In the strong breadwinner model countries, there is a firm dividing line between public and private responsibility for caregiving.

"Modified" male breadwinner policy logics are present in societies such as France and Belgium. Such societies are characterized by a moderate level of women's full-time labor market participation and better social security protection, because women have social protection as either workers or mothers. In these states, the government accepts some responsibility for helping families provide care for children while parents are employed. There are "weak" male breadwinner policy logics in Sweden and Denmark. Here a high level of women's full-time labor market participation combines with individual tax and social security arrangements, and individual rights to public childcare and parental leave. This is also called the "dual breadwinner policy logic" (Bussemaker 1998; Lewis, 1997; Ostner & Lewis, 1995).

The concepts of welfare regimes and policy logics are not only used to characterize national welfare states, but also to predict the development of European social policy. Ostner and Lewis (1995) argue that the EU would be unwilling to expand into the sphere of care provision because strong male policy logics prevail among the European member states. Moreover, the emphasis on economic integration would prevent the EU from becoming involved in care policy (Plantenga, 1997).

In this article we explain why, in contrast to these expectations, the EU became involved in childcare policy in the 1990s. Moreover, we explain why childcare policies appeared in the same period on the political agenda in three welfare states characterized as having strong male breadwinner policy logics. To describe and explain these developments, we turn to the actors involved in the policy debates and the arguments they used to justify their claims. At the European level, the major actors are the member states in the Council of Ministers and in European institutions such as the European Commission and the European

Parliament. At the national level, the main actors are political parties inside and outside the government. Other actors participate at both levels; for example, the women's movement is organized at the national and European level, as are trade unions and employers' organizations.

METHOD

Our research method was content analysis of primary and secondary sources on European social policy. We reconstructed the European and national debates on the basis of official documents, archival research, using Departmental archives at the Dutch Ministry of Social Affairs, the Hague, and the Archives of the European Communities at the European University Institute in Florence. We also conducted semi-structured interviews with key figures in the policy process and a literature review of secondary sources.

We first reconstructed the policy debates on childcare on the basis of policy documents, periodicals and archival sources. We performed content analysis of the material by organizing the arguments on the issues of inclusion, equality, responsibility and activity. After that, we selected arguments that we intuitively found to be the most outspoken and different from each other. By placing them in chronological order, we revealed the pattern of argumentation in the development of the debate. To enhance the intersubjectivity of the analysis, we presented our reconstruction to a select group of key figures in the policy process on the Childcare Recommendation, allowing them to correct misinterpretations and give additional information. We based our definitive reconstruction on these interviews.

By analyzing the development of the policy debates on childcare, we found three basic arguments on childcare. They include concern for children's well-being, equal opportunities for men and women, and economic efficiency (see also Bussemaker, 1998). Political actors use these arguments to justify different assumptions about the sectors of society primarily responsible for the care of children: the state, the market, non-governmental organizations, or parents. All three lines of reasoning are articulated to either defend or combat the expansion of childcare facilities. First, we discuss and analyze arguments on children's well-being. They might be used to encourage state involvement, claiming that public childcare enhances the development of young children. But arguments on children's well-being might also be used to oppose state involvement with childcare, claiming that children are best served by being cared for at home by parents.

Second, we elaborate on arguments based on equal opportunities. A reference to equal opportunities may be used to defend female labor market participation and women's economic independence, as well as the collective public responsibility for providing childcare facilities. Equal opportunities may also be used to emphasize fathers' childcare responsibility and thus focus on the sexual re-division of labor at home.

Third, we examine arguments pertaining to economic efficiency. The central concern is whether day care facilities can be expected to keep the welfare state affordable in the long term, for example, by enlarging the labor force in times of low population growth. This argument may be used to emphasize the common responsibility of the state, trade unions and employers to invest in public care facilities. Arguments of economic efficiency may, however, also be used to oppose state investments in childcare. To restrict public expenditure and reduce labor costs, the responsibility may be left to the private sector, emphasizing the individual responsibility of parents and the role of private agencies in civil society. We compared the use of these three arguments during the policy preparation process with the final content of the policy, investigating what arguments came to be dominant and how this can be explained.

RESULTS

We first analyze the European debates on childcare and then compare them with the debates at the national level. The childcare debate began in the 1980s, when a European policy network of women emerged and feminists ("femocrats") came to work at the European Commission and European Parliament (Hoskyns, 1996). The Commission was the first to mention the need for government action in the field of childcare in its first Equal Opportunities Action Programme for 1982-1985 (Commission of the European Communities, 1981). In this period, five Directives on Equal Treatment of Women and Men were developed; European Commission "femocrats" put the topic of childcare on the agenda in an effort to broaden equal treatment policy from labor market policy to the broader field of welfare provisions. On the initiative of its Committee on the Rights of Women, in 1986 the European Parliament joined the European debate on childcare policies. Arguments on children's well-being dominated its contribution. In a resolution on childcare, the European Parliament stated, "One of the fundamental features of childcare centres is that they provide nursery education for all children, and that this education can offset inequalities experienced by certain socially and culturally disadvantaged groups, giving them a basic level of equal opportunity" (Official Journal of the European Communities, 1986, p. 22).

In the resolution, the European Parliament encouraged state responsibility for care facilities, primarily to increase social equality among children. In particular, the members of the Committee for Women's Rights and the European Socialist Party (the present-day PSE) argued that childcare could be provided by public and private organizations, but the national state should have final responsibility. Access to childcare facilities should be a basic social right and the European Commission should develop a draft Directive on equal access to childcare facilities. These arguments are in keeping with dual caregiver policy logics.

However, opponents to European childcare policy also refer to children's well-being. In the European Parliament, the main opposition is from the Christian Democrats, unified in the European People's Party (PPE). In the debate on the resolution text, Mr. Estgen, a member of the PPE for Luxembourg, argued that children are best cared for by their close relatives. His line of reasoning fits a strong male breadwinner policy logic:

> The family provides the most suitable framework for children to grow up in because it is the most natural. That is not a reactionary retreat into Conservative ideology, but an open-minded reaction to scientifically supported findings. Childcare institutions, even at their best, are and always will be a third best solution for very young children. The best is always being cared for by the parents, the second best is being cared for by relatives such as grandparents, and in my view communal social facilities should come only as a last resort." (Debates of the European Parliament, 1986, p. 20)

From this standpoint, the PPE argued against a basic right to childcare facilities and wanted to leave childcare to the family and private companies. The state should financially support these initiatives and have budgetary authority over them. This was a minority standpoint. With an overwhelming majority, the European Parliament adopted a resolution to order the European Commission to present a draft directive on childcare (Official Journal of the European Communities, 1986).

The political climate in the 1980s was, however, not conducive to an expansion of European social policy. Feminists at the European Commission and European Parliament called for action, but the Council of Ministers opposed any expansion of European social legislation. Hedy D'Ancona, former Dutch minister of Welfare, Health and Culture (personal communication, June 16, 1999), claims there was a strong fear of opposition from the Thatcher government. It was probably because of this opposition that in its second Equal Opportunities Programme (1986-1990), the European Commission decided to first build more support for the topic by announcing the foundation of a Childcare Network and not presenting a proposal. The Network with experts from all the twelve member states was asked to examine the situation in each member state and formulate recommendations (Commission of the European Communities, 1985).

Starting in 1987, the Childcare Network was extremely productive in presenting reports on the situation in the various countries. Arguments on behalf of children's well-being dominated their contributions. The reports the Network published in the late 1980s explicitly refer to childcare as a "citizenship right" (European Commission Childcare Network, 1990, p. 2; Moss, 1988, p. 292). Children are not only future citizens, they should be treated as European citizens in their own right. Co-ordinator Peter Moss (personal communication, July 10, 2002) explained that the Childcare Network felt it was society's responsibility to protect children from harm and distress and ensure that their care does not depend on their parents' income, but on their own needs.

Much as the European Parliament did in its 1986 Resolution, the Childcare Network advocated a childcare Directive. Its standpoint on state responsibility was even more explicit. Public authorities should provide equal access to childcare for all children. Leaving childcare to the social partners would exclude children of non-employed parents from its benefits. Moreover, the state should be responsible for the quality of the services and the appropriate wages and working conditions of childcare workers (European Commission Childcare Network, 1990). So based on arguments on children's well-being, the European Parliament and European Commission's Childcare Network both favored public childcare as a central welfare provision to be guaranteed by the state.

In Childcare Network publications from 1988, arguments on equal opportunities for men and women were also prominent. Increasing the number of childcare facilities should contribute to a more equal division of labor between men and women and expand freedom of choice. The sexual re-division of domestic care responsibilities entered the discussion at this point. In 1990, the Childcare Network explicitly advocated a greater involvement of men in the care of children:

> Childcare is a "men's issue" as much as a "women's issue." No formula can be applied uniformly in all families–how responsibilities are shared may vary between families and, within the same family, may vary over time with one parent doing more at one stage and less at another. Having acknowledged this, there is still plenty of scope, and an urgent need, for greater involvement by men in childcare (particularly in families but also as workers in services) and for policies to encourage and support this process. (European Commission Childcare Network, 1990, p. 3)

When the European Commission presented a draft Council Recommendation on Childcare in 1991 (Commission of the European Communities, 1991), the discussion became more pragmatic. Notwithstanding appeals from the European Parliament and its own Childcare Network, the Commission chose to present a draft recommendation instead of a directive. In an official statement to explain this choice, a Commission official referred to the risk of a directive countering the dominant ideas of subsidiarity (Debates of the European Parliament, 1991, p. 365). The Commission obviously didn't want to face the risk of the United Kingdom using its veto right at the Council of Ministers to block a Childcare Directive, as it did with earlier proposals for directives on parental leave and atypical work (see Rutherford, 1989).

To justify the policy, the European Commission took a less controversial approach than the Childcare Network and European Parliament had in the past. It replaced the argument on behalf of children's well-being by one on economic efficiency to better suit the EU's general goal to establish a European market. It stated that a need for women's growing labor market participation is needed for demographic reasons. In addition, the Commission held that improving the level of childcare facilities in the member states would facilitate the free movement of workers in the labor market.

This argumentation on economic efficiency was supported with references to equal opportunities, but only in a restricted sense. Equal opportunities were interpreted in a one-sided way as opportunities for both sexes to participate in the labor market, but no references were made to the sexual re-division of domestic care responsibilities. Only article 6 mentions the need for increasing men's participation in caring for children. This reference was controversial enough to be the topic of serious debate at the working group preparing the Council of Minister's meetings. The issue was state responsibility to intervene in how care responsibilities were divided at home. The original proposal of the European Commission noted ". . . in relation to the responsibilities arising from the care and upbringing of children, it is recommended that member states promote and encourage increased participation by men to achieve a more equal sharing of parental responsibilities between men and women" (Commission of the European Communities, 1991, p. 17).

The European Parliament proposed making this formulation more concrete (Official Journal of the European Communities, 1991), but at the Council working group, the British opposed this formulation and argued that the division of caring tasks is a family responsibility, not a state one. On the request of the British, a statement was added that men should always have freedom of choice with regard to caring activities. To meet further British objections, the Dutch president proposed adding a sentence to explain that men's care was needed to enable women to participate on the labor market (Departmental archive, Dutch Ministry of Employment and Social Affairs [DAMESA], 1992 the Hague, file aanbeveling 92/241/EEG inzake kinderopvang 31/03/1992). So the Recommendation defended men's care for its instrumental value and no longer for its intrinsic value. The chair of the Council working group at the time, Frank Schumacher, emphasized that this change was supported by the other countries (personal communication, September 10, 2001).

Men's participation in care was a controversial issue in the Council of Ministers, but improving women's participation in the labor market was not, although there was a slight shift in justification. The European Parliament and Economic and Social Committee had been concerned with substantive equality, emphasizing women's growing need to earn their own income due to the rising divorce rate and growing number of single parents (Official Journal of the European Communities, 1991; 1992b). The Council of Ministers combined a more formal approach to gender equality with arguments concerning economic efficiency, emphasizing the growing need for women's labor due to the ageing population. A reference to women's opportunities in the labor market was obviously less controversial than a reference to their economic needs. Female employment was needed to keep the welfare state affordable. Whether or not it gave individual women enough income to support their family was not discussed.

With the growing presence of economic and demographic arguments, the assumptions concerning the role of the state also changed.

References to children's well-being may have promoted state responsibility (as was argued by feminists and Social Democrats in the European Parliament) or the responsibility of the family and civil society (as was argued by Conservatives and Christian Democrats), but with the introduction of economic and demographic arguments, attention shifted to the social partners. Here the British and the Dutch played a role in the Council of Ministers. In the autumn of 1991, the Dutch president of the Council of Ministers proposed responding to the British objections to public responsibility for childcare by putting a greater emphasis on the shared responsibility of national, regional and local governments, social partners, non-governmental organizations and individuals. This change in formulation helped overcome British objections. The German government emphasized the need to guarantee the quality of services, but wasn't supported by the other countries (DAMESA, 1992 the Hague, file aanbeveling kinderopvang). References to public quality control and the working conditions of childcare workers were left out of the final recommendation. The Council of Ministers was thus able to adopt the Childcare Recommendation on March 31, 1992.

Though the Recommendation was criticized by feminist authors as being non-binding (Ostner & Lewis, 1995), it could also be seen as a departure from the dominant views at the time on European social policy (see Hoskyns, 1996). Childcare and the division of domestic care were no longer strictly a national affair, but were acknowledged as the common responsibility of all the national and European actors. As Agnes Hubert, the head of the EC Equal Opportunities Unit, noted (personal communication, June 24, 2002):

> At the time it was a revolutionary text. It put something on the EU agenda that had never been there before. It was the first time the European Union made an explicit reference to the involvement of fathers in the upbringing of children. And there was something on state and public responsibility for the care for children. Of course the final result was less than the Childcare Network had initially proposed, but we took the Recommendation as fairly progressive, considering the context of the discussion.

In the European debate on childcare, arguments on children's well-being became less important, while references to economic efficiency increased. References to equal opportunities were present throughout the discussion, although the emphasis on the role of fathers in care lost ground because it was given an instrumental rather than a principal value. In contrast, women's labor market participation was felt to serve a wider goal such as economic and fiscal policies. This shift in argumentation corresponded with a shift in the actors considered responsible for providing services. The single emphasis on the role of either the state (dual breadwinner policy logic) or the parents (male breadwinner policy logic) was replaced by a policy logic on the shared responsibility of the state, social partners, civil society and parents. To legitimize European involvement in childcare policies, it was necessary to emphasize the common responsibility of the various social and political actors.

Let us now examine whether the European childcare policy logic resembles the national policy logics and vice versa. The three welfare states in question are characterized as having strong male breadwinner policy logics (Bussemaker, 1998; Lewis, 1997; Ostner & Lewis, 1995). Historically, public childcare is poorly developed in these countries, and in part as a result, the labor market participation of women is very low. Being welfare states with traditionally limited public involvement with childcare services, why did the issue enter national political agendas in the 1990s? And how did these countries implement the European childcare recommendation?

The UK

In the 1980s and early 1990s, Conservative governments dominated politics in the United Kingdom. The successive Conservative governments, headed by Margaret Thatcher and John Major (1979 -1997), were against state responsibility for childcare. Even the marginal public childcare that existed in the early 1980s became a subject of discussion (Hansard, Col 150, 12-7-1988). Public childcare was among the poorest in Europe and decreased even further (see Moss, 1991). The opposition to traditional family policies was weak. Labor and trade unions held traditional views on childcare based on a male breadwinner ideology and assumptions on the private nature of the family. Moreover, the feminist movement was internally divided on paid work for women and public childcare (Lovenduski & Randall, 1993).

Although the government didn't want to be directly involved, it felt that childcare services would support female labor market participation. It formulated the explicit goal of increasing voluntary and private childcare initiatives (Dwyer, 1998; Land & Lewis, 1998). To support employer involvement in childcare, in 1991 the British introduced tax relief plans for employers who provided workplace nurseries. The effects were limited though because high costs kept employers from providing the facilities. In addition, the Conservative government tried to stimulate employer childcare initiatives by launching the Opportunity 2000 project. The central aim was to create win-win situations that served the interest of employers and (female) employees alike (Gauthier, 1996). In addition to measures directed at employers, the government wanted to stimulate other private services, like child-minders and nannies. The 1989 Children's Act regulated some of the private initiatives at a minimal level. The Act obliged local authorities to develop systems for registering private services and to provide childcare for children in need (Land & Lewis, 1998).

Up until then, the Conservative government had maintained the emphasis on private responsibility for childcare that it had also advocated at the European level. It feared any European social legislation, and in the preparations for the Childcare Recommendation in the Council working group, it argued that the division of caring tasks is the responsibility of the family, not the state (DAMESA, 1992 file kinderopvang). The British argument was successful in changing the proposed emphasis on public responsibility for childcare to a shared responsibility of local and national governments, social partners, non-governmental organizations and individuals. As a result, the recommendation no longer challenged the poor British childcare policies. Nevertheless, the Conservatives began to cautiously recognize some public responsibility for childcare. In the 1992 election campaign, the Conservative government announced that there would be more out-of-school care sites starting in 1993 (Gauthier, 1996). Overall, in the early 1990s, public childcare developed step-by-step in the United Kingdom, usually linked to labor market policy (see O'Connor, Orloff & Shaver, 1999).

The fundamental shift in childcare policy logic occurred in 1997 with the change in political power at the national level. With New Labour in power, public as well as private childcare facilities were expanded. In contrast to the old Labour Party, where the male breadwinner ideology still dominated, New Labour was explicitly committed to gender equality and state support for working women and their families (Sassoon, 1996; Siim, 2000). The Blair government formulated the explicit aim of ensuring free facilities of good quality for all 4-year-olds whose parents wanted them (Land & Lewis, 1998). The Blair government stated that expanding childcare facilities serves both economic efficiency and children's well-being, calling childcare a shared responsibility of the state, the social partners and private agencies. This argument was perfectly in keeping with the approach of the European Childcare Recommendation and resulted in an increase in facilities in the next years.

The Netherlands

The turning point in Dutch childcare policy was around 1990, when the expansion of childcare facilities became state policy. Until late into the 1980s, the notion that private care was fundamental to children's well-being dominated the public debate. Public childcare was seen as something immoral in a well-developed welfare state. Mothers were supposed to stay at home and take care of their children. Since the 1970s, the state had only provided part-time playgroups for two- and three-year-olds ("peuterspeelzalen"). Feminists and left-wing parties were the only ones in favor of childcare services as a basic provision.

As in the UK, the Dutch Social Democrats (PvdA) had a longstanding tradition of protecting traditional family and gender relations, and until the late 1980s they had an ambivalent approach towards public childcare. The Christian Democrats (CDA), in power with the Conservative Liberals (VVD) in the 1980s, dominated the political debate on childcare. They advocated a neo-Conservative ideology on the caring society as opposed to state involvement. Christian Democrat Minister of Welfare Elco Brinkman, known for his neo-Conservative ideas on the family, noted that childcare should never become a general public service (Bussemaker, 1997). In his opinion, state-funded childcare embodied the evils of government interference and control in private life as well as the indifference and selfishness of individual citizens who allowed their own interests to prevail over those of their children.

It was only in the late 1980s that the male breadwinner policy logic lost ground in the Netherlands. The implementation of the five European Directives on Equal Opportunities in Dutch social policy made the principle of equal opportunities more influential. A growing consensus emerged on the need for an economic restructuring of the welfare state. Politicians started to defend women's labor market participation with arguments of economic efficiency and to present childcare as a means to increase competitiveness.

This development can be explained by two factors. First, in 1989 a new Cabinet of Social Democrats and Christian Democrats came into power. The Social Democrats, like Labour in the UK, argued that public childcare might contribute to children's well-being and equal opportunities for men and women. Entering the Cabinet, they were able to influence the policy process. Secondly, a report by the influential Scientific Council for Government Policy (WRR, 1990) provided arguments to legitimate public childcare to other political parties as well. It noted that women's labor market participation should be stimulated to ensure welfare provisions such as pensions in the long run. Childcare was an important requirement in this connection. It was no longer the division of responsibility between the family and the state that was the issue, but the shared responsibility of employees, companies and the state.

The new coalition of Christian Democrats and Social Democrats developed the first Dutch policy program to increase childcare, the Stimulation Measure, in 1990. It introduced financial support for public and private services. Since then, childcare has become a booming business in the Netherlands. In particular, the historically unique coalition Cabinet of Liberals (VVD and D66) and Social Democrats (1994-2002) made the expansion of childcare arrangements an important policy goal. To stimulate companies setting up their own childcare facilities, in 1995 the Cabinet introduced tax incentives for employers. It argued financing childcare should be a shared responsibility of the state, employers and trade unions. Under the influence of European legislation, the Cabinet also developed legislation on unpaid parental leave and introduced fiscal measures to establish paid parental leave.

Thus arguments on economic efficiency, strategically combined with arguments on equal opportunities for men and women, dominated the Dutch public debate on childcare in the 1990s. The post-1990 expansion of childcare facilities was more an effect of alterations in labor market policy and the need for fiscal restructuring than of co-ordinated policy on gender equality. In this respect, Dutch social policy was in keeping with the changes in the European childcare debate, advocating policy logics of economic efficiency.

Germany

Like the Netherlands, Germany witnessed a turning point around 1990 in the public childcare debate, though for very different reasons. Germany's reunification in 1989 suddenly confronted it with two very different childcare systems. Former Communist East Germany had ample state facilities for childcare, but in West Germany public facilities were very rare and only supplemented by a few private efforts on the part of the parents themselves.

As in the Netherlands, a strong male breadwinner policy logic prevailed in West Germany in the 1970s and 1980s. The argument that children were best cared for at home by their mothers dominated the public debate. The Conservative Cabinets in the 1980s dominated by the Christian Democrats (CDU and CSU) saw little reason to question this approach. The only policy instrument which rose sharply in the

1970s, public subsidies to host parents ("Tagesmütter"), declined in the early 1980s (Ergas, 1990).

It was only after German unification in 1989 that childcare became an important political issue. The government had to face the challenge of combining two totally different systems into one. Christian-Democrats did not want the expansion of public childcare to be linked to totalitarianism, state control or state education, as they described the East German situation. As the CDU stated in a pamphlet:

> It was socialist but not social to wake small children from their sleep at five in the morning and transport them in crowded vehicles to institutions ("Einrichtungen"). At all these institutions . . . children were exposed to a one-sided ideological model of control. (CDU, Die Sozialpolitische Entwicklung in Deutschland-Familien Förderung, date unknown)

In 1991 the Christian-Democrat government introduced a new Federal Act on Children and Youth Support ("Kinder-und Jugendhilfegestz"). One of its aims was to create a comprehensive and coherent system of facilities for children in the 0-6 age group, regulating day care centers, kindergartens, out-of-school care facilities and childminders. The Act facilitated procedures for becoming a childminder, devoting attention to the educational value of childcare. The basic argument for increasing childcare was not economic efficiency, but children's well-being and a balanced family life. Men and women should decide freely whether or not they wanted a career. In a debate about the new Act in 1991, Bundeskanzler Köhl spoke in terms of a right to childcare, although he noted it should always be a free choice:

> We want every person, male or female, to be able to choose freely between family and a career or a combination of the two. Therefore, . . . public childcare facilities and other forms of childcare should increase. The German government will really do its best to secure a right to childcare in the Law on Children and Youth Support. (Verhandlungen 1990-1991, vol. 155, 12/5, p. 81)

When Kohl made this statement in the Bundestag, members of some political parties broke out laughing. However, a year later they all backed the new regulation. The Act on Children and Youth Support committed the German state to guarantee public childcare for all children in the 3-6 age group at nursery schools ("Kindergartens"), to take effect in 1996 (European Commission Childcare Network, 1996). Because not all the Länder [states] were able to implement the new law, in 1996 a transitional measure was to go into effect until 1999 (Ditch, 1996).

To a far greater extent than the Dutch and British debate, the political debate in Germany echoed the arguments of the European Parliament and European Childcare Network on childcare as a basic right for parents and children. With the historical presence of public childcare services in parts of the republic, arguments on the well-being of children were relatively important. This also explains the German position in the Council of Ministers, emphasizing the quality of services rather than the majority argument of economic efficiency (DAMESA, 1992).

The Children and Youth Support Act represented a major step in German childcare policy. Under a Christian-Democrat Cabinet, Germany created a basic right to childcare. Apart from Bavaria, all the Länder accepted this right. In 1993 there was also a gradual expansion of partly paid parental leave to 36 months. Combining work and family life gradually reached a higher position on the German political agenda.

The three strong male breadwinner states started important changes in their childcare policies in the early 1990s. In all three cases, welfare state restructuring and the influence of European equal opportunities policies helped make childcare a topic of public policy. In addition, specific political factors played a role. In Germany the reunification process put childcare on the political agenda. In the Netherlands the entrance of Social Democrats in the Cabinet pushed for change. In the United Kingdom the threat of a demographic time bomb put childcare on the political agenda. In the UK as well as the Netherlands, the expansion of childcare under the Conservatives and Christian Democrats (in the Netherlands in coalition with Social Democrats) was combined with more (the UK) or less (the Netherlands) market-driven provisions. In Germany, a Christian Democrat Cabinet introduced a basic right to childcare and generous paid parental leave. Here the rather atypical emphasis of Christian Democrats on public childcare was the result of a specific historical situation, the reunification of East and West Germany.

The changes in the European debate on childcare were reflected in the shifts in national policy logics. In all three countries, arguments concerning the well-being of children and a traditional gender ideology dominated social policy in the 1970s and 1980s. It was not until the end of the 1980s that arguments concerning equal opportunities and combining work and family life emerged. In the Netherlands and the UK, they were combined with references to economic efficiency. Childcare facilities could facilitate the female labor market participation that was needed to compensate for the ageing population, as was noted by advisory boards. In Germany concerns for children's well-being remained relatively important, combined with references to equal opportunities (a legacy from East Germany and EU policy). So, in the 1990s, in all three countries political debates showed a shift from a male breadwinner policy logic towards a policy logic of shared responsibility for caregiving. It would take a decade longer before the policy became effective.

DISCUSSION

The 1992 EU Childcare Recommendation represents a shift in the European policy debate on childcare. The Council of Ministers replaced arguments concerning the well-being of children, introduced by the European Parliament and the European Childcare Network, with arguments concerning economic efficiency and equal opportunities in the labor market. This shift was also expressed in the policy debates at the national level. In the United Kingdom, the Netherlands and Germany there was growing pressure to expand public childcare from social and political actors (political parties, especially left-wing ones, trade unions, employers and women's groups) and from intellectuals (advisory boards or networks of experts). However, the forces for change were very different in the individual states. In the UK, strong Labour opposition and the demographic need for women's labor market participation, an effective argument for employers, were important factors stimulating public and private childcare. In the Netherlands, the Social Democrats in the Cabinet in 1989 pushed for change, supported by arguments on economic efficiency. German reunification confronted the country with two different systems of childcare, stimulating the government to formulate a new starting point for childcare and youth policy. Here references to children's well-being were used to replace the extensive collective childcare services of the former East German regime by a more voluntary right to public childcare.

So in the three member states, there were pushes for change from below. There was also pressure from above, from the European level. In the EU, there was a strong feminist call for equal opportunities at the European Parliament and European Commission. In the 1970s and 1980s, equal treatment policies had a legitimizing function in the project of European integration. With the transition to a common European

Market in 1992, political pressure to develop European social policy increased. The formulation of common policy aims on childcare at EU level reconciled common economic interests (demographic changes and the need for shaping an internal market), the need for equal opportunities for men and women and space for variety. The policy logic advocating shared responsibility of employers and trade unions, governments and families for childcare linked perfectly to the logic of European economic integration.

Our analysis reveals interesting similarities between the debates in states with former male breadwinner logics and the EU. There is a clear interdependence between the policy logics on childcare at the national and the European levels. It is difficult to say which direction the influence goes. The member states still seem to dominate the development of European social policy. The opposition of one member state, the UK, changed plans for a Childcare Directive into a less perilous Recommendation. But, notwithstanding the absence of legal force, after the Recommendation public involvement in childcare in three countries with formerly strong male breadwinner policy logics grew. The most striking growth was visible in the UK. By 2000, in the United Kingdom, 34% of children in the 0-3 age group were in formal childcare. In the same period in Germany and the Netherlands formal childcare provision increased to 10% and 6%[2] (OECD, 2001, p. 144). The focus on economic integration did not prevent European social policy from covering the issue of caregiving, as had been predicted (Ostner and Lewis, 1995). On the contrary, the need for women's labor market participation came to be the main justification for European involvement in childcare. Common pressure from social and political actors in the member states and feminist actors at European institutions forced a break in the dominant conception of European social policy (see Bleijenbergh, 2004).

European involvement in childcare was to be further expanded a decade later when European member states formulated clear target figures for the expansion of childcare in Barcelona in 2002. By 2012, 33% of all children in the age group 0-3 should be in formal childcare (European Commission, 2002)

Our results are in keeping with the explanation of earlier unexpected developments in European social policy based on common efforts of actors inside and outside EU institutions (Hoskyns, 1996; Vleuten, 2002). The acknowledgement of the common responsibility of political actors, social partners and non-governmental actors is also in line with Falkner's argument that the process of European integration came to exhibit a more corporatist pattern in the 1990s (Falkner, 1998). The 1992 Childcare Recommendation anticipated a new phase in European social policymaking. The Maastricht Treaty, signed several months later, confirmed a greater involvement of social partners and national political actors in the development of European social policy. Although emphasizing shared responsibility with member states, social partners, non-governmental organizations and parents, the Childcare Recommendation first shows EU responsibility for childcare provision. And although stimulating men's role in childcare is only defended for instrumental reasons, the Recommendation also exhibits a historically new involvement in the sexual re-division of tasks in the private sphere.

NOTES

1. The then twelve member states of the EU were Belgium, Denmark, France, Germany, Greece, Ireland, Italy, Luxembourg, the Netherlands, Portugal, Spain and the United Kingdom. Since then the EU has widened to 25 countries.
2. The Dutch figure refers to 1998 instead of 2000.

REFERENCES

Bleijenbergh, I. (2004). *Citizens who care–European social citizenship in EU debates on childcare and part-time work*. Amsterdam, The Netherlands: Dutch University Press.
Bussemaker, J. (1997). *Recent changes in European welfare state services: A comparison of childcare politics in the UK, Sweden, Germany and the Netherlands*. Minda de Gunzburg Center for European Studies. Working Paper Series. Cambridge, MA: Harvard University.
Bussemaker, J. (1998). Rationales of care in contemporary welfare states: The case of childcare in the Netherlands. *Social Politics, 18*, 71-96.
Bussemaker, J., & van Kersbergen, K. (1994). Gender and welfare states: Some theoretical reflections. In D. Sainsbury (Ed.), *Gendering welfare state* (pp. 8-25). London: Sage.
Commission of the European Communities (1981). *A new community action programme on the promotion of equal opportunities for women 1982-1985*. Brussels, Belgium, 9 December (COM (81) 758).
Commission of the European Communities (1985). *Equal opportunities for women–Medium term community programme 1986-1990*. Brussels, Belgium, 19 December (COM (85) 801).
Commission of the European Communities (1991). *Proposal for a recommendation on childcare*. Brussels, Belgium, 28 August (COM (19) 233).
Debates of the European Parliament (1986). *Resolution on childcare infrastructures*. No. C 88/21-24, 14 April.

Debates of the European Parliament (1991). *Debate on childcare.* No. 3-411/362-367, 22 November.

Ditch, J. (1996). *European Observatory on National Family Policies, Developments in national family policies in 1994.* York, UK: University of York Social Policy Research Unit.

Dwyer, P. (1998). Conditional citizens? Welfare rights and responsibilities in the late 1990s. *Critical Social Policy, 18,* 493-518.

Ergas, Y. (1990). Childcare policies in comparative perspective. In OECD, *Lone parent families.* Paris, France: OECD.

Esping-Andersen, G. (1990). *Three worlds of welfare capitalism.* Cambridge, UK: Policy Press.

European Commission (2002). *Impact evaluation of the EES–Equal opportunities for women and men–background paper,* EMCO/29/060602/EN_REV.

European Commission Childcare Network (1990). *Childcare in the European Community 1985-1990.* Brussels, Belgium: Commission of the European Communities.

European Commission Childcare Network (1996). *A review of services for young children in the European Union, 1990-1995.* Brussels, Belgium: Commission of the European Communities.

Falkner, G. (1998). *EU Social policy in the 1990s: Towards a corporatist policy community.* New York, NY: Routledge.

Gauthier, A. H. (1996). *The state and the family. A comparative analysis of family policies in industrialized countries.* Oxford, UK: Clarendon Press.

Hansard Parliamentary Proceedings, House of Commons, various years.

Hoskyns, C. (1996). *Integrating gender: Women, law and politics in the European Union.* London, UK: Verso.

Land, H. & Lewis, J. (1998). Gender, care and the changing role of the state in the UK. In J. Lewis (Ed.), *Gender, social care and welfare state restructuring in Europe* (pp. 51-84). Aldershot, UK: Ashgate.

Lewis, J., & Hobson, B. (1997). Introduction. In J. Lewis (Ed.), *Lone mothers in European welfare regimes: Shifting policy logics* (pp. 1-20). London and Philadelphia: Jessica Kingsley Publishers.

Lewis, J. (1992). *Women and social policies in Europe.* Aldershot, UK: Edward Elgar.

Lewis, J. (1997). *Lone others in European welfare regimes: Shifting policy logics.* London and Philadelphia: Jessica Kingsley Publishers.

Lovenduski, J. & V. Randall (1993). *Contemporary feminist politics. Women and power in Britain.* Oxford, UK: Oxford University Press.

Moss, P. (1988). *Childcare and equality of opportunity.* Consolidated report to the European Commission, Brussels, Belgium: European Commission Childcare Network.

Moss, P. (1991). Day care for young children in the United Kingdom. In E. Melhuis and P. Moss (Eds.), *Day care for young children* (pp. 121-141). London, UK: Tavistock / Routledge.

O'Connor, J., Orloff, A.S., & Shaver, S. (1999). *State, markets, families. Gender, liberalism and social policy in Australia, Canada, Great Britain and the United States.* Cambridge, UK: Cambridge University Press.

Official Journal of the European Communities (1986). *Resolution on childcare infrastructures.* No. C 88/21-24, 24 April.

Official Journal of the European Communities (1991). *Proposal for a council recommendation on childcare by the European Parliament approved with the following amendments.* No. C326/274-279, 16 December.

Official Journal of the European Communities (1992a). *Council recommendation of 31 March 1992 on childcare.* No. L123/16-18, 8 May.

Official Journal of the European Communities (1992b). *Opinion of the Economic and Social Committee on the proposal for a Council recommendation on childcare.* No. C40/88- 91, 17 February.

Orloff, A.S. (1993). Gender and the social rights of citizenship –The comparative analysis of gender relations and the welfare state. *American Sociological Review 58,* 303-328.

OECD (2001). *OECD employment outlook,* Paris, France: Organisation for Economic Co- operation and Development.

Ostner, I. & Lewis, J. (1995). Gender and the evolution of European social policies. In S. Leibfried & P. Pierson (Eds.), *European social policy. Between fragmentation and integration* (pp. 159-193). Washington DC: The Brookings Institution Press.

Phillips, A. & Moss, P. (1989). *Who cares for Europe's children? The short report of the European Childcare Network.* Luxembourg: Office for Official Publications of the European Communities.

Plantenga, J. (1997). European constants and national particularities–The position of women in the EU labour market. In A. Dijkstra & J. Plantenga (Eds.), *Gender and economics–A European perspective* (pp. 86-103). New York, NY: Routledge.

Rutherford, F. (1989). The proposal for a European directive on parental leave: Some reasons why it failed. *Policy and Politics 17,* 301-310.

Sainsbury, D. (Ed.), (1999). *Gender and welfare state regimes.* Oxford: Oxford University Press.

Sassoon, A. Showstack (1996). Beyond pessimism of the intellect: Agendas for social justice and change. In M. Perriman (Ed.), *The Blair agenda.* London, UK: Laurence & Wishart.

Siim, B. (2000). *Gender and citizenship: Politics and agency in France, Britain and Denmark.* Cambridge: Cambridge University Press.

Verhandlungen des Bundesrates (Records of proceeding of the German Parliament). 1990-1991.

Vleuten, A. van der (2002). Dure vrouwen, dwarse staten: de Europese sandwich en de nationale boomerang [Expensive women, perverse states: The European sandwich and the national boomerang]. *Nemesis 4,* 89-96.

WRR [Wetenschappelijke Raad voor Regeringsbeleid: Scientific Council for Government Policy] (1990). *Een werkend perspectief. Arbeidsparticipatie in de jaren negentig [A Working perspective: Labour market participation in the 1990s].* The Hague, The Netherlands: SDU uitgevers.

Family Well-Being Between Work, Care and Welfare Politics: The Case of Norway

Kjersti Melberg

SUMMARY. This article examines how policy-relevant aspects such as gender equality, work load and relationship qualities affect family well-being. The analysis aims at identifying the constellation of factors that can explain family life satisfaction using data drawn from the International Social Survey Programme (ISSP). Despite the fact that Norwegian welfare policies have a strong emphasis on supporting gender equality and mothers' employment, the study finds a gendered pattern in parents' work and family lives. Family well-being is shown to be influenced by family internal factors, such as time pressure, the quality of close relations, and level of conflict. This in turn provides input for national policy-making. *[Article copies available for a fee from The Haworth Document Delivery Service: 1-800-HAWORTH. E-mail address: <docdelivery@*

Kjersti Melberg is affiliated with Rogaland Research, Stravanger, Norway.
Address correspondence to: Kjersti Melberg, Senior Research Scientist, Rogaland Research, P.O. Box 8046, 4068 Stavanger, Norway (E-mail: kjersti.melberg@rf.no).

This work is part of the research project "Life quality in the family," funded by the Norwegian Research Counsel, the program for Welfare Research. Thanks to Professor Knud Knudsen and two anonymous reviewers for their useful comments, and to Gunnar Thesen for technical assistance.

[Haworth co-indexing entry note]: "Family Well-Being Between Work, Care and Welfare Politics: The Case of Norway." Melberg, Kjersti. Co-published simultaneously in *Marriage & Family Review* (The Haworth Press, Inc.) Vol. 39, No. 3/4, 2006, pp. 337-358; and: *Families and Social Policy: National and International Perspectives* (ed: Linda Haas, and Steven K. Wisensale) The Haworth Press, Inc., 2006, pp. 337-358. Single or multiple copies of this article are available for a fee from The Haworth Document Delivery Service [1-800-HAWORTH, 9:00 a.m. - 5:00 p.m. (EST). E-mail address: docdelivery@haworthpress.com].

KEYWORDS. Family, gender relations, Norway, welfare policy, well-being, work-life balance

INTRODUCTION:
THE IMPORTANCE OF FAMILY WELL-BEING

The focus of this article is on the well-being of Norwegian family households with dependent children, with its purpose being to identify policy-relevant dimensions of close relations. The research question is: How is satisfaction with family life influenced by aspects such as gender equality, integration of work and family responsibilities and parenting? Family life satisfaction is understood as a person's overall cognitive appraisal of his/her family life situation (Lewinsohn, Redner & Seeley, 1991; Næss, 2001), here also labelled family well-being.

The concept of subjective well-being is multidimensional, captures elements of both cognition and affect, and is situationally and historically bound to the role expectations which shape self-evaluation (Bryant & Veroff, 1982). This study is based on the understanding that family members affect each others' well-being through a network of personal resources, personal characteristics and social interaction. The aim is to gain a better understanding of the way the well-being of families is influenced by goals promoted by allegedly family-friendly policies.

Understanding the quality of married and family life has long been a concern of family sociology (Mancini, 1979), and the importance of family situation in promoting happiness has been demonstrated in a large number of studies (Andrews & Withey, 1976; Campbell, 1981; Campbell, Converse & Rodgers, 1976; Hellevik, 2003). Research typically has focused upon the marital dyad (Hayes & Bean, 1982; Knudsen, 2001; Knudsen 2005; Knudsen & Melberg, 1999; Spitze & Waite, 1981); the more general area of family life satisfaction in Norway has been left underresearched (Blom & Listhaug, 1988). One aim of this work is to contribute to the empirical literature on the topic of contemporary family life as well as to the broader sociological literature on well-being.

Currently, the state of the family is being debated as never before as the past four decades have yanked the rug out from under patterns of family, work and sexuality. Also in Norway, contemporary family living arrangements are diverse with the future of the family being questioned (Knudsen & Wærness, 2001). The objective of this study is to grasp the connection between political targets and outcomes in people's everyday life. The purpose is to identify domains which explain different aspects of husbands' and wives' well-being and to investigate how contemporary family life determines exposure to dissatisfaction. The main substantive point of this work concerns the central question of whether the family life of people in Norway is influenced by aspects related to the political process or by interpersonal circumstances.

FAMILIES AND FAMILY POLICIES:
THE NORWEGIAN SETTING

With a gender equality-friendly policy model on one side, and transitional gender practices and apparently persistent, traditional social values on the other (Ellingsæter, 1998), Norway is an interesting and ambiguous case. First, the Norwegian family picture is increasingly diverse and complex. The nuclear family of the 1950s and 1960s was reshaped relatively late, but rapidly by high rates of nonmarital childbearing, sharp increases in the divorce rate, postponed marriage and childbearing, and dual-earner marriages. In response to changing sexual attitudes and behavior, national family and gender politics are in a process of continuous reform. The Nordic welfare states have a long tradition of extensive social policies directed at the family, such as providing services and social transfers. Moreover, a hybrid family policy model that covers both general family support and dual earner support is employed (Korpi, 2000), combining cash transfers to families with dual earner support (Ellingsæter, 2003).[1]

More specifically, family policy in Norway is extensive. All employees have a right to parental leave, an extensive cash-for-care reform was implemented in 1998, family allowance and child benefits are universal, the parliament keeps passing public child care guarantees, and institutionalization of parental maintenance is promoted. All these political incentives have formed different societal contexts for the modernization of gender relations (Ellingsæter, 1998; St.meld, 2002-2003). From an international point of view, gender equalization has come far in Norway; women are above the international average in their representation in parliament and other political organizations, committees and boards.

A May 15, 2005 report presented by the World Economic Forum put Norway (behind Sweden) in second place in gender equalization when it comes to the gap between women and men in politics, society, working life and education. Female employment is close to reaching the level of male employment. However, a majority of women work part-time, many in typically women-dominated occupations. Among those with children 1 or 2 years old, 70% of the mothers are wage earners (see <http://www.ssb.no> for these statistics).

The concept of part-time work generally refers to a contract of employment on 1-36 working hours per week (Kjeldstad & Nymoen, 2004). An exception is when the employee works 32-36 hours in an occupation where this is regarded as full-time employment. Thus a traditional male breadwinner norm still seems to influence the choices of families. The "junior partner" family, where the father is the main provider while the mother works part-time and is in charge of care, is often practiced.

These changes are partly due to a welfare system that promotes a more equal division of work between mothers and fathers at home and in the labor market (Knudsen & Wærness, 2001). A family model where both spouses work and share household tasks equally is the implicit ideal in public and political debate on the family. Public policy integrates normative arguments in favor of equal opportunities for women. A main line of argument in political rhetoric is that transformation of the gender division of labor has realized the dual-earner, gender-equalized family form. Indirectly, this is assumed to increase family well-being. Families in which both spouses are employed and share family responsibility on an equal basis are indirectly thought of as well-functioning families. This study explores this assumption.

LITERATURE REVIEW

Understanding the quality of married and family life has long been a concern of sociological analysis and political discourse. One reason for this is the recognition that the family is still an important institution of socialization and welfare. Moreover, the importance of family situation for happiness has been demonstrated in a large number of studies (Diener, Suh, Lucas & Smith, 1999). It is consistently indicated that satisfaction with family life, relationships with children and spouse are substantial contributors to the overall feeling of well-being (Andrews & Withey, 1976; Campbell et al., 1976; Hellevik, 2003). The family, its internal arrangements, strategies and well-being appear to be a crucial factor to be taken into account, and how well families deal with the dual needs of income and care is essential to policy formation.

In Norway, extensive maternal employment has led to a greater focus on the importance of unpaid work in the household and on various ways of combining family life and employment among parents (Kitterød, 2002). Changes in family practice are often seen as the result of public policies transforming the gender division of labour, indicating the existence of a policy model of integrating mothers into the labor force (Ellingsæter, 1998), and encouraging fathers to be actively involved in caring and domestic tasks. Equal opportunities for women and men are promoted in policy as an ideal for which to strive (St.meld. 17, 2002-2003). But in real life, gender inequality is said to be persistently practiced in Swedish families (Björnberg, 2004), while Norway is described as the more gender traditional case in Scandinavia (Ellingsæter, 2003). This study assumes that political rhetoric has influenced public opinion, i.e., *both men and women promote values of gender equalization* (H_1), but that *this has not led to equal status between the genders in the practical division of unpaid work in Norwegian families* (H_2).

There are a variety of reasons to expect gender differences in the way men and women experience relationships, and the concept of stress presents one opportunity to observe how deeply family well-being is affected by the structured arrangements of people's lives and by the repeated experiences that stem from these arrangements (Pearlin, 1989). First, occupations affect exposure to stress by the way they organize the timing and placement of demanding tasks (Elder, George, and Shanahan, 1996). The demands that seem to be most ubiquitously shared among occupations are work load (the amount of work to be done in a given amount of time), role conflict (the incompatibility of various work and family roles), and issues pertaining to pay, salary, and economic viability. In the analyses, I expect to find negative relationships between family well-being and work load in paid and unpaid work and the experience of time pressure and role conflict.

Mancini (1979) found husbands and wives are similar in regard to primary indicators of satisfaction with family life, which for both is positively related to satisfaction with friendship, marriage, and leisure. In addition, spousal employment status influences family life satisfaction. A Finnish study concluded that health effects of worktime control were particularly evident among women with families (Ala-Mursula, Vahtera, Pentti & Kivimäki, 2004). These demands may be of relevance to this study's understanding of gender differences in well-being.

Indeed, the debate between men and women over who works more hours, performs more domestic tasks, and gets paid more money is the frequent subject of research.[2] A Norwegian study demonstrated that while women clearly dislike long working days and having too little time off, a man's satisfaction is high regardless of how much time he and his wife spend on paid work (Dagbladet, <www.dagbladet.no> November, 18, 2002).

Because many social roles are differentially allocated by gender, men and women differ in their potential for exposure to role-bound stress. There is an increasing concern regarding how to balance work and family for both husbands and wives in all sectors of society. Many parents with small children face incompatibilities between their roles of mother/father and employee because the institutional and family support necessary to fulfill both roles often does not exist. In this way, work-family overload may be an important stress source. Because women still seem to be the most central part of family life and child care, the described structures call for more study. As a third hypothesis, I argue that the *quality of relationship with partner and children, and the conflicts spouses have in combining work and family responsibilities, will affect individual's satisfaction with family life–though in different ways for men and women* (H_3). Further, the inclusion of sex, age, education and income in the analyses is a way to look at variations in social background.

Gender differences are assumed to exist in the formation of family satisfaction, as it is likely men and women still hold divergent social roles and experience different kinds of work overload. Flexibility in the work organization and in the work schedule is often seen as an opportunity for both women and men to handle the conflicts between work, care and family obligations. However, patterns of work are highly gendered in the labor market, as is seen in a recent Swedish study that confirms the flexibility which is controlled by the employees is male-dominated (Grönlund, 2004). Nonetheless gender relations and roles should affect the experience of family satisfaction. Men and women hold different positions in family and society, and I expect to find that their family well-being is affected differently.

THE STUDY

Sample

The data are drawn from the "Attitudes towards Family and Gender-roles" (2002) module of the International Social Survey Programme

(ISSP), an international consortium of survey organizations that collect precisely comparable cross-national data on social attitudes and values (Davis & Jowell, 1989). The gross national sample included 2500 individuals, which with a response rate of 60.4% (due to adjusted sample size) gives a total sample of 1,475 individuals. The data quality is considered satisfactory with little missing data. Analyses performed here include a total of 519 persons, 252 men and 267 women, who are married or cohabiting and have dependent children between 2 and 16 years. The Norwegian Social Science Data Services (NSD) made the data available.[3]

Even though the topic of family life satisfaction could have been researched with other methods, for instance qualitative, in-depth interviews, this study makes use of survey data, the product being a quantitative description of the population. The main argument for this methodological approach is that it may provide background information on context and subjects, i.e., it allows the researcher to establish relationships among variables. Also, employing quantitative research may provide results that make it possible to generalize (in a statistical sense) to a larger population (Brannen, 1992). Such an analysis may in turn help with the choice of subjects for a qualitative investigation, i.e., it can be used to explain the factors underlying the broad relationships that are established.

Measures

The main dependent variable is *satisfaction with family life*. It was measured by individuals' responses to a question asking them to rate "how satisfied are you with your family life?" on a six-point scale from "completely dissatisfied" to "completely satisfied."

The independent variables in the analyses included gender attitudes, the division of work, relations with spouse/partner, relations with children, and conflicts with spouse/partner regarding work and family.

A scale measuring *gender attitudes* included five variables on gender equalization, measured on five-point scales (ranging from "strongly agree" (1) to "strongly disagree" (5) with "don't know" registered as a mid-category). Statements included, "Both the man and the woman should contribute to family income; A man's job is to earn money, a woman's job is to look after the home and family; Men should do more housework than they do today; and Men should take more responsibility in bringing up children." Factor analyses of the data clearly point toward a one-factor solution, and an additive index with good reliability (Cronbach's alpha = .66) was constructed on this basis.

Division of work was measured with four items. The first was the respondent's estimate of hours (*time*) *spent on domestic work* (for themselves and their partner). The second variable was the respondent's perception of the *fairness of the division of work*, obtained by asking "What alternative best describes the distribution of housework between you and your partner"– "I do a lot more housework than what is fair" to "I do a good deal less housework than what is fair" (on a four-point scale). The third variable was the respondent's report concerning *work time*, which refers to their estimate of paid hours worked by themselves and their partner in "an ordinary week." *Income distribution* measured whether respondent or his/her partner had the highest income, using six categories ranging from "I have a lot higher income" to "we have about the same income," to "I have no income."

Relations with spouse/partner was measured with two multi-item scales. *If you hadn't been married* was the first scale, made up of responses to six items (Cronbach's alpha = .75). Respondents were asked, "Although it seems unlikely, think about how your life would be if you had/hadn't been married or lived in a cohabitating relationship. Would it be much better, slightly better, just about the same, slightly worse or a lot worse regarding your (1) living standard, (2) social life, (3) sex life, (4) job and career, (5) life quality and (6) life as a parent." The second four-item scale, *quality of marriage/cohabitation,* was developed with responses to these questions, "To what degree do you feel that your spouse/partner (1) supports you and cares about you; (2) is willing to listen to your problems and worries; (3) makes too many demands on you; (4) is critical of you and what you do?" Replies varied between (0) in high degree to 3 = not at all. Factor analysis indicated a one-dimensional scale, which had good reliability (Cronbach's alpha = .76).

Relations with children includes three measures, *activities with children*, *negative behavior toward children* and *positive behavior toward children.* A four-item scale with good reliability (Cronbach's alpha = .74), was developed by asking parents, "How often do you do the following activities with your children? (1) leisure time activities outside the home; (2) play together at home; (3) talk privately together; (4) help with homework." Replies could vary between (0) almost every day to (4) almost never or seldom. *Negative behavior towards children* refers to combined frequency of spanking/smacking and shouting, and *positive behavior towards children* refers to combined frequency of praising children and allowing children to take part in setting limits. Frequency categories ranged from (0) often to (3) never.

Conflicts with spouse/partner regarding work and family was measured in three areas, the distribution of domestic tasks, experience of time pressure, and perception of the *family as obstacle* to work success. Disagreement about the distribution of domestic tasks was measured by asking "How often do you and your partner disagree about the distribution of domestic tasks?" Answers ranged from (0) several times a week (high conflict) to (4) never (low level conflict). Time pressure was measured by asking, "How often during the last three months have you (1) come home from work too tired to do daily tasks, (2) felt that it is hard to meet family obligations, (3) come to work too tired to function properly because of all the domestic work I've done, (4) had difficulties concentrating on work due to family obligations?" Replies formed a reliability index (Cronbach's alpha = .83). The *family as obstacle measure* asked "How much has your family responsibility stood in the way of your work opportunities?" with answers ranging from (0) a lot to (4) not at all.

Six *control variables* were included: (1) *age* is coded in years; (2) *marital status* is a dichotomous variable–married and cohabitant; (3) *education* was measured by the number of years beyond mandatory level, for respondent and partner; (4) *income* is treated as a categorical variable, ranging from zero in Norwegian kroner, measured for both the respondent and partner; (5) *household income* was calculated by dividing the amount of income of both partners divided by the number of household measures; (6) *number of dependent children* varies from one to nine.

In addition to looking at factors associated with family well-being, the study measured gender attitudes with these questions: "We have some statements about women. To what degree do you agree or disagree?" (Values ranged from 1 = strongly agree to 5 = strongly disagree): (a) "Both men and women should contribute to domestic economy"; (b) "Men should earn money, while women should take care of the home"; (c) "Men should take greater responsibility in domestic work"; (d) "Working mothers should have paid maternity leave;" (e) "To have a job is the best way for a woman to be independent"; and (f) "It is not good that a man is at home and takes care of children and the wife is working."

Perceptions of the division of household labor were measured with these questions: "Who does the following tasks in your household?" (Values ranged from 1 = always me, 2 = usually me, 3 = share between us/usually together, 4 = usually my spouse/cohabitant, 5 = always my husband/cohabitant, 6 = is being done by a third partner): (a) does the laundry; (b) does minor repairs; (c) cares for ill family members; (d) does the grocery shopping; (e) cooks; (f) pays bills; (g) keeps an overview over the family economy; (h) makes decisions regarding upbringing of children.

Analysis Techniques

Descriptive statistics and appropriate correlations and regressions were computed using SPSS, version 13. I begin by examining the bivariate differences in gender attitudes (Table 1) and practices (Table 2), and satisfaction (Table 3), running t tests to examine differences in women's and men's responses (testing hypothesis 1 and 2). Correlations referred to in Table 4 are Pearson's r. The third hypothesis is tested through ordinary least squares (OLS) regression analysis. In multiple regression, the sum of squared differences between observed and predicted scores is minimized, and the relative influence of each predictor variable on the outcome variable (family life satisfaction) is estimated (data presented in Table 5).

Results

Gendered attitudes and practices. Table 1 displays men's and women's attitudes on gender equalization. Most respondents of both genders agree or strongly agree that "both men and women should con-

TABLE 1. Indicators of Attitudes on Gender Equalization. Mean, Standard Deviation and t-test for Difference of Means. N = 337. (From 1 = "Strongly Agree," to 6 = "Strongly Disagree")

	Men Mean (std.dev.)	Women Mean (std.dev.)	t
"Both men and women should contribute to domestic economy."	2.30 (1.01)	2.42 (1.13)	−1.07
"Men should earn money, while women should take care of the home."	4.09 (0.97)	4.33 (0.86)	−2.42*
"Men should take greater responsibility in domestic work."	2.66 (1.16)	2.22 (0.81)	4.02**
"Working mothers should have paid maternity leave."	1.79 (0.95)	1.36 (0.74)	4.73**
"To have a job is the best way for a woman to be independent."	3.14 (1.49)	3.03 (1.28)	0.75
"It is not good that a man is at home and takes care of children and the wife is working."	3.72 (0.94)	4.07 (0.84)	−3.60**

Two-tailed test of significance: * = significant at 0.02-level and ** = significant at 0.01-level.

TABLE 2. Sharing of Household Tasks. Percent That "Always" or "Usually" Perform Different Tasks. (Men N = 156, Women N = 181)

	Men			Women		
	Him	Her	Share	Her	Him	Share
Laundry	3.8	73.7	22.4	85.5	3.4	11.1
Minor repairs	89.7	1.9	7.7	7.2	72.7	26.7
Unpaid care	3.8	32.0	59.0	50.8	1.7	45.3
Shopping	10.9	41.0	48.1	58.3	6.7	33.0
Cleaning	1.3	62.8	34.0	75.6	4.5	20.0
Cooking	10.9	51.3	37.8	64.8	5.6	29.6
Pay bills	40.3	21.9	27.7	23.5	44.1	32.4
Family economy	39.7	19.2	41.0	24.6	33.6	41.9
Raise children	0	7.7	91.6	12.4	0	87.7

TABLE 3. Satisfaction with Family Life, Partner and Child Relationships. Mean, Standard Deviation and t-test for Difference of Means. (From 0 = "Completely Dissatisfied," to 6 = "Completely Satisfied")

	Sex	N	Mean	Std. Dev.	t
Satisfaction with family life	M	156	4.68	0.80	0.44
	F	181	4.64	0.81	
Satisfaction with partner	M	156	4.66	0.97	−0.52
	F	179	4.72	0.95	
Relationship with child(ren)	M	155	5.34	0.72	−2.52*
	F	176	5.54	0.71	

Two-tailed test of significance: * = significant at 0.02-level and ** = significant at 0.01-level.

tribute to domestic economy" and "to have a job is the best way for a woman to be independent." However, when it comes to sharing domestic tasks, there is a significant sex difference: Fewer women than men agree that "men should earn money, while women should takes care of the home" and "it is not good that a man is at home and takes care of children and the wife is working." Also, more women than men agree that working mothers should have paid maternity leave. In this way, the first hypothesis stating that both genders promote values of gender equalization is confirmed, but we see a tendency that women are more concerned with the question of gender equalization than men are.

Table 2 illustrates that these attitudes are evidently not transferred to the practical sharing of tasks. While a majority of women say that they always or usually do the laundry (86%), shopping (58%), cleaning

TABLE 4. Descriptive Statistics and Correlations for Variables in the Analysis. 1 = age, 2 = marital status, 3 = education (self), 4 = income, 5 = household income/members, 6 = work time, 7 = partner's education, 8 = work time (partner), 9 = number of children, 10 = activities with children, 11 = negative behavior, children, 12 = positive behavior, children, 13 = time, domestic work (self), 14 = time, domestic work, partner, 15 = division, domestic work, partner, 16 = disagreements, domestic work, 17 = time pressure, 18 = family as obstacle, 19 = gender attitudes, 20 = income distribution, 21 = if you hadn't been married, 22 = quality of partnership.

	M	SD	1	2	3	4	5	6	7	8	9	10	11	12	13	14	15	16	17	18	19	20	21
1	20	6.2																					
2	0.2	0.4	-.16**																				
3	3	1.9	.10	.00																			
4	0.2	0.4	-.11*	.02	-.04																		
5	145	137	.02	.00	.11	-.17**																	
6	37.5	12.6	.10	.12*	-.03	.02	.04																
7	3.3	1.6	.03	-.08	.45**	-.02	.20**	-.06															
8	33.6	10	-.08	.03	.06	.14*	.09	-.15**	.09														
9	1.4	0.7	.00	-.13*	-.02	.08	-.14*	.07	-.02	.00													
10	11.3	2.7	-.30**	.05	.04	.11	-.02	-.10	.08	.08	-.01												
11	0.6	0.6	-.05	.03	-.01	.06	-.09	.04	-.09	-.04	-.04	-.08											
12	1.2	0.8	.06	.04	-.11	.01	.03	.00	-.05	-.03	.11	-.28**	.08										
13	8.9	7.2	-.02	-.04	-.01	.29**	.13*	-.26**	.09	.37**	.18**	.12*	.01	-.05									
14	7.7	7.8	.13*	-.08	-.06	-.11*	-.03	.29**	-.03	-.22**	.05	-.09	.00	.01	-.08								
15	0.6	0.5	.05	.05	.06	-.04	-.01	.03	-.06	.05	-.04	-.15**	-.07	.05	.00	.03							
16	1.5	1.1	-.02	-.02	.12*	-.03	-.04	.01	.08	-.04	-.07	.05	-.02	-.05	-.01	.03	.31**						
17	7.6	2.9	-.12*	.01	-.10	.45**	.07	-.18**	-.07	.19**	.11	.24**	-.06	-.03	.27**	-.23**	-.16**	-.18**					
18	2.8	1.1	-.04	.04	-.08	-.08	.08	.10	-.05	-.17**	-.06	-.11	.02	-.01	-.25**	.12*	-.06	-.11	.02				
19	4.9	2.4	-.07	-.05	-.19**	.17**	.08	.09	-.11*	-.10	.13*	.00	.07	.14*	.04	.21**	-.20**	-.15*	.09	.25**			
20	3	1.6	-.20**	-.01	-.05	.27**	.10	-.43**	.10	.44**	.06	.17**	-.02	-.08	.43**	-.45**	-.07	-.04	.38**	-.17**	-.07		
21	10.4	3.1	-.04	-.10	.11	.01	.10	-.05	.06	.07	-.04	.07	-.01	.06	-.03	.03	.02	-.13*	.11	.13*	.01	.08	
22	4.7	1.6	-.01	.11	-.09	.16**	-.03	-.13*	-.13*	.07	-.04	-.06	.02	.03	.13*	-.14*	-.05	-.10	.19**	-.06	-.01	.23**	.02

Two-tailed test of significance: * = correlation significant at 0.05-level and ** = correlation significant at 0.01-level.

348

TABLE 5. Satisfaction with Family Life - Multiple Regression Results. Standardized and Unstandardized Coefficients. Married Men and Women with Children. (Men N = 156, Women N = 181)

Satisfaction with family life, multiple regression						
	Men			Women		
	B	beta	t-verdi	B	beta	t-verdi
Constant	4.60		5.41	3.81		4.32
Age	−.03**	−.24	−2.48	−.01	−.09	−0.90
Marital status	−.10	−.05	−0.55	.36*	.18	1.83
Education	−.07	−.17	−1.57	−.10**	−.22	−2.11
Partner's education	−.04	−.08	−0.74	.07	.15	1.38
Income	.19	.06	0.64	.19	.10	0.80
Household income/members	.00	.12	1.09	.00	−.03	−0.28
Number of children	.15	.11	1.08	.08	.06	0.61
Gender attitudes	.02	.06	0.64	−.01	−.02	−0.19
Time spent on dom. work, self	.01	.03	0.32	−.01	−.12	−1.04
Time spent on dom. work, partner	.00	−.04	−0.41	.01	.06	0.62
Division of domestic work	.16	.10	1.01	−.01	−.01	−0.06
Work time, self	.01	.10	1.00	−.01	−.10	−1.00
Work time, partner	−.01	−.10	−1.10	.00	.01	0.06
Income distribution	.03	.04	0.35	−.02	−.03	−0.25
If you hadn't been married…	.08***	.31	3.25	.09***	.33	3.63
Quality of marriage/coh.	−.07	−.12	−1.18	−.04	−.08	−0.85
Activities with children	−.01	−.04	−0.40	.07**	.24	2.33
Negative behavior	−.12	−.09	−0.96	.07	.05	0.48
Positive behavior	−.21**	−.21	−2.02	.11	.11	1.25
Disagreements, domestic work	−.10	−.13	−1.31	−.14**	−.20	−2.03
Time pressure	.09***	.27	2.67	−.02	−.06	−0.52
Family as obstacle	.00	.00	0.02	.04	.05	0.55
	R²	Adj. R²	F	R²	Adj. R²	F
Model summary	.38	.23	2.51	.39	.24	2.59

* = significant at 0.10-level; ** = significant at 0.05-level; *** = significant at 0.01-level.

(76%) and cooking (65%), men claim they have responsibility for minor repairs (90%) and paying bills (40%), and also that they take care of the family economy (40%). None of the men always or usually raise children, while this goes for 12% of women. Many of both sexes do, however, agree that both spouses share responsibilities such as caring for family members, grocery shopping and raising children. Although attitudes reflecting equal opportunities for women and men are widespread among Norwegian parents, they shape relatively traditional, gendered patterns in their everyday practices, as expected in the second hypothesis. As also stated by Knudsen and Wærness (2001), this study indicates that Norwegian women are more positive to gender equalization then men are.

As Taylor-Gooby (1991) points out; in promoting equal opportunities and gender equality, the division of both paid and unpaid work becomes crucial. Despite the fact that most men and seven of ten women in this survey are employed, many of the employed mothers are working part-time while their spouse works full-time (not shown). When asked who earns most in the couple, eight of ten women say their partners earn more than they do. This confirms the view that there has been a slow integration of Norwegian women into the labor market (Skrede, 1984).

Family life satisfaction. Both the subjective assessments of work-family factors and objective characteristics of employment and family life may foster strain. Survey results in Table 3 demonstrate that most married and cohabiting people are generally happy with their family life, their spouse and their relationship with minor children. Men and women on average rate their satisfaction with partner and family life highly.[4] A total of 65% say they are "completely" or "very satisfied" with their family life and their spouse. There is, however, a difference in how men and women evaluate their relationship with their children; mothers are significantly more satisfied with this relation than fathers are. This may be due to particularly close relations and frequent contact between mothers and their offspring, or it may reflect a social expectation of such a connection.

Two findings of this study are that the quality of close relations influences family life satisfaction, and that work-family overload is a primary stress source which diminishes well-being. Table 4 presents the means and standard deviations for the variables in the analysis.

Table 5 illustrates how the main dependent variable, family well-being, is being affected by factors such as work load at home and work, attitudes and the quality of close relationships. Analyses are performed separately for women and men to test the claim that men's and women's family satisfaction is formed in different ways (H_3).

For men, family well-being is related to age; as husbands and fathers get older, their satisfaction with family life increases. Possibly this is linked to the fact that for many, as children get older, the work load diminishes and domestic economy improves, which in turn may increase men's satisfaction with family life. This confirms one of the established social patterns of emotional well-being and distress. Well-being is relatively low and depression is relatively high during periods when family income is low (Mirowsky & Ross, 1989). Men's family satisfaction is in this analysis, however, not significantly related to factors such as education, income, working hours, domestic work time or number of children. The latter finding is supported in earlier works; although being valued and loved, the presence of children in the home is not correlated with psychological well-being of mothers and fathers (Blom & Listhaug, 1988).

According to the expectations of this study, positive relations with the children has a positive effect on fathers' well-being. Also, the feeling of time pressure has an effect on how they experience family life; if fathers spend too much time at work or come home from work too tired to fulfill family responsibilities, or if they are tired and have difficulties concentrating on work tasks due to family and home commitments, their family satisfaction is likely to decrease. Finally, if men imagine that their lives would be better if they did not have a partner, their family well-being is likely to be fairly low. The quality of relations with spouses/partners is also of some importance to fathers' family satisfaction; if their spouses/partners support and listen to them, don't make too many demands and avoid criticism, this has a positive effect on men's family well-being.

For women, the pattern is slightly different, confirming the third hypothesis of this study. First and somewhat surprisingly, the analysis indicates that cohabiting mothers are more satisfied with their family life than married women are. Such a difference in family satisfaction between married and cohabiting mothers is unexpected, mainly because cohabitation and marriage in Norway is understood as similar modes of living. This also stands somewhat in contrast to other recent studies, which find that both married and cohabiting women report better mental health than unmarried (Lau, Moum, Sørensen & Tambs, 2002). Further, working mothers' family satisfaction increases with education; the higher their education level, the higher is the satisfaction. A common finding is that the higher a person's socioeconomic status (education, job, and income), the lower that person's level of distress. Higher education is regarded as a central resource in handling stressors mainly through crucial individual characteristics, including instrumentalism (the belief that you control your own life) and flexibility (the ability to imagine complex solutions to a problem) (Mirowsky & Ross, 1989). In the case of Norwegian women, such characteristics seem of importance in handling stressful everyday situations. Although the number of children does not influence family satisfaction, mothers' well-being increases when they engage in activities with their children. Negative or positive behavior towards them, however, is not associated with level of family satisfaction. As to the effect of work load and partners' conflicts on well-being, there is a correlation (though not significant) between the feeling of domestic work overload and well-being, and a significant correlation between disagreements over domestic work and women's family well-being. Variables measuring the level of time pressure have a negative, but weak impact on women's satisfaction with family life. If they feel life is stressful, either at work or at home, or if obligations in one arena hinder their efforts in the other arena, the women's family well-being is likely to decrease. As for men, the experience that they are satisfied with married/cohabiting life economically, sexually, and socially, increases family well-being. Attitudes toward gender do not influence family well-being for either men or women, which differs from earlier studies which conclude that traditional family values have a positive effect on family well-being (Blom & Listhaug, 1988).

A finding which also goes for both men and women is that although only a few variables have a significant influence on family well-being, the explained variances are relatively high. Earlier research demonstrates that satisfaction with family life is strongly linked to satisfaction with other domains of life, such as life in general and satisfaction with spouse and children (Campbell et al., 1976; Melberg, 2004; Næss, 2001). When a person's family satisfaction is so clearly bound up with the fundamental experience of well-being, other factors, although they obviously have an effect on people's everyday life, will have a relationship to the subjective evaluation of family life that is statistically weak. If this is taken into account, the level of adjusted R^2 is as could be expected. While the data are cross-sectional, meaning it is not feasible to conclude which are causal relationships, the theoretical basis of this study does support the chosen direction of causation.

CONCLUDING REFLECTIONS

This article has examined how policy-relevant aspects such as gender equality, work load and relationship qualities affect family well-being. The aim has been to explore if Norwegian parents' experience of family life is influenced by current family policy or if satisfaction relates principally to the private sphere. As the family is at the center of many policy issues, family policy has been an expanding field in Norway. Indirectly, the main aim of family and welfare policy is to steer a course and adjust for demographic and societal developments, thereby creating a safety net for family members in general and for children in particular.

Taken together, this study suggests that there is a gap between political objectives on the one side and individuals' attitudes on gender and family policy and the organization of family lives on the other. In Norway, which promotes a family policy that supports the two-earner family and legally defends women's rights in the labor market, the mainstream political idea is that parents with dependent children should share domestic tasks and have equal work opportunities (St.meld., 2002-2003). Hochschild (1989) found that men share domestic work equally with their wives in only 20% of American dual-income families. In Norway, one would expect a close to equal division of work between the sexes.

Corresponding attitudes are in this study only partly reflected in public opinion on parents' employment and family responsibility. Mean values for indicators of attitudes on gender equality show that more women than men are positive toward working mothers, dual-income families and an equal division of work between mothers and fathers. The results provide some other insights into contemporary sex roles. Findings indicate that men's and women's labor market participation and domestic work efforts are more traditional than expected. Partly, this confirms earlier findings. Norway has one of the most gender-segregated labor markets (Ellingsæter & Leira, 2004; Frønes, 1996), and traditional norms are perceived to dominate among Norwegian parents (Ellingsæter, 1998; Knudsen & Wærness, 2001).

One relevant observation is that much of the systematic growth in female employment is part-time, making it possible–and even necessary–for a group of men to prioritize work, regardless of the values and norms they express. The argument is that women's part-time employment preserves gender roles in Norwegian families. This distinction between policy intent and policy outcome is said to be essential in understanding the mixed Norwegian family policy model (Ellingsæter, 2003). It highlights the complexity of the Norwegian case. The country has been characterized as having a policy regime distinguished by separate gender roles (in which men claim benefits as earners and women as carers), which does not capture the duality and complexity in contemporary family life.

However, this study confirms that the domain of family life is extremely diverse and encompassing in the lives of many people. It is probably impossible for any one theory to adequately outline the content domain of family life. Although this work illustrates the challenges in explaining the subjective dimension of family well-being, it does provide some insight into how mothers and fathers experience their family lives. Higher age (for men), better education (for women), a positive relation with child and partner, low level of time pressure and a certainty that life is good in married/cohabiting life are all connected with family well-being. Therefore, this study gives some input to the family policy area. For policymakers, providing families with time control can save considerable costs through lower health risks. Possibly the major subject of concern is that of child care. Readily available, affordable, childcare, which is a policy area of major interest in Norway, may ease the strain on employed mothers and fathers.

Politics may matter, but first and foremost the study indicates that close relations within the family are still a powerful source of tending, supporting, and well-being. It is essential for who we are and how we live (Taylor, 2002). As Beck and Beck-Gernsheim (1995) say it, love is our secular religion. A good marriage or cohabiting relationship provides the sense of being cared for, loved, esteemed, and valued as a person. Love for children is understood as an eternal and natural bond: Because most parents love their children, see them as one of the great joys and blessings of life, and spend much time with them, many people believe that children increase parents' sense of well-being. These aspects are, however, not easy to examine with a quantitative approach.

We can say that the human ability to tend, nurture and care for other persons will remain internal to the family system, but that politics and institutions stay crucial in understanding the structuring of relations in society. "Politics matter," but the ways in which welfare state policies interact with other structural and cultural mechanism in generational change are complex (Ellingsæter, 1998, p. 71) and not easily captured in survey data; politics and their outcomes are embedded in complicated processes. Much like marriage satisfaction, family life quality requires considerable additional research. At least two methodological approaches may be worth further research. First, the relationship between policy and well-being can be fruitfully examined doing a comparative analysis using cross-country data. Secondly, in-depth discussions with respondents would contribute to our understanding of this topic. Research and theory provide a strong justification for further exploration of the familial and extra-familial exchange processes contributing to adult well-being.

The worlds of home and work have undergone momentous changes over the last thirty years, with trends suggesting the variety of work-family arrangements will increase (Hochschild, 1997, 1989). Work time is in transition in Western societies, with the major trends being toward work hours becoming differentiated, individualized, and made more flexible. The policy areas of family, gender and work should be seen in connection; the lack of readily available child care and still limited practice of shared responsibility for children put stress on families–not employment per se (Mirowsky & Ross, 1989). There is also reason to expect the complexity of Norwegian family policy to increase; minority and/or coalition governments have dominated political life, and the instability of politics is likely to continue in the future. It is a challenge to policymakers in Norway, as in most European countries, to know how to adjust welfare policy to a situation of even greater diversity of family practices and commitments to the labor market.

NOTES

1. General family support includes cash allowance to minor children, family tax benefits to minor children and to an economically non-active spouse, and public day care services for children from 3 years up to school age. Dual-earner support includes public day care services for children 0-2 years of age, paid maternity and paternity leave, and public home health to the elderly (Korpi, 2000, pp. 145-146).

2. Because women in Michigan face gender and wage discrimination that exceeds the national average, they are unlikely to escape poverty without an education, according to a University of Michigan study (see website www.umich.edu).

3. Neither NSD nor Statistics Norway are responsible for the data analyses or the interpretations presented here. The use of data is the author's responsibility.

4. Around 50% of all parents engage in leisure-time activities with their children, as close to 70% play with them at home, 75% talk intimately with them, and close to 80% help their children with reading and/or homework ("almost every day" or "several times a week").

REFERENCES

Ala-Mursula, L., Vahtera, J., Pentti, J., & Kivimäki, M. (2004). Effect of employee worktime control on health: A prospective cohort study. *Occupational Environmental Medicine, 61*, 254-264.

Andrews, F.M., & Withey, S.B. (1976). *Social indicators of well-being.* New York, NY: Plenum Press.

Beck, U. & Beck-Gernsheim, E. (1995). *The normal chaos of love.* Cambridge, UK: Polity Press.

Björnberg, U. (2004). Making agreements and managing conflicts: Swedish dual-earner couples in theory and practice. *Current Sociology, 52*, 33-52.

Blom, S., & Listhaug, O. (1988). Familie og livskvalitet [Family and quality of life]. *Tidsskrift for samfunnsforskning, 29*, 5-28.

Brannen, J. (Ed). (1992). *Mixing methods: Qualitative and quantitative research.* Aldershot, UK: Avebury.

Bryant, F. B., & Veroff, J. (1982). The structure of psychological well-being: A sociohistorical analysis. *Journal of Personality and Social Psychology, 43*, 653-673.

Campbell, A. (1981). *The sense of well-being in America.* New York, NY: McGraw-Hill.

Campbell, A., Converse, P., & Rodgers, W.L. (1976). *The quality of American life.* New York, NY: Russell Sage Foundation.

Davis, J.A. & Jowell, R. (1989). Measuring national differences. An introduction to the International Social Survey programme (ISSP). In R. Jowell, S. Witherspoon & L. Brook (Eds.), *British social attitudes: Special international report*, pp. 1-13. Aldershot, UK: Gover.

Diener, E., Suh, E., Lucas, R.E., & Smith, H.L. (1999). Subjective well-being: Three decades of progress. *Psychological Bulletin, 125*, 276-302.

Elder, G.H., George, L.K., & Shanahan, M.J. (1996). Psychosocial stress over the life course. In H.B. Kaplan (Ed.), *Psychosocial stress: Perspectives on structure, theory, life course and methods* (pp. 247-292). Orlando, FL: Academic Press.

Ellingsæter, A.L. (1998). Dual breadwinner societies: Provider models in the Scandinavian welfare states. *Acta Sociologica, 41*, 59-73.

Ellingsæter, A.L. (2003). The complexity of family policy reform. *European Societies, 5*, 419-443.

Ellingsæter, A.L., & Leira, A. (2004). *Velferdsstaten og familien: Utfordringer og dilemmaer* [The welfare state and the family: Change and dilemmas]. Oslo, Norway: Gyldendal.

Frønes, I. (1996). Revolusjon uten opprør: Kjønn, generasjon og sosial endring i Norge på 80-tallet [Gender, generation & social change in Norway in the 1980s]. *Tidsskrift for samfunnsforskning, 1*, 71-85.

Grönlund, A. (2004). *Flexibitetens gränser* [The limits of flexibility]. Umeå, Sweden: Borea *Förlag.*

Hayes, B.C., & Bean, S. (1982). The impact of spousal characteristics on political attitudes in Australia. *Public Opinion Quarterly, 56*, 524-529.

Hellevik, O. (2003). Economy, values and happiness in Norway. *Journal of Happiness Studies, 4*, 243-283.

Hochschild, A. (1997). *The time bind: When work becomes home and home becomes work.* New York, NY: Henry Holt.

Hochschild, A. (1989). *The second shift.* New York, NY: Avon Books.

Kitterød, R.H. (2002). Mothers' housework and childcare: Growing similarities or stable inequalities? *Acta Sociologica, 45*, 127-149.

Kjeldstad, R. & Nymoen, E.H. (2004). *Kvinner og menn i deltidsarbeid: Fordeling og forklaringer* [Women and men in part-time work: Distribution and explanations]. *Report 2004/29.* Oslo, Norway: Statistics Norway.

Knudsen, K. (2001). Samspill i paret: Tilfredshet med livet for ektefeller på norske gårdsbruk [Interaction in the dyad: Life satisfaction for spouses on Norwegian farms]. *Sociologisk forskning, 38*, 67-90.

Knudsen, K. (2005). Sosiologisk grep på dyaden: Par-analyse med structural equation modeling (SEM) [Sociological understanding of the dyad: Couple-analysis with structural equation modeling (SEM)]. *Sosiologisk tidsskrift, 13*, 133-156.

Knudsen, K., & Melberg, K. (1999). Livet i par: Subjektiv livskvalitet for henne og han på gården [Subjective quality of life for spouses on Norwegian farms]. *Sosiologisk tidsskrift, 7*, 91-111.

Knudsen, K., & Wærness, K. (2001). National context, individual characteristics and attitudes on mothers' employment: A comparative analysis of Great Britain, Sweden and Norway. *Acta Sociologica, 44*, 67-79.

Korpi, W. (2000). Faces of inequality: Gender, class and patterns of inequalities in different types of welfare states. *Social Politics, 7*, 343-371.

Lau, B., Moum, T., Sørensen, T., & Tambs, K. (2002). Sivilstand og mental helse [Marital status and mental health]. *Norsk Epidemiologi, 12*, 281-290.

Lewinsohn, P., Redner, J., & Seeley, J. (1991). The relationship between life satisfaction and psychosocial variables: New perspectives. In F. Strack, M. Argyle & N. Schwarz, (Eds.), *Subjective well-being—An interdisciplinary perspective* (pp. 141-169). International Series in Experimental Social Psychology, Vol. 21, Oxford, UK: Pergamon Press.

Mancini, J.A. (1979). Social indicators of family life satisfaction: A comparison of husbands and wives. *International Journal of Sociology of the Family, 9*, 221-231.

Melberg, K. (2004). Jeg er tilfreds med levekårene mine, men har jeg det faktisk godt [The level of living standards and the quality of life]? *Tidsskrift for velferdsforskning, 7*, 131-149.

Mirowsky, J., & Ross, C.E. (1989). *Social causes of psychological distress.* New York, NY: Aldine de Gruyter.

Næss, S. (2001). *Livskvalitet som psykisk velvære* [Life quality as psychological well-being]. Rapport 3/01. Oslo, Norway: NOVA.

Pearlin, L.I. (1989). The sociological study of stress. *Journal of Health and Social Behavior, 30*, 241-256.

Skrede, K. (1984). Familieøkonomi og forsørgerlønn [Domestic economy and provider salary]. *Tidsskrift for samfunnsforskning, 25*, 359-388.

Spitze, G., & Waite, L.J. (1981). Wives employment: The role of husbands' perceived attitudes. *Journal of Marriage and the Family, 43*, 177-224.

St.meld. 29 (2002-2003). Om familien. Forpliktende samliv og foreldreskap [About the family. Obligatory cohabitation and parenthood]. White paper, Norwegian Ministry of children and family affairs.

Taylor, S.E. (2002). *The tending instinct: How nurturing is essential for who we are and how we live.* New York, NY: Times Books/Henry Holt.

Taylor-Gooby, P. (1991). Welfare states regimes and social citizenship. *Journal of European Social Policy, 1,* 93-105.

The Evolution of Family Policy in Spain

Gerardo Meil

SUMMARY. The aim of this article is to trace the evolution of Spanish family policy from its beginning in the 1930s to the present, showing the shifting role played by the State in defining and supporting family formation and functioning. Different periods are considered according to the objectives and characteristics of this policy as well as according to the support it received from the political forces ruling in each period. For each period, objectives, mechanisms, output and outcome are analyzed. The evolution over the whole period has been, on one hand, away from support of the patriarchal family to the recognition of family pluralism, and, on the other, evolution from a government provided family salary to a policy intended to combat poverty. *[Article copies available for a fee from The Haworth Document Delivery Service: 1-800-HAWORTH. E-mail address: <docdelivery@haworthpress.com> Website: <http://www.HaworthPress. com> © 2006 by The Haworth Press, Inc. All rights reserved.]*

KEYWORDS. Family allowances, family policy, reconciliation of family and working life, Spain

Gerardo Meil is affiliated with the Department of Sociology, Universidad Autónoma de Madrid.

Address correspondence to: Gerardo Meil, Departamento de Sociología, Facultad de CC. Económicas y Empresariales, Universidad Autónoma de Madrid, c/ Francisco Tomás y Valiente, 5 28049 Madrid, España (E-mail: gerardo.meil@uam.es).

[Haworth co-indexing entry note]: "The Evolution of Family Policy in Spain." Meil, Gerardo. Co-published simultaneously in *Marriage & Family Review* (The Haworth Press, Inc.) Vol. 39, No. 3/4, 2006, pp. 359-380; and: *Families and Social Policy: National and International Perspectives* (ed: Linda Haas, and Steven K. Wisensale) The Haworth Press, Inc., 2006, pp. 359-380. Single or multiple copies of this article are available for a fee from The Haworth Document Delivery Service [1-800-HAWORTH, 9:00 a.m. - 5:00 p.m. (EST). E-mail address: docdelivery@haworthpress.com].

There is no common definition of family policy, although a host of researchers have approached the topic. In fact, some researchers doubt whether it can be defined at all, given the heterogeneity in time and space of the measures labeled as such (Pitrou, 1994). Problems in defining family policy may stem from the policy point of view itself, but also from the meaning of family. From the policy point of view, one of the difficulties is that in Spain there is no institutional public body responsible for this type of policy: it is rather a task cutting across many State agencies as well as many other public policies. One alternative to the institutional definition is to examine the motives behind public intervention. Family policy could be then understood as everything done by State agencies for the well-being of families (Dumon, 1987; Kamerman & Kahn, 1978). The problem with this approach is that most public policies affect families directly or indirectly. Economic policy could be considered an important part of family policy, as is education policy and so on. With the plurality of forms that families now take, and the shifting policy objectives concerning intervention in family life, the very concept of family has also gained ambiguity. Over time, family policy has abandoned its goal to provide legal and social protection for the institutional family form, and has begun to concentrate on supporting family functions (Wingen, 1997).

In this article, family policy will be understood as a package of public policy measures, or instruments, articulated to varying degrees, that aim to define family ties and to protect and/or replace the social functions performed through family life. Family policy then implies a set of policy objectives, as well as certain values in relation to family life, serving to legitimate public intervention. Depending on how articulated values, objectives, and measures are, family policy will be defined more or less clearly. Following Kamerman and Kahn (1978), we will use explicit and implicit family policy concepts to refer to different degrees of articulation of such measures or instruments.

It has become common to view family policy in terms of three main dimensions (Kamerman & Kahn, 1978; Kaufmann, Herlth & Strohmaier, 1982; Wingen, 1997; Zimmerman, 1988). The first dimension concerns the legal definition of the establishment and dissolution of family ties as well as of the rights and obligations of the different actors as role incumbents, mainly endorsed in family law, but also in other areas like labor law. The second dimension concerns economic intervention, meaning income transfers aimed at compensating to some extent the costs deriving from certain family obligations, typically child rearing. The third dimension concerns intervention through services with the aim of improving families' social milieu, by supplying resources or enhancing competencies that facilitate or make it possible for families to function. Because space is limited, this article focuses mainly on the first two dimensions.

THE CHURCH, THE STATE AND THE FAMILY IN THE 1930s

Family policy, in the sense of an articulated set of measures for redistributing income in favor of families, was born in Spain with the establishment of General Franco's dictatorship (1939-1975). One of the basic ideological foundations of this dictatorship was the "recognition, exaltation, and protection of the family as society's original cell," "the basis of society . . . endowed with inalienable rights" (Girón de Velasco, 1951, p. 8, 15). A wide range of instruments were developed for this purpose. These instruments, accompanied by a radical reform in family law, marked the social policy of the new State with a profound family orientation. In fact, Franco's dictatorship presented itself as the solution to the (Christian) "family crisis" postulated by right-wing ideological positions. This crisis of "the family" was also considered, according to conservative social theory (Cicchelli-Pugeault & Cicchelli, 1998), to be at the very root of the social crisis that brought about the civil war (1936-1939).

The causes of the family crisis were attributed, first, to the reform in family legislation that was undertaken after the downfall of the monarchy and the establishment of the Second Republic (1931). In effect, as a result of the new Republican Constitution, which introduced a clear separation between Church and State, family law as a whole was completely removed from ecclesiastical legislation. At the same time, profound legislative reform was undertaken, establishing obligatory civil marriage, the possibility of divorce by mutual consent, the equality of spouses, the equality of children born within wedlock and those born outside of wedlock, as well as the regulation of legal abortion (Alberdi, 1978; Campo, 1995; Iglesias de Ussel, 1998). With these changes, republican family legislation was, in many aspects (such as divorce by mutual consent or the regulation of abortion), more than three decades ahead of the reforms in family law in many western European countries.

The price of this advancement, though, was that it outdistanced social reality at that moment (Alberdi, 1978). The immense majority of the population did not actually live according to these principles and this cost the Republic a radical confrontation with the Catholic Church and with the political parties and social groups under its influence (Iglesias de Ussel, 1998). In fact, the Church considered these reforms, as well as others meant to limit its enormous political and social influence, as a direct attack, and it responded with verbal virulence, social mobilization, and explicit support from the majority sector for the forces that rose up against the Second Republic and unchained the civil war (1936-1939).

Although the crisis of the family was blamed on the Second Republic's family legislation, the deepest roots of the (Christian) "family crisis" were actually attributed to liberalism, in its economic, social, and political aspects. This criticism came from within the general framework of the Catholic Church's social doctrine. The most evident manifestations of this crisis were, it was affirmed, the drop in the birthrate on one hand (which became systematic at the start of the 20th century as a result of the beginning of the demographic transition), and increases in mothers' paid work, on the other. From this perspective, married women's paid work undermined the family's functionality, forcing the mother to abandon the care of her home, of her children, and of her spouse, and so renouncing her educational and socializing functions (Aznar, 1932; Jordana de Pozas, 1938).

Within the context of the Catholic Church's traditional criticism of liberalism, the deepest cause of the working family's "crisis," and the reasons for women taking outside jobs, was to be found, above all, in the commodification of work, that is to say, in salaries being set uniquely and exclusively according to the supply and demand dynamics of the labor market, foregoing any consideration of the worker's family situation. This argument essentially states that, given the fluctuations in the labor market and the low level of salaries imposed by market dynamics, the conversion of work into a commodity eroded the family institution's stability by not providing sufficient material resources and by forcing women into paid work, thus causing a lower birthrate. The solution advocated by certain Catholic sectors, supported by different encyclicals and by the evolution of Social Security policies in France, Belgium, and Italy, was the controversial idea of the "family salary." In Spain, this idea was defended by Social Catholics, and taken up also by the Falange, one of the principal political groups Franco used to support his fight for power. The Social Catholics conceived the idea of the "family salary" as being achieved through the establishment of social insurance for family responsibilities (Aznar, 1947), financed by workers and employers. The Falangists, however, considered that it would best be achieved by bonuses financed from compensation funds established by the companies (Arrese, 1940), as had been done during the 1920s in some industrial sectors in Germany, France and in Belgium.

The principal social forces that supported Franco's dictatorship also defended the need for an ideological crusade and a legal reform of family law in favor of the traditional family, as well as an active family policy that would actually make the idea of the family salary real. These same groups were the ones that, once the dictatorship was established (1939), would occupy the key positions to undertake the implementation of these ideas; the Social Catholics controlled the management organ of Social Security (the so-called National Institute of Prevision–Instituto Nacional de Previsión) and the Falangists controlled the Ministry of Work, in charge of regulating the labor market.

The international reference for family policy's emergence in Spain was, accordingly, the developments then taking place in Europe, particularly in France, Belgium, and Italy. Its conceptual reference framework was the so-called "social question," that is, preoccupation with workers' living conditions and their consequences for the established order as interpreted by the social Catholic doctrine and the Falange. The implantation of a large-scale family policy after the civil war was not, then, a simple diffusion of international developments in the area of social insurance. It was, rather, "an act of ideological affirmation," as the preamble to Family Subsidies law stated, because classic social insurances (sickness, retirement, and injuries) had hardly been developed at all when the first family policy instruments were established (Cruz Roche, 1984). The main initial motivation for family policy was compensatory and was destined more to avoid poverty derived from the existence of family obligations than to promote fertility (Meil, 1995). It was argued that a higher birthrate was a consequence of families' higher standards of living, but not its source of legitimacy (Aznar, 1947). The demographic motivation afterwards eclipsed the initial compensatory motivation, at times acquiring greater rhetorical dominance and even creating different benefits specifically destined to reward higher birthrates.

FAMILY POLICY AS INCOME POLICY, 1940-1959

The end of the civil war and the establishment of General Franco's dictatorship (1939-1975) meant the annulment of all republican family legislation and the restoration of ecclesiastic law's primacy in these matters, with the new State expressly declaring itself Catholic (Iglesias de Ussel, 1998). Equality between legitimate and illegitimate children was annulled, and contraceptives, as well as adultery and non-matrimonial cohabitation, were penalized (Alberdi, 1995). Obstacles were put in the way of women who wished to work (especially married women). Co-education was prohibited, large families were encouraged, and religious marriage was made obligatory for people who were baptized. The Church was made competent to judge separations and matrimonial annulments, and inequality of rights according to sex was reinstituted. While the majority of these counter-reforms were justified by Catholic doctrine concerning the family, naturalist-type arguments were also cited to legitimate the reestablishment of the patriarchy. Following this line, the Law of April 24, 1958 affirms that (the family) "requires a directing power that Nature, Religion, and History attribute to the husband." Parallel to these legislative reforms, an active family policy and a propaganda campaign in favor of the traditional family and, in particular, the large family, were promoted.

The first instrument that embodied this active family policy was the social insurance called Family Subsidies (1938). These subsidies gave family allowances for dependent children (up to 14 years of age) from the second child on, varying according to rank, and, starting in 1941, included short-term widow's pensions and orphan's pensions for families without resources. Financing this social insurance fell mainly to the employers; farmers and self-employed were excluded from coverage. During the decade of the 1940s, these benefits, destined to make the "family salary" a reality, within the framework of an explicit pro-natalist and pro-marriage policy, were enacted with other complementary measures addressed to newlyweds and large families (Campo, 1974). Along this line, the 1943 Large Family law established a 10% additional supplement in family subsidies for families with 4 to 7 children and a 20% supplement for families with more than 7 children. In addition, high tax reductions benefited large families with higher incomes, with more reductions the higher the income. It is true, though, that the Spanish Ministry of Finance's capacity to collect income taxes was very limited until the 1980s; this resulted in widespread tax evasion. This law also conceded to large families preferential treatment in the areas of education, transportation, housing, and employment. Together with this law, 1941 saw the introduction of prizes for the families with the greatest number of children. This measure had a purely propagandistic component because, apart from benefiting very few families and being a one-time prize, these prizes were often given by General Franco himself and were widely publicized by the media. These prizes continued until democracy was re-established in 1976. To promote marriage, given the enormous difficulties of forming an independent family after the war (housing and food were very scarce), marriage loans were also introduced. These were awarded to couples with low incomes and could be repaid by having children. There were also one-time subsidies for each child born.

This whole set of instruments was inspired by the evolution of family policy in France, Belgium, and Italy (Hoffnes, 1940; Meil, 1995). Except for the prizes for large families, the rest of these benefits existed, with more or less intensity, in these countries. Nevertheless, we must point out one difference: family allowances came into being in Spain directly as social insurance, not as an integral part of collective bargaining between employers and unions, as happened in these other countries. This was basically because the dictatorship did not allow collective bargaining. The family subsidy was, however, always conceptually linked to paid work, which together constituted the "family salary." The object to be protected was, as in the other countries, the traditional family, promoting women's remaining at home to care for the children and relatives who lived with and were dependent upon the person insured.

Given the absence of a re-evaluation of these benefits according to the loss of buying power and the high inflation registered in Spain during the post-war years, these benefits soon lost their compensatory capacity. In the political context of the moment, union organizations defending workers' interests were prohibited and severely punished and the government set salaries by ministerial orders with almost no adjustment for inflation, which led to the erosion of salaries. To deal with this, the Labor Ministry established a second income-transfer instrument called the family bonus (Plus familiar) (Rull Savater, 1974a). The "family bonus" consisted of the distribution of a family fund among each company's workers, according to amount of family obligations (wife and number of dependent children). This family fund came from the resources generated by applying a certain percentage to the volume of real wages paid in each company and was financed almost wholly by the employers. The percentage to be applied to the salaries varied from one productive sector to another, as well as through time. In the 1940s, the percentages varied between 5% and 20% (Toharia, 1943, p. 813), with 15% being the most frequent figure, while from 1954 on the most frequent figure was 25% (Blanco, 1964, p. 340). Family obligations were translated into points through a legally established scale (which gave greater value to more children). The value of a point was then obtained by dividing the total volume of the fund by the number of points accumulated by the company's staff. Each worker received a bonus for family obligations (called the "Plus") according to the number of points he could accredit and the value of each point at that moment; this last was dependent upon the percentage applied as well as the family obligations of the company's total workforce.

The introduction of this bonus was justified in terms of reinforcing the family salary, as interpreted by the Falangists, in spite of the fact that the establishment of the family subsidy, as we have seen, already embodied the idea of the family salary. The implementation of the bonus was really, however, a cheap method, consistent with the regime's ideological position, for selectively raising salaries that were otherwise subject to an iron-handed control, being legally regulated through work regulations, in a context of rapid price growth. The family salary constituted, therefore, a mechanism destined to facilitate a rapid accumulation of capital, keeping individuals' salaries down and compensating the loss of buying power by partially socializing salaries. Family policy during this stage can be depicted as a large-scale policy to fight, or rather to limit, poverty, with strong regressive components (Meil, 1995).

These family allowances represented about two thirds of the income redistributed by Social Security during the 1940s. During the 1950s, this proportion decreased as the other types of social insurance matured, reaching little more than 50% at the beginning of the 1960s. In terms of gross domestic product (GDP), and including the estimates on the volume of resources redistributed by the Family Bonus, family allowances represented between 3% and 2.5% of the GDP. This proportion doubled the amount allocated to public health and situated Spain, in the 1950s, among the countries that redistributed the most income according to family criteria (Bikkal, 1954; Rull Savater, 1974a).

The impact on families' disposable income was quite varied, due as much to the heterogeneity of the instruments applied as to the fact that this protection was basically directed only to salaried workers. This left out self-employed workers and a great many farmers, in a country with a large farming population (50% of the labor force was working in the agriculture at the beginning of the 1950s). The degree of coverage was, consequently, limited; in 1950, only 49% under the age of 14 were beneficiaries of the subsidies for dependent children. Among the salaried workers with family obligations, the importance of family allowances for the family's disposable income depended, in turn, on whether or not the worker had the right to receive the Family Bonus; the principal groups excluded from this bonus were salaried agricultural workers and public employees. In the 1950s, among those who did not receive the Family Bonus, the benefits for a family with three children were only 8% of per capita income and only became a significant amount (between 90% and 130% depending on the year) for a very large family (10 or more children). Among those who did receive the Family Bonus, a worker with average earnings, a wife, and three dependent children, received an increase in his income equivalent to 50% to 70% of his base salary (which was, during those years, at about the level of per capita income) (Alonso Olea, 1953, 1954,1956).

THE RATIONALIZATION OF FAMILY POLICY, 1963-1975

Economic stagnation and economic and tax crises, along with the social discontent generated by the restrictive social and economic policy practiced by the dictatorship, all brought about the questioning of the model of economic growth established after the war. This questioning was settled by re-balancing the power within the groups that supported the dictatorship and by an in-depth reform of the State's intervention in the economy (Ros Hombravella, Clavera, Esteban, Monés & Montserrat, 1973). As far as family policy goes, its reform took place in the context of an in-depth reform of the Social Security system. The objective of this general reform was to integrate the heterogeneous set of social insurances established during the 1940s and 1950s. Many of these insurances duplicated one another and gave very different degrees of protection according to the influence of the different power groups, and the purpose was to form a coherent universalistic system with no duplications and no preferred clientele (Cruz Roche, 1984). Spain's model of economic growth continued, nevertheless, to be based upon a policy of low salary costs and low levels of social protection that would attract labor-intensive foreign investments.

Within this framework, this period's reorientation of family policy constitutes a rationalization of family social protection by making it compatible with the functional principles and requisites of a market economy. To understand this reorientation, we must look at it in the wider framework of the institutional reforms carried out to dismantle the bases on which the unsuccessful model of economic and social development had been founded and to establish the necessary foundations for developing capitalism in Spain.

This reform essentially involved the suppression of the Family Bonus Regime, because of its distorting effects on the relation between work rendered and remuneration received. It also involved the reform of family subsidies, raising and standardizing the allowances for dependent children and eliminating subsidies for the insured person's economically dependent cohabiting relatives. With this reform, family allowances were aimed only at the conjugal (nuclear) family (wife and dependent children), leaving the other members of the kinship network outside of coverage. At the same time, retirement pensions were increased with wider coverage, with the introduction of entitlement to pensions for widows, orphans, and for economically dependent relatives (del Peso, 1967). The model of the conjugal family that was protected continued to be the traditional family, with the woman's place being at home caring for the members of her family.

The family policy instruments that were implemented and in effect until 1991 were periodic allowances for dependent spouses and children. The allowances for dependent children were equal for all beneficiaries, regardless of the company in which the insured person worked (200 pesetas monthly, 11% of the 1963 minimum wage, raised to 250 in 1971, 6% of the minimum wage), although the effect of the law protecting large families was to give these families higher allowances. But this aid did not benefit all insured individuals. Since it was still conceived more implicitly than explicitly to be a family salary, only salaried workers were acknowledged, leaving self-employed workers in all sectors unprotected (Rull Savater, 1974b). There was no real universal protection for dependent children, in accordance with the principle of "equal protection for equal family responsibility" that the law sought to introduce. The allowance for a dependent spouse (wife or incapacitated husband) was reformed according to the same criteria, presenting, therefore, similar coverage problems. The amount of this allowance was set at 300 pesetas per month (17% of the 1963 minimum wage), that is to say, 50% more than the allowance per dependent child. This quantity was raised to 375 pesetas in 1971 (9% of the minimum wage). As this benefit was collected whether the couple had children or not, in reality the family social protection system prioritized women's remaining at home. The allowances for marriage and for children's births were also adapted to the new system, standardizing them and establishing the amounts of 5,000 and 2,500 pesetas (2.8 and 1.4 times the 1963 monthly minimum wage) respectively (6,000 and 3,000 pesetas from 1971 onwards, representing 1.5 and 0.75 times the monthly minimum wage). On the other hand, the prizes for large families were not affected by the reform and continued to be held yearly until the transition to democracy (Meil & Iglesias de Ussel, 2001).

The reform of family policy reduced the volume of social resources designed to compensate for family obligations, despite the greater coverage attained by the new system and the substantial improvement it meant for the people who had not benefited from the Family Bonus system. This relative loss of importance was due partly to the expansion of the other branches of Social Security, particularly of health benefits and retirement benefits in a strongly inflationary context. One exception occurred in 1971, when these benefits were brought up to date with inflation, but the effect was quickly neutralized by the acceleration of the inflationary process. On the other hand, the spectacular economic growth during this period situated Spain among the group of developed industrial societies during the 1970s. Social Security's economic benefits for family support decreased from values close to 3% of the GDP at the beginning of the 1960s to around 1% halfway through the 1970s, while the value fluctuated around 2.5% in Belgium and around 2.7% in France during the same period, showing no similar trend (Meil & Iglesias de Ussel, 2001).

As a consequence of the increase in disposable income derived from the spectacular economic growth during the 1960s, and the absence of re-evaluations for inflation, family benefits kept losing importance in family economies. Consequently, in the mid-1950s a family with three children could obtain family supplements representing two-thirds of the per capita income or average wage, while one decade later these supplements were less than one-third of the per capita income. By the 1970s they were less than 10% of the average wage. In comparison with other European Union countries, Spain was one of the countries that redistributed a greater volume of income according to family criteria in the decade of the 1950s and most of the 1960s. By the mid-1970s, however, Spain was among the countries that earmarked a rather scanty amount of income for public compensation for family obligations, in spite of the fact that this public compensation continued to hold a prominent place in political rhetoric. (See Table 1.)

POLITICAL DEMOCRATIZATION AND THE TRANSFORMATION OF FAMILY POLICY, 1976-1995

Modernization of Family Law

In 1975, General Franco's death paved the way for a modern democracy, which brought about profound changes at all levels of social and

TABLE 1. Social Security Expenditure in the Function of Family in Some European States as a Percentage of GDP, 1955-1974

	AU	BE	DK	FR	GE	IR	IT	NL	NO	SW	UK	SP
1955	1.4	1.8	0.6	3.4	0.2	1.1	2.2	1.4	0.5	1.1	0.6	2.7*
1960	1.4	2.1	0.4	3.0	0.3	1.2	2.1	1.5	0.6	1.4	n.d.	2.8
1965	2.0	2.5	1.0	2.9	0.4	1.1	1.8	2.0	0.5	1.2	0.5	2.6
1970	1.9	2.8	1.1	n.d.	0.6	1.0	1.4	2.0	1.5	0.9	0.8	1.6
1974	1.6	2.6	1.2	2.7	0.4	1.3	1.7	1.9	1.0	1.2	0.5	1.2

n.d.: non disposable; *1958
Key: AU = Austria, BE = Belgium, DK = Denmark, FR = France, GE = Germany, IR = Ireland, IT = Italy, NL = The Netherlands, NO = Norway, SW = Sweden, UK = United Kingdom, SP = Spain.
Source: Own calculations based on Banco de Bilbao (1979), Banco de España (1979), and Flora (1983).

political life, including family policy and other aspects highly relevant for family formation. The first big change in family policy took place with the establishment of a new democratic Constitutional Law in 1978, which established the lay character of the State. This meant that civil marriage was no longer considered to have less status than religious (Catholic) marriage, and that citizens could choose the form of their marriage according to their religious beliefs.

The Constitution also shaped a new marriage model based on the equality of the spouses' rights and obligations and the spouses' full autonomy, subject, nevertheless, to the family's common interests. Thus woman's traditional legal subordination to man was eliminated. In addition, the Constitution radically changed the relationship between parents and children, first by making children born in wedlock and children born out of wedlock equivalent and proclaiming their equality of rights with respect to their parents, and, second, by establishing that paternal authority corresponded to both progenitors together (Alberdi, 1995; Campo, 1995; Picontó-Novales, 1997).

The 1981 Civil Code reform (laws 11/81 and 30/81), besides reforming family law according to constitutional precepts, once again regulated divorce. Given the social controversy that the reintroduction of divorce caused in its day, and attending to pressure from anti-divorce groups headed by the Catholic Church (Iglesias de Ussel, 1998), a two-step divorce procedure was enacted. Legal separation was the first step to divorce; couples or individuals who wanted to divorce had to go through two legal processes, with corresponding emotional and economics costs. As a consequence many couples separated without following through on the divorce.

Other legal changes included eliminating penalties for non-matrimonial sexual relations, and lifting the prohibition on selling birth control devices. Unlike the situation in the 1930s, all these changes occurred without raising important conflicts or tensions in society (Iglesias de Ussel, 1994).

The Evaporation of Economic Protection for the Family

Although the 1978 Constitution established the government's obligation to protect the family, the buying power of these benefits "evaporated." These benefits were not re-evaluated to keep up with inflation in a strongly inflationary context, nor was there any eagerness to modify the instruments inherited from the previous period to adapt them to the new family reality that was emerging. One exception to this was the prizes for large families, which the first democratic government abolished. Other social problems like the very low amount of public pensions and the rapidly increasing levels of unemployment, together with rapidly growing social expenditures and growing fiscal deficit, came to the forefront of the political arena.

The lack of adaptation of the earlier family policy instruments to the new family reality was regularly criticized during the successive Social Security reform attempts that followed one another during the democratic transition. This criticism centered especially on allowances for dependent wives, marriage, and births, which were considered inadequate to the new family reality. In spite of this criticism, however, the political incapacity to go ahead with reform of Social Security, given the weakness of the first democratic governments, prevented approval for new allocations. This situation was not resolved until the Socialist party (PSOE) achieved an absolute majority in Parliament in 1982, when the 1985 Social Security Reform Law (Law 26/1985) was approved. During the period 1975-1985, the matter of updating family benefits was raised in Parliament on many occasions, but these proposals were systematically denied or simply ignored by the government, without generating controversy (Meil & Iglesias de Ussel, 2001). Thus, the essence of family policy dissipated with inflation. This absence of a political will to protect the family economically can also be seen in the income tax treatment of the family.

The combined effect of Social Security benefits and tax deductions for family reasons are hardly noticeable in families' disposable income. Thus, during the whole decade of the 1980s and the greater part of the 1990s, the difference in disposable income after taxes and family transfers of an average-income wage-earner with a wife and two dependent children, compared to a wage-earner with equal income but no family obligations, was only between 5% and 6% of the gross salary. So a single worker with no children and with an average income had the use of 82.7% of his gross salary in 1991, while a worker with a wife and two dependent children and an equal salary had the use of 87.8%. These percentages varied very little during the period under consideration. Compared to other central and northern European Union countries, the tax treatment of earned income in Spain was characterized by a relatively low tax burden for workers with no family obligations as well as for those with family obligations; public compensation of family obligations was, therefore, very low (Meil, 1994).

The Transformation of the Economic Protection of the Family into Means-Tested Benefits

Parallel to this "evaporation" of the family's economic protection, a concept of social solidarity developed that put special emphasis on guaranteeing an existential minimum to under-protected groups. In these cases, the family situation became an important criterion for defining access to a greater degree of protection. This consideration of family situation as a qualifier for access to aid benefits was introduced first in unemployment benefits (1980), later in retirement benefits (1983), in mean-tested social salaries established in the Regions (starting in the second half of the 1980s), and finally in the area of family allowances (1985 and 1990). The objective of increases in pension was to guarantee a vital minimum for married pensioners, as well as to make economic independence with respect to their children's generation possible. This is, then, an implicit family policy of promoting residential independence for the different generations, in accordance with prevailing family values.

After 1990 benefits for dependent children became recognized for all families with a yearly income under a yearly established threshold (one million pesetas, or 56% of the average wage in 1991, plus a 15% for every child after the first), independently of whether or not they are in the Social Security system; when handicapped persons are involved, there is no upper income limit. The families with dependent children receive an allowance when their children are under 18 years of age or if they are older children with disabilities. The greater the disability, the larger the allowance. The amount of the allowance for children under 18 was set at 36,000 pesetas yearly (5% of the minimum wage or 2% of the average wage); this quantity doubles if there is a 33% or higher handicap. These allowances were not adapted on a yearly basis to the rhythm of inflation until the year 2000. This exemplifies once more the reluctance towards increasing family protection.

The Emergence of the Reconciliation of Family and Working Life

Following the deep political and social changes after democracy, and in the context of the growing influence of European Union developments as well as the institutionalization of feminism (Valiente, 1996), both an equal opportunity policy and a non-discrimination policy regarding gender emerged. Within the framework of these developments, a new sensibility emerged regarding the social costs of maternity, and new instruments additional to maternity leave were introduced. This later evolved into a policy of promoting work-life balance. This type of policy is understood to be the articulation of several instruments aimed at facilitating time for child rearing while maintaining one's labor market involvement.

The first measures that go beyond maternity leave date from 1980 when legal regulation of the job market was undertaken in order to adapt it to constitutional imperatives (López, 1996). This reform consisted of several measures. The first was an extension of maternity leave (from 12 to 14 weeks, with a substitution salary equivalent to sick leave, that is, 75% of the salary). Another measure was the establishment of the possibility of reducing the workday because of maternity from one-half to one-third with no economic compensation. Other measures included the reduction of the workday by one hour for nursing, and the introduction of a one year parental leave for maternity reasons, with no economic compensation and without holding the job open. Except for maternity leave, men as well as women could opt for these measures. The women, however, were the ones who, given traditional family role definitions, probably ended up benefiting most from these possibilities. However, they also had to take on the costs that using these benefits implied (reduced income, risk of losing the job, and lower social benefits, among others).

Since 1980, the leave legislation has been modified on three occasions, in 1989, 1995, and 1999, mostly as a consequence of recommendations or directives from the European Union. Coverage was extended in 1989, by including leave for adopted or foster children, by extending maternity leave to 16 weeks and lengthening parental leave up to three years. In 1999, coverage was extended by establishing the possibility of requesting one year leaves to care for relatives who, due to age or illness, cannot care for themselves and do not carry out any paid economic activity. Fathers were also given the possibility of taking up to four weeks of maternity leave.

Job guarantees after leave were strengthened in 1989, when the right to have one's job reserved during the first year of leave was established, and since 1995, when the reservation was extended to 3 years. In 1999, dismissal because of maternity was prohibited. Partial reduction of the costs derived from using leaves, for the worker as well as for the employer, occurred first in 1995, when maternity insurance was shaped as an aspect of Social Security, with a right to a substitution salary of 100%, instead of the previous 75%, with more flexible qualifying conditions (180 days of Social Security contributions in the previous 5 years). The costs of leaves for workers were also reduced by counting the first year of parental leave for seniority and Social Security benefits. The costs for the companies were reduced, starting in 1999, by exonerating companies from social benefit costs for substitution contracts (temporary employment) for workers on leave for childcare. Starting in 2002, this was also extended to the substitutions for workers on leave caring for relatives (López & Valiño, 2004).

This leave policy was accompanied by advancing the school entrance age for children to three years of age in the 1990 education reform. The motives for advancing the school entrance age, however, had nothing to do with the policy of promoting the reconciliation of family life and work life, but rather with the objectives of education policy. So although the age for mandatory entrance into school is still six years of age, the public authorities are obliged to provide educational openings, independent of the parents' work status, for all children three and over if parents request this. The consequence of this policy has been the generalized entrance into school of children between 3 and 6 years of age, going from 71% in 1988 to 97% in 2005. As for children up to two years of age, the 1990 education reform has also defined this as an educational period. As a result, the private nursery school services on the market have been forced to undergo a reform to become infant schools, with educational projects and quality requirements in line with the European Union's recommendations, but without becoming part of the public education system. Today, many have still not met such requirements. In fact, the supply of public services or publicly subsidized services for the

0-2 year age group is very low, with the rate of schooling in this type of center at 13.5% in 2005.

The work-family reconciliation policy that has, little by little, been designed in Spain has consisted, therefore, of facilitating more time for taking on family responsibilities while trying to guarantee job security. This has been done through legal instruments as well as incentives for companies, but always privatizing the costs derived from the options in favor of family care. The idea that those who care for children or relatives are providing something of value to society and thus should be publicly compensated, has not formed part of the evaluation of social reality considered when designing social policy. One example in particular will serve to illustrate this fact. Between 1994 and 1998, part of the costs derived from placing children under three years of age in private daycare centers could be deducted from income tax, but before and after these dates, this type of expense is not considered necessary tax-wise in order to obtain earned income and therefore is not deductible.

Of the benefits available, most used is paid maternity leave, with only 2.5% of men taking a portion of this (Instituto de la Mujer, 2005) and most having no intention to use it (Eurobarometer, 2004). Taking unpaid parental leave, on the contrary, is infrequent. According to a survey done in 2004, the proportion of working parents who have ever used parental leave is 2.4% (3.1% of the mothers and 1.4% of the fathers) while those who reduced their working time was 7.4% (8.8% of the mothers and 5.8% of the fathers) (Instituto de la Mujer, 2005). The majority of families resort to informal services, especially family members (specifically grandmothers) to solve the problems of reconciling family life and work life (Tobío, 2005).

NEW SENSITIVITIES TOWARD LOW FERTILITY AND FAMILY CHANGE (1995-2005)

With the conservative party's arrival in government in 1995 (1995-2004), there has been a timid reorientation of family policy, framed in an increasing sensibility toward the potential costs derived from low fertility. This change in attitude shows itself first in public declarations and political speeches. Parliament officially declared itself to be in favor of the preparation of an "Integral Support Plan" for the family in 1997, but the government did not launch the Plan until 2001. Even the opposition socialist party has shown the same change of attitude, once new leaders stopped identifying social protection for the family with conservatism. It is no longer politically incorrect to speak of family policy in terms of the government's explicit commitment to facilitate families' decisions to take on family responsibilities (to have children or to care for disabled members), by partially compensating the personal costs incurred from these options.

The materialization of this new sensitivity does, however, have its lights and large shadows. On one hand, tax treatment of the family improved. As a consequence of the reform, the disposable income of an average income family with two dependent children increased to an after-tax amount of 95% of the gross income, compared to 90% under previous legislation. The family's disposable income went up 5 percentage points, compared to an improvement of only 2 percentage points for a single person, a difference which roughly persists in the present. On the other hand, the direct Social Security allowances, assigned almost exclusively since 1991 to those families under the income threshold to pay income tax, have been brought up to date with inflation only once, in 2000. Their low amounts (2.3% of a worker's average wage in 1991 and 2.2% in 2000) have not been increased, even though they are meant for "poor" families. In 2000, a new one-time allowance for low-income families was introduced for the birth of third and successive children, equivalent to 3.4% of a worker's average wage in 2000. In 2000, exceptional one-time payment allowances were also introduced for families with multiple births. The last new allowance introduced in 2003, amounting to 1200 euros a year, is paid only to working women until a child reaches age three (provided the working mother pays social security fees over this amount, otherwise it is reduced accordingly). The aim is to compensate for the (undefined) costs working women have to bear when they have to reconcile working and family life. Non-working mothers and mothers on parental leave after the sixteenth week are not entitled to such an allowance.

In general, there has been improvement in public compensation for family obligations, along with an improvement in the instruments for reconciling family life and work life. Although family benefits (excluding tax benefits) as a percentage of total social protection expenses grew from 1.7% in 1994 to 2.5% in 2002, the social protection of the family in Spain continues to be the lowest one in the EU (Abramovici, 2003). Perhaps the greatest change has been the explicit declaration of a family policy by the central government, which launched this policy at the end of 2001 within the framework of an Integral Support Plan for the Family (2001-2004), but without substantial improvements in the policy instruments themselves. This Plan superseded the Integral Support Plans for the Family that some regions had designed during the second half of the 1990s, although these regional plans had great limitations.

Government change in 2004 brought the socialist party into power, whose policy program in family matters, despite the rhetoric of the challenges derived from low fertility, has been reoriented towards recognizing family change. This policy reorientation has taken the form of two legislative proposals concerning divorce and same sex marriage. The reform of the divorce proposal aims to facilitate divorce by reducing the two step process to one, allowing divorce without previous separation of the spouses as well as in cases when one spouse opposes it. Further, it introduces the possibility of shared custody of children. In the context of this reform, a State Guarantee Fund for the custody payments of divorced parents has been proposed, an old demand previously rejected by the ruling government on cost grounds. The reform of marriage law aims to introduce the right to marry to same sex couples on the same terms as heterosexual couples, with the same rights and obligations, including the right to adopt children as a couple.

CONCLUSION

The evolution of Spanish family policy is closely intertwined with the deep social, economic and political transformations that occurred during the 20th century. An explicit family policy was first established by the Dictatorship of General Franco at the end of the 1930s as an ideological affirmation of the so-called New State, a means of gaining social support. Its explicit objective was to reestablish the economic, legal as well as ideological foundations of the patriarchal family, which was considered the basis of the social order and hence of the Dictatorship. The contradictions that characterized its structure and functioning weren't resolved until the late 1950s when a new institutional framework was established to facilitate capitalist development. The adaptation of family policy to the requirements of a capitalist labor market didn't change the objective of supporting the patriarchal family, but its economic importance decreased with inflation during the rapid economic development of the 1960s.

The transition to democracy brought about a dramatic change in family policy. The legal regulation of family ties changed profoundly toward recognition of the pluralism of family forms and the equal treatment of all family members, although the idea of an explicit family policy lost its legitimacy since it was identified with support of the patriarchal family and the social policy of the Dictatorship. Nevertheless, an implicit family policy evolved, as family status became an indicator of need in areas of social policy such as public pensions and social protection in cases of unemployment or poverty. Over time, family allowances lost their capacity to improve income and were redirected later to low-income families. By the late 1980s, family policy was seen only as a part of a social policy against poverty.

In parallel with this evolution, a new policy grew slowly to promote the reconciliation of family and working life, not as labor market policy to guarantee enough working population, as unemployment was always structurally high, but as a means to promote equal employment opportunities to men and women, in line with developments in other western countries. The instruments of this policy were designed to facilitate time for caring, but the costs of using parental leaves after maternity leave have been supported by families themselves. Concerns about very low fertility rates grew during the 1990s, awakening a new sensibility for the need to support care giving performed by families. Although this new sensibility is evident in the political arena and the media, little has been done so far to compensate individuals for the costs of assuming family responsibilities.

During the period covered by this article, family policy in Spain has evolved from support for the patriarchal family to the recognition of family pluralism and from the evolution of the family salary to a policy aimed to combat poverty and to promote the reconciliation of family and working life.

REFERENCES

Abramovici, G. (2003). Social protection: Cash family benefits in Europe. *Eurostat. Statistics in Focus,* theme 3-19/2003.

Alberdi, I. (1978). *Historia y sociología del divorcio en España* [History and sociology of divorce in Spain]. Madrid, Spain: Centro de Investigaciones Sociológicas.

Alberdi, I. (Ed.). (1995). *Informe sobre la situación de la familia en España* [Report on the social situation of the family in Spain]. Madrid, Spain: Ministerio de Asuntos Sociales.

Alonso Olea, M. (1953). Salarios y Seguridad Social [Salaries and social security]. *Revista Iberoamericana de Seguridad Socia* [*Journal of Iberoamerican Social Security*], 2, 225-271.

Alonso Olea, M. (1954). Salarios y Seguridad Social, 1954 [Salaries and social security, 1954]. *Revista Iberoamericana de Seguridad Social, 3,* 442-475.

Alonso Olea, M. (1956). Salarios y Seguridad Social, 1956 [Salaries and social security, 1956]. en *Revista Iberoamericana de Seguridad Social, 2,* 237-368.

Arrese, J. L. (1940). *Obras completas* [Complete Works]. Madrid, Spain: Edit. Nacional.

Aznar, S. (1932). *El seguro de maternidad* [Maternity insurance]. Madrid, Spain: Instituto Nacional de Previsión.

Aznar, S. (1947). *Los seguros sociales* [Social insurance]. Madrid, Spain: Instituto de Estudios Políticos.

Banco de Bilbao (1979). *Informe económico 1978* [Report on the economic situation 1978]. Madrid, Spain: Banco de Bilbao.

Banco de España (1979). *Boletín estadístico* [Statistical Bulletin]. Madrid, Spain: Banco de España

Bikkal, D. (1954). La seguridad social en España [Social security in Spain]. *Revista Iberoamericana de Seguridad Social, 3*, 409-452.

Blanco, J.E. (1964). Planificación de la seguridad social española [Planning of Spanish Social Security]. Barcelona, Spain: Editorial Marte.

Campo, S. del (1974). *La política demográfica en España* [Spanish demographic policy]. Madrid, Spain: Edicusa.

Campo, S. del (1995). *Familias: Sociología y política* [Families: Sociology and politics]. Madrid, Spain: Editorial Universidad Complutense.

Cicchelli-Pugeault, C. & Cicchelli, V.1998. *Les théories sociologiques de la famille* [The sociological theories of the family]. Paris, France: La Decouverte.

Cruz Roche, I. (1984). *Análisis económico de la Seguridad Social, 1972-1982* [Economic analysis of Social Security]. Madrid, Spain: Instituto de Estudios Laborales y de la Seguridad Social.

Del Peso, C. (1967). *De la protección gremial al vigente sistema del Seguridad Social* [From the guild protection to the present Social Security system]. Madrid, Spain Hijos de E. Minuesa.

Dumon, W. (1987). La politique familiale en Europe occidentale. Une réflexion sociologique [Family policy in western Europe. A sociological approach]. *L'Année sociologique* [Annual Review of Sociology], *37*, 291-308.

Eurobarometer (2004). European's attitudes to parental leave, *Special Eurobarometer 189*, wave 59.1. Brussels, Belgium: European Comission, Directorate–General Employment and Social Affairs

Flora, P. (1983). *State, economy, and society in Western Europe 1815-1975*. Frankfurt, Germany: Campus Verlag.

Girón de Velasco J.A. (1951). *Quince Años de política social dirigida por Franco* [Fifteen years social policy of Franco]. Madrid, Spain: Ediciones O.I.D.

Hoffnes, C. (1940). La legislación de los subsidios familiares durante los últimos años [Family subsidies legislation during the last years)] *Revista de Trabajo* [Labor Journal], *2*, 628-643.

Iglesias de Ussel, J. (1994). La familia [The family]. In Fundación FOESSA (Ed.). *V Informe sociológico sobre la realidad social de España* [5th sociological report on the Spanish social situation] (pp. 415-547), Madrid, Spain: Euroamérica.

Iglesias de Ussel, J. (1998). *La familia y el cambio político en España* [Family and political change in Spain]. Madrid, Spain: Tecnos.

Instituto de la Mujer (2005). Estudio sobre la conciliación de la vida familiar y laboral: Situación actual, necesidades y demandas [Reconciliation of family and working life: Present situation, needs and demands]. Available: http://www.mtas.es

Jordana de Pozas, L. (1938). *La política familiar del Nuevo Estado* [Family policy of the New State]. Santander, Spain: Aldus Artes Gráficas.

Kamerman, S. & Kahn, A. (1978). Family policy as a field and perspective. In S. Kamerman & A. Kahn (Eds.). *Government and families in fourteen countries* (pp. 476-503). New York, NY: Columbia University Press.

Kaufmann, F.X., Herlth, A., & Strohmaier, H.P. (1982). *Staatliche sozialpolitik und familie* [Social policy and the family]. München, Germany: Oldenbourg.

López, I. (1996). Evolución en España de la normativa sobre los permisos parentales [The evolution of the legislation on parental leaves in Spain]. *Infancia y sociedad* [Childhood & society] *34-35*, 313-320.

López, M. T. & Valiño, A. (2004). *Conciliación de vida familiar y laboral* [Reconciliation of family and working life]. Madrid, Spain: Consejo Económico y Social.

Meil, G. (1994). L´évolution de la politique familiale en Espagne: du salaire familial à la politique contre la pauvreté [The evolution of Spanish family policy: From family salary to a policy against poverty]. *Population, 4-5*, 959-998.

Meil, G. (1995). La política familiar española durante el franquismo [Family policy during Franco´s dictatorship]. *Revista Internacional de Sociología* [Internacional Journal of Sociology] *11*, 47-87.

Meil, G. & Iglesias de Ussel, J. (2001). La política familiar en España [Family policy in Spain]. Barcelona, Spain: Ariel.

Picontó-Novales, T. (1997). Family law and family policy in Spain. In J. Kurczewski & M. MacClean (Eds.), *Family law and family policy in the New Europe* (pp. 109-127). Dartmouth, UK: Aldershot.

Pitrou, A. (1994). *Les politiques familiales. Approches sociolgiques.* [Policies towards the families. Sociological approaches]. Paris, France: Syros.

Ros Hombravella, A.; Clavera, J.; Esteban, J.; Monés, M.A. & Montserrat, A. (1973). *Capitalismo español: De la autarquía a la estabilización (1939-1959)* [Spanish capitalism: From autocracy to stabilization, 1939-1959]. Madrid, Spain: Cuadernos para el Diálogo.

Rull Savater, A. (1974a). La política social de España. Examen del pasado y perspectivas [Spanish social policy. Review of the past and future perspectives]. *Revista de Trabajo, 46*, 2-39.

Rull Savater, A. (1974b). *Instituciones y economía de la Seguridad Social española* [Social security institutions and economy in Spain]. Madrid, Spain: Confederación española de Cajas de Ahorro.

Tobío, C. (2005). *Madres que trabajan. Dilemas y estrategias* [Mothers who work. Dilemmas and strategies]. Madrid, Spain: Cátedra.

Toharia, L. (1943). El plus de cargas familiares [The family bonus]. *Revista de Trabajo, 8*, 792-829.

Valiente, C. (1996). Olvidando el pasado: la política familiar española, 1975-1996 [Forgetting the past: Spanish family policy, 1975-1996]. *Gestión y Análisis de Políticas Públicas* [Management and Analysis of Public Policies] *5-6*, 156-161.

Wingen, M. (1997). *Familienpolitik* [Family policy]. Stuttgart, Germany: Lucius & Lucius.

Zimmerman, S. (1988). *Understanding family policy. Theoretical approaches*. Newbury Park, CA: Sage.

Index

T - #0464 - 101024 - C0 - 212/152/22 - PB - 9780789032409 - Gloss Lamination